T0139145

Simultaneous Global New Drug Development

Chapman & Hall/CRC Healthcare Informatics Series

Series Editors

Christopher Yang, Drexel University, USA

For more information about this series, please visit: https://www.routledge.com/ Chapman–HallCRC-Healthcare-Informatics-Series/book-series/HEALTHINF

Simultaneous Global New Drug Development

Multi-Regional Clinical Trials after
ICH E17

Edited by
Gang Li, Bruce Binkowitz
William Wang, Hui Quan, and
Josh Chen

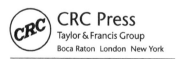

CRC Press
Taylor & Francis Group
Boca Raton London New York

CRC Press is an imprint of the
Taylor & Francis Group, an **informa** business
A CHAPMAN & HALL BOOK

First edition published 2022
by CRC Press
6000 Broken Sound Parkway NW, Suite 300, Boca Raton, FL 33487-2742

and by CRC Press
2 Park Square, Milton Park, Abingdon, Oxon, OX14 4RN

© 2022 selection and editorial matter, Gang Li, Bruce Binkowitz, William Wang, Hui Quan, and Josh Chen; individual chapters, the contributors

CRC Press is an imprint of Taylor & Francis Group, LLC

Reasonable efforts have been made to publish reliable data and information, but the author and publisher cannot assume responsibility for the validity of all materials or the consequences of their use. The authors and publishers have attempted to trace the copyright holders of all material reproduced in this publication and apologize to copyright holders if permission to publish in this form has not been obtained. If any copyright material has not been acknowledged please write and let us know so we may rectify it in any future reprint.

Except as permitted under the US Copyright Law, no part of this book may be reprinted, reproduced, transmitted, or utilized in any form
by any electronic, mechanical, or other means now known or hereafter invented, including photocopying, microfilming, and recording, or
in any information storage or retrieval system, without written permission from the publishers.

For permission to photocopy or use material electronically from this work, access www.copyright.com or contact the Copyright Clearance Center, Inc. (CCC), 222 Rosewood Drive, Danvers, MA 01923, 978-750-8400. For works that are not available on CCC please contact mpkbookspermissions@tandf.co.uk.

Trademark notice: Product or corporate names may be trademarks or registered trademarks and are used only for identification and explanation without intent to infringe.

Library of Congress Cataloging-in-Publication Data
Names: Li, Gang, editor.
Title: Simultaneous global new drug development : multi-regional clinical trials after ICH E17 / edited by Gang Li, Eisai Inc., USA [and four others].
Description: First edition. | Boca Raton : Chapman & Hall, CRC Press, 2022. | Series: Chapman & Hall/CRC biostatistics series | Includes bibliographical references and index.
Identifiers: LCCN 2021028873 (print) | LCCN 2021028874 (ebook) | ISBN 9780367565602 (hardback) | ISBN 9780367625795 (paperback) | ISBN 9781003109785 (ebook)
Subjects: LCSH: Drug development. Classification: LCC RS420 .S57 2022 (print) | LCC RS420 (ebook) | DDC 615.1/9--dc23
LC record available at https://lccn.loc.gov/2021028873
LC ebook record available at https://lccn.loc.gov/2021028874

ISBN: 978-0-367-56560-2 (hbk)
ISBN: 978-0-367-62579-5 (pbk)
ISBN: 978-1-003-10978-5 (ebk)

DOI: 10.1201/9781003109785

Typeset in Palatino
by MPS Limited, Dehradun

Contents

Preface

Following the 2016 book titled "Multiregional Clinical Trials for Simultaneous Global New Drug Development," development has continued on the best practices and methods for multiregional clinical trials (MRCTs). The recognition of the crucial role and necessity in the development of innovative medical products of global clinical development strategy for MRCTs continues to grow, and this growth was codified by the International Committee on Harmonization (ICH) E17 Guidance. The ICH E17 guidance and the associated training materials are proof that studying patients from different regions within a single trial under a single protocol is an efficient and desirable method of trial design and medical product development. ICH E17 recognizes the challenges in the design, conduct, and interpretation of MRCTs, and offers guidance towards overcoming those challenges.

This book is intended to continue to educate practitioners of MRCTs, expand on the 2016 MRCT book, and follow up, and continue beyond, ICH E17. This book is a collection of chapters contributed by different authors, and these authors cover a wide scope with their backgrounds and experience, across industry, academia, and health authorities. Section I expands on the ICH E17 guidance, with more insight from the experts who were involved with creating ICH E17. The reader will greatly benefit from these chapters expanding on ICH E17. Section II brings examples from real MRCT trials and discusses the issues that arose, providing the reader with results that may be familiar and can translate to the reader's own trial experience. Sections III and IV are about the continuing development of a methodology to improve the design and analysis of MRCTs. Section III focuses on analysis methods, while Section IV focuses on design methods.

This book is of particular interest to biostatisticians working in the late-stage clinical development of medical products. It will also be helpful to statisticians, clinicians, and regulatory experts in the biopharmaceutical industry, at regulatory agencies, and at medical research institutes. Expanding well past the scope of the 2016 book, this book adds examples, new methodology, and serves as an expansion of the concepts introduced in ICH E17. In doing so, this book provides the reader with additional information and expertise on the topic of MRCTs, which continue to grow in importance as medical product development continues to become more global.

Editor Biographies

Dr. Gang Li is Senior Director, Real World Evidence (RWE) and Medical Value, the Neurology Business Group of Eisai Inc. He received his PhD in Mathematical Statistics from the State University of New York at Binghamton. He co-authored over 60 publications on statistical methodologies, and research on psychiatry, obesity, and diabetes. He served as the Executive Director of the International Statistical Association (2017–2019). Dr. Li is a Fellow of the American Statistical Association.

Dr. Hui Quan is currently the global head of the Statistical Research group of the Biostatistics and Programming Department of Sanofi. He received his PhD degree in statistics from Columbia University in 1990. He has 30 years of pharmaceutical industry experience in many therapeutic areas. He has published 108 papers including 84 statistical papers. He is a co-author and co-editor of three books. He has served as an associate editor for two journals. He is a fellow of the American Statistical Association.

Dr. William (Bill) Wang is Executive Director in the Department of Biostatistics and Research Decision Sciences (BARDS), Merck Research Laboratories. He has 25+ years of experience in clinical trial design, bio-statistics, data management, and regulatory filings across multiple TAs including vaccine and oncology. From 2007 to 2014, Bill had led the design, build-up, and day-to-day oversight of global biometrics operations in China. From 2014 to the present, Bill has led the establishment of the clinical safety statistics group to support the clinical safety model. He is currently responsible for managing the global clinical safety statistics operation and the late development statistics in the Asia Pacific region. Through his 20+ years tenure at Merck & Co, Inc, Bill has led the study design, execution, filing, and approval by multi-regional regulatory agencies.

Bill has served as the deputy topics-leader for the ICH E17 working group. The ICH E17 is an ICH efficacy guidance for designing multi-regional clinical trials in global simultaneous drug development and regulatory approval. Bill has also co-founded and co-chaired an American Statistical Association (ASA) Interdisciplinary Safety Working Group. Dr Bill Wang received the DIA Inspire Award in 2017 and was elected as a Fellow of the American Statistical Association in 2018.

Bruce Binkowitz earned his PhD from what is now named the Rutgers School of Public Health. He is the Vice President of Biometrics at Arcutis Biotherapeutics in Westlake, California. Bruce has more than 30 years of pharmaceutical industry experience across many therapeutic areas as well as from early phase through phase IV clinical trials. He has experience in study design, conduct, analysis, and interpretation of results for clinical trials, as well as many interactions with health authorities worldwide. Dr. Binkowitz is active in the Statistical Community, having served many leadership roles including a 3-year term on the ENAR Regional Board of Advisors; as a part of the DIA Statistics Core Community including a 3-year term as the industry representative responsible for organizing the Statistics Track for the DIA Annual Meeting; and has served the statistical community as a member of the American Statistical Association including as a 5-year member of the steering committee for the ASA Biopharmaceutical Section FDA/Industry Statistics Workshop, culminating as the 2013 Workshop Industry Chair. Most recently Bruce was honored to be elected as the 2020 chair of the ASA Biopharmaceutical Section. Bruce is currently in his second term as co-leader of the cross-industry MutliRegional Clinical Trial Consistency Working Group.

Bruce has taught numerous short courses on MultiRegional Clinical Trials, has been the lead or co-author on more than 40 published papers across the Statistical and Medical Literature as well as lead author or co-author on more than 45 conferences and workshop presentations.

Dr. Binkowitz was elected a fellow of the American Statistical Association in 2015.

Dr. Yonghua (Joshua) Chen received his PhD in Statistics from the University of Wisconsin-Madison, and his Master's and Bachelor's degrees in Probability and Statistics from Peking University. He is currently the Head of Global Biostatistical Sciences at Sanofi Pasteur. Before joining Pasteur, Josh worked on the clinical development of small molecules, biologics, and vaccines at Merck Research Labs. His experience spans many therapeutic areas with a major focus on human vaccines and antiviral drugs. He has extensive experience in study design, conduct, and reporting of international clinical trials from proof-of-concept through regulatory approvals and life cycle management. His primary research interest is clinical trial designs, including group sequential methods, adaptive designs, and multiregional clinical trials (MRCTs). He was a co-lead of the across-industry MRCT Consistency Working Group under PhRMA (2008–2011) and Society for Clinical Trials (2012–2014). Dr Chen is a Fellow of the American Statistical Association.

Contributors

Yoko Aoi
*Pharmaceuticals and Medical Devices
 Agency*
Japan

Vibeke Bjerregaard
Novo Nordisk

Aloka Chakravarty
US FDA, USA

Chi-Tian Chen
StatPlus, Inc.
Taiwan

Yu-Chieh Cheng
*Institute of Population Health Sciences
 National Health Research Institutes*
Taiwan

Paul Gallo
Novartis Pharmaceuticals
USA

Hua Guo
 Allergan
USA

Xiang Guo
BeiGene, Ltd.
China

Toshimitsu Hamasaki
George Washington University
USA

Kun He
R&G US Inc.
USA

Shintaro Hiro
Pfizer

Chinfu Hisio
*Institute of Population Health Sciences
 National Health Research Institutes*
Taiwan

Chin-Fu Hsiao
*Institute of Population Health Sciences
 National Health Research Institutes*
Taiwan

Ya-Ting Hsu
*Institute of Population Health Sciences
 National Health Research Institutes*
Taiwan

Shuji Kamada
*Pharmaceuticals and Medical Devices
 Agency*
Japan

Seung-Ho Kang
Yonsei University
Korea

Saemina Kim
Yonsei University
Korea

Armin Koch
Hannover Medical School
Germany

Osamu Komiyama
Pfizer

K.K. Gordon Lan
Brightech International
USA

Fang-Jing Lee
*National Institute of Infectious Diseases
 and Vaccinology, National Health
 Research Institutes*
Taiwan

Min Li
*National Medical Products
    Administration*
China

Jason Liao
Incyte Corporation
USA

Nobushige Matsuoka
Pfizer

Yasuto Otsubo
 *Pharmaceuticals and Medical Devices
    Agency*
Japan

Soo Peter Ouyang
SPO Consulting LLC
USA

Weining Z Robieson
AbbVie Inc.
USA

Yaru Shi
Merck & Co., Inc
USA

Joe Shih
Rutgers University
USA

Rominder Singh
Pfizer

Ming Tan
Georgetown University
USA

Yoko Tanaka
Daiichi Sankyo, Inc.
USA

Hsiao-Hui Tsou
*Institute of Population Health Sciences
    National Health Research Institutes*
Taiwan

Yoshiaki Uyama
*Pharmaceuticals and Medical Devices
    Agency*
Japan

Jun Wang
*National Medical Products
    Administration*
China

Zhaoyun Wang
*National Medical Products
    Administration*
China

Hsiao-Yu Wu
*Institute of Population Health Sciences
    National Health Research Institutes*
Taiwan

Meng-Hsuan Wu
*Institute of Population Health Sciences
    National Health Research Institutes*
Taiwan

Yuh-Jenn Wu
Chung Yuan Christian University
Taiwan

Tai Xie
*Brightech International & CIMS Global
    LLC*
USA

Hideharu Yamamoto
Chugai Pharma
Japan

Zhimin Yang
*National Medical Products
    Administration*
China

Jingjing Ye
BeiGene, Ltd.
China

Shilin Yu
Georgetown University
USA

Ziji Yu
AbbVie Inc.
USA

Ao Yuan
Georgetown University
USA

Sammy Yuan
Marinus Pharmaceuticals
USA

Xin Zeng
National Medical Products

Administration
China

Lanju Zhang
 AbbVie Inc.
USA

Hongjie Zhu
BeiGene, Ltd.
China

1

General Introduction of E17

Yoshiaki Uyama, Yasuto Otsubo, Shuji Kamada, and Yoko Aoi

1.1 Paradigm Shift of the Drug Development Strategy

In the past, clinical trials for the purpose of regulatory approval of a drug in Japan were conducted independently from those in the United States (US) or European Union (EU) because of concerns that ethnic differences between the Japanese and the Western populations might affect drug responses (efficacy and safety). This strategy made it possible to obtain clinical trial data specifically for the Japanese population. However, in general, the strategy initiating development in one region following up with similar studies in subsequent regions would result in duplication of studies and delayed development with late market access in the subsequent regions. This situation was actually seen in Japan before 2010 known as the drug lag (a situation in which a drug is not available in Japan for several years even after its first launch in the Western countries) (Uyama et al. 2005; Hirai et al. 2010). To increase the efficiency of drug development and to minimize the duplication of clinical trials, the E5 guideline entitled "Ethnic factors in the acceptability of foreign clinical data" was established in February 1998 by the International Conference on Harmonisation of Technical Requirements for Pharmaceuticals for Human Use (ICH), followed by regulatory implementation in March 1998 in the EU, June 1998 in the US, and August 1998 in Japan (see Chapter 7).

Since 1998 several drugs have been approved in Japan based on the ICH E5 guideline (Uyama et al. 2005). In such approvals, a bridging study, which is typically designed as a pharmacokinetic study and comparative dose-response study, is usually included in the clinical data package for regulatory submission to allow both an examination of the impact of ethnic factors on drug responses and extrapolation of foreign

DOI: 10.1201/9781003109785-1

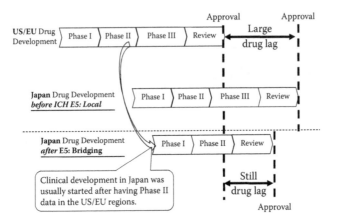

FIGURE 1.1
Limited impact of the bridging strategy based on the ICH E5 guideline on the drug lag.

clinical data to the Japanese population (Uyama et al. 2005). Drug development via a bridging study is helpful to shorten the duration of clinical development in Japan by minimizing the clinical trials that have to be conducted in the country (e.g., phase III trials could be skipped), but it does not completely resolve the drug lag caused by the delayed initiation of drug development in Japan (Figure 1.1) (Uyama et al. 2005; Hirai et al. 2010).

The drug lag still exists because the initiation of drug development in Japan is usually started only after phase II data have been obtained in the US or the EU.

In 2007, a new guideline entitled "Basic principles on global clinical trials" was published in Japan to promote simultaneous drug development and resolve the drug lag, followed by two related guidelines published in 2012 ("Basic Principles On Global Clinical Trials (Reference Cases) (PFSB/ELD Administrative Notice)" 2012) and 2014 ("Basic Principles for Conducting Phase I Trials in the Japanese Population Prior to Global Clinical Trials (PFSB/ELD Administrative Notice)" 2014). Through these efforts, the number of multi-regional clinical trials (MRCTs) conducted in Japan has increased markedly (Asano, Uyama and Tohkin 2018). In fact, the percentage of drug approval for which an MRCT provided pivotal clinical data for regulatory review increased from approximately 1% in 2007 to approximately 48% in 2019 (Figure 1.2). Relative to local drug development, the drug lag has also been significantly shortened in the case of global drug development using MRCTs (Ueno et al. 2014).

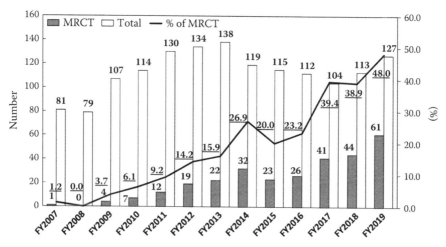

FIGURE 1.2
Trends in MRCT-based approved drugs in Japan.

1.2 Backstory of the ICH E17 Expert Working Group

1.2.1 Why Were the ICH E17 Guidelines Established?

In recent years, global development, including MRCTs, has been widely happening in populations from different parts of the world (Japan, the US, the EU as well as other regions and countries) (Thiers, Sinskey and Berndt 2008; Asano, Uyama and Tohkin 2018). Regulatory authorities have faced challenges in evaluating data from MRCTs for drug approval (Ichimaru, Toyoshima and Uyama 2010; Asano et al. 2013). In the later 2000s, guidelines and other related documents relating to MRCTs were published in Japan and the EU ("Basic Principles On Global Clinical Trials (PFSB/ELD Notification No. 0928010)" 2007 "Basic Principles on Global Clinical Trials (PFSB/ELD Notification No. 0928010)" 2007; "Reflection Paper On The Extrapolation Of Results From Clinical Studies Conducted Outside The EU To The EU-Population" 2009 "Reflection Paper on the Extrapolation of Results From Clinical Studies Conducted Outside The EU To The EU-Population" 2009). The US Food and Drug Administration (FDA) also published a perspective regarding regulatory and scientific issues on the use of foreign data in support of new drug applications (Khin et al. 2013). At that time, however, there were no internationally harmonized guidelines on MRCTs, especially one focusing on scientific issues in the planning and/or design of MRCTs. Although the Q&A section of the ICH E5 guideline partly covers issue relating to MRCTs, more specific guidelines on MRCTs was expected to further promote the conduct of MRCTs in a harmonized way and to increase the efficiency of drug development, thereby avoiding duplicative works in drug development and enabling better regulatory decisions.

1.2.2 The History of the ICH E17 Guideline

In 2014, the Pharmaceuticals and Medical Devices Agency (PMDA) submitted to the ICH a concept paper proposing new harmonized guidelines on general principles for planning and design of MRCTs ("Final Concept Paper E17: General Principle On Planning/Designing Multi-Regional Clinical Trials" 2014). In June 2014, an ICH-steering committee endorsed the concept paper and decided to establish a new expert working group (EWG), known as "E17 EWG", for creating the new internationally harmonized guideline entitled "General Principles for Planning and Design of Multi-Regional Clinical Trials." As shown in Figure 1.3, after the establishment of E17 EWG, the members actively discussed the proposed guidelines through face-to-face meetings, regular web conferences, and e-mails. Consensus on the draft ICH E17 guideline was reached within the E17 EWG in June 2016, and the guideline was then published in each region for comments. More than 1000 comments were received from many regions during the public consultation period. The E17 EWG carefully reviewed all comments and discussed the best solutions to reflect the points raised in the comments. Active and constructive

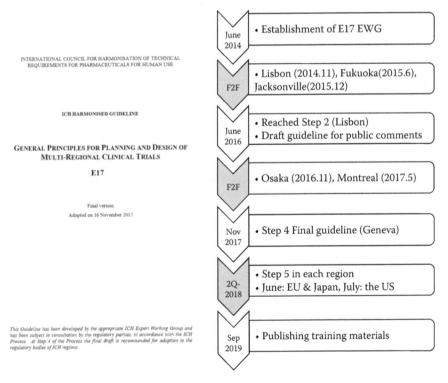

FIGURE 1.3
A history of the ICH E17 guideline.

discussions were again made through face-to-face meetings, as well as regular web conferences and e-mails. Ultimately, consensus on the final ICH E17 guideline was reached at a meeting in Geneva in November 2017 ("ICH E17 Guideline" 2017). Each regulatory authority subsequently worked to implement the ICH E17 guideline under local legislation. Importantly, the ICH E17 guideline was officially implemented in many regions including the EU and Japan in June 2018, followed by the US in July 2018, the Republic of Korea in October 2018, Canada in April 2019, Brazil in May 2019, and China in November 2019.

After the establishment of the ICH E17 guideline, ICH continued to work to provide training materials aiming for proper implementation of the ICH E17 guideline on the correct understanding of the E17 principles. Standardized training materials aid the implementation of the ICH E17 guideline consistently across regions. The final training materials were published in August 2019 and are available on the ICH website (https://www.ich.org/page/efficacy-guidelines). They describe more practical details about the key principles of the ICH E17 guideline, such as pre-consideration of regional variability, selection of doses, sample size allocation, pooling strategies, evaluation of consistency, and selection of comparators (see Chapters 3, 4, 5, and 6 for more details).

1.3 Key Principles of the ICH E17 Guideline

The ICH E17 guideline describes practical issues relating to MRCTs, such as common points to consider in their planning and design and how to minimize conflicting opinions from regulatory authorities. This guideline should be used together with other ICH guidelines, including E5, E6, E8, E9, E10, and E18.

As shown in Figure 1.4, the ICH E17 guideline is based on seven key principles (known as the "Lucky 7 Principles" that make your drug development more efficient and successful). These principles, which highlight the key considerations in MRCTs, are described below.

1. Strategic use of MRCTs in the drug development programs

Strategic use of MRCTs in drug development programs, properly designed and executed according to this guideline, can increase the efficiency of drug development. MRCTs may enable simultaneous submission of marketing authorization applications (MAA) and support regulatory decision-making in multiple regions, allowing earlier access to new drugs worldwide. Although MRCTs may generally become the preferred option for investigating a new drug for which regulatory submission is planned in

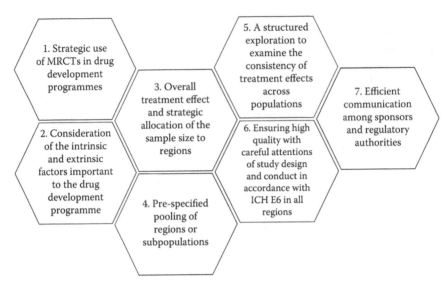

FIGURE 1.4
Key principles of the ICH E17 guideline.

multiple regions, the potential for regional differences to impact the interpretability of study results should be carefully considered.

2. Consideration of the intrinsic and extrinsic factors important to the drug development program

The intrinsic and extrinsic factors important to the drug development program should be identified early. The potential impact of these factors could be examined in the exploratory phases before the design of confirmatory MRCTs. Information about them should also be collected during the confirmatory trial for evaluation of their impact on treatment effects.

3. Overall treatment effect and strategic allocation of the sample size to regions

MRCTs are planned under the assumption that the treatment effect applies to the entire target population, particularly to the regions included in the trial. Strategic allocation of the sample size to regions allows an evaluation of the extent to which this assumption holds.

4. Pre-specified pooling of regions or subpopulations

Pre-specified pooling of regions or subpopulations, based on established knowledge about similarities, may help to provide flexibility in sample size allocation to regions, facilitate the assessment of consistency in treatment effects across regions, and support regulatory decision-making.

5. A structured exploration to examine the consistency of treatment effects across populations

A single primary analysis approach for hypothesis testing and estimation of the overall treatment effect should be planned so that it will be acceptable to all concerned regulatory authorities. A structured exploration to examine the consistency of treatment effects across regions and subpopulations should be planned.

6. Ensuring high quality with careful attention to study design and conduct in accordance with ICH E6 in all regions

In light of diverse regional practices, ensuring the high quality of study design and conduct in accordance with ICH E6 (Good Clinical Practice) in all regions is of paramount importance to ensure the study results are interpretable. Careful attention to quality during trial planning, investigator training, and trial monitoring will help achieve a consistently high trial quality that is required for a successful MRCT.

7. Efficient communication among sponsors and regulatory authorities

Efficient communication among sponsors and regulatory authorities is encouraged at the planning stage of MRCTs, with the goal of obtaining acceptance of a global approach to study design across the different regulatory regions.

More details of the key principles are described in other chapters.

➤ *Promote international harmonization*
  • A globally harmonized approach to drug development should be considered first.
➤ *Earlier access to innovative therapies*
  • Provide an innovative drug earlier to patients by synchronizing the timing of clinical drug development across different regions
➤ *Avoid duplication*
  • Reduce the need to conduct standalone regional or national studies.
➤ *Provide better evidences for drug approval in each region*
  • Encourage better planning and design of MRCTs based on the latest scientific knowledge and experiences
➤ *Longitudinal build-up of capability and infrastructure for global drug development*
  • Planning and conducting high quality MRCTs throughout drug development will build up trial infrastructure and capability

FIGURE 1.5
Roles of the ICH E17 guideline in drug development.

1.4 Roles of the ICH E17 Guideline in Drug Development

The ICH E17 guideline is expected to promote international harmonization in conducting MRCTs and contribute to multiple aspects, as described below (Figure 1.5), including earlier access to innovative therapies, avoidance of study duplication, provision of better evidence for drug approval in each region, and longitudinal building of capability and infrastructure for global drug development.

1.5 Concluding Remarks

In conclusion, for the efficient and successful development of a new drug, MRCTs should be planned and designed in accordance with the principle of the ICH E17 guideline. An MRCT based on the ICH E17 guideline will facilitate simultaneous MAAs to different regulatory agencies and drug approval without the drug lag in different regions. Accumulation of experiences in the conduct of MRCTs in many regions will further promote international harmonization and will build up the capability and infrastructure suitable for MRCTs.

References

Asano, K, A Tanaka, T Sato, and Y Uyama. 2013. "Regulatory Challenges in the Review of Data from Global Clinical Trials: The PMDA Perspective". *Clinical Pharmacology & Therapeutics* 94 (2): 195–198. 10.1038/clpt.2013.106.

Asano, K, Y Uyama, and M Tohkin. 2018. "Factors Affecting Drug-Development Strategies in Asian Global Clinical Trials for Drug Approval in Japan". *Clinical and Translational Science* 11 (2): 182–188. 10.1111/cts.12520.

"Basic Principles for Conducting Phase I Trials in the Japanese Population Prior to Global Clinical Trials (PFSB/ELD Administrative Notice)". 2014. *Ministry-of-Health-Labour-and-Welfare*. https://www.pmda.go.jp/files/000157777.pdf.

"Basic Principles on Global Clinical Trials (PFSB/ELD Notification No. 0928010)". 2007. *Ministry-of-Health-Labour-and-Welfare*. https://www.pmda.go.jp/files/000153265.pdf.

"Basic Principles on Global Clinical Trials (Reference Cases) (PFSB/ELD Administrative Notice)". 2012. *Ministry-of-Health-Labour-and-Welfare*. https://www.pmda.go.jp/files/000208185.pdf.

"Final Concept Paper E17: General Principle on Planning/Designing Multi-Regional Clinical Trials". 2014. *ICH*. https://database.ich.org/sites/default/files/E17EWG%20Final%20Concept%20Paper%20June%202014.pdf.

Hirai, Y, H Kinoshita, M Kusama, K Yasuda, Y Sugiyama, and S Ono. 2010. "Delays in New Drug Applications in Japan and Industrial R&D Strategies". *Clinical Pharmacology & Therapeutics* 87 (2): 212–218. 10.1038/clpt.2009.215.

"ICH E17 Guideline". 2017. *ICH.* https://database.ich.org/sites/default/files/E17EWG_Step4_2017_1116.pdf.

Ichimaru, K, S Toyoshima, and Y Uyama. 2010. "Effective Global Drug Development Strategy for Obtaining Regulatory Approval in Japan in the Context of Ethnicity-Related Drug Response Factors". *Clinical Pharmacology & Therapeutics* 87 (3): 362–366. 10.1038/clpt.2009.285.

Khin, N A, P Yang, H M J Hung, K Maung-U, Y-F Chen, A Meeker-O'Connell, and P Okwesili et al. 2013. "Regulatory and Scientific Issues Regarding Use of Foreign Data in Support of New Drug Applications in the United States: An FDA Perspective". *Clinical Pharmacology & Therapeutics* 94 (2): 230–242. 10.1038/clpt.2013.70.

"Reflection Paper on the Extrapolation of Results From Clinical Studies Conducted Outside The EU To The EU-Population". 2009. *European-Medicines-Agency.* https://www.ema.europa.eu/en/documents/scientific-guideline/reflection-paper-extrapolation-results-clinical-studies-conducted-outside-european-union-eu-eu_en.pdf.

Thiers, F A, A J Sinskey, and E R Berndt. 2008. "Trends in the Globalization of Clinical Trials". *Nature Reviews Drug Discovery* 7 (1): 13–14. 10.1038/nrd2441.

Ueno, T, Y Asahina, A Tanaka, H Yamada, M Nakamura, and Y Uyama. 2014. "Significant Differences in Drug Lag in Clinical Development among Various Strategies Used for Regulatory Submissions in Japan". *Clinical Pharmacology & Therapeutics* 95 (5): 533–541. 10.1038/clpt.2013.223.

Uyama, Y, T Shibata, N Nagai, H Hanaoka, S Toyoshima, and K Mori. 2005. "Successful Bridging Strategy Based on ICH E5 Guideline for Drugs Approved in Japan". *Clinical Pharmacology & Therapeutics* 78 (2): 102–113. 10.1016/j.clpt.2005.04.001.

2

New Principles in Global Development Using ICH E 17 Guideline

Vibeke Bjerregaard and Rominder Singh

The mission of ICH (The International Council for Harmonisation of Technical Requirements for Pharmaceuticals for Human Use) is to achieve worldwide harmonisation to ensure that safe, effective, and high-quality medicines are developed and registered in the most resource-efficient manner. Regulations in different parts of the world, impact the conduct and the oversight of clinical trials. Since 1990, ICH has worked as a tripartite organisation. However, in 2015, ICH reorganised in order to become a more inclusive global harmonisation effort. ICH is now expanding its membership and inviting global organisations to join. Multiple new regulatory bodies and industry organisations have joined since 2015, and the number of new members continues to grow. This change from a tri-partite to a more inclusive global organisation is crucial for the success and acceptability of the ICH E17 guideline. These guidelines aim at truly global development and authorisation of new treatments. Since the ICH E17 guideline was published in 2017, the number of multiple-region clinical trials (MRCTs) supporting marketing authorisations has gradually increased. Most applications for new drugs are now supported by data generated from MRCTs applying many of the ICH E17 principles (see also Chapter 1, 7; FDA: Drug trials snapshots 2015–2019; Zhou et al. 2021). The COVID-19 crisis also demonstrated how much the world is interconnected, and many MRCT principles have been used for the development of both treatments and vaccines.

The ICH E17 guideline on the conduct of MRCTs is aimed at the pivotal phases of development with the goal of including populations from different parts of the world within a single protocol. The scope of drug development has broadened from local to global to provide clinical data supporting marketing in all relevant parts of the world. For more details, see the ICH E17 training material video and Module 1 (Chapter 1). Going global requires several new and more complex considerations, including early planning of the overall development programme and/or the design of each MRCT. The ICH E17 seven principles (Chapter 1) support global development and allows for the utilisation of MRCTs covering all parts of the world, where populations that may benefit from the new treatment are prevalent. The planning and design phases of the confirmatory MRCTs are facilitated by the studies preceding the late phase MRCTs. It is critical to a successful global development plan, that the overall clinical programme is planned with end in mind, i.e., the global plan for marketing of the investigational drug. This means that the pharmacology studies and exploratory studies are preferably planned to support the design of the global, confirmatory MRCTs. Ultimately, the development plan is aimed at associability of the drug to the broader population of the world that may benefit from the new treatment.

Thus, ICH E17 promotes simultaneous development and near-simultaneous marketing authorisations across the world. The aim of each MRCT is to show the overall treatment effect with the assumption that drug effects, efficacy, and safety, apply to all concerned populations across regions, and thereby also be able to understand both similarities and differences in how the new treatment performs in different regions and different populations.

Content:

2.1. Aspects of Strategic Planning

2.2. Pre-considerations of Regional Variability

2.3. The Targeted Population and Definitions

2.4. Global Drug Development and Business Perspectives

2.5. Identify Influential Ethnic Factors (Effect Modifiers) and Mitigation Strategies

2.6. Consultation with Regulatory Authorities

2.7. Overcoming Regional Variabilities

2.8. Concluding Remarks

2.9. Case Examples; liraglutide, insulin and gefitinib, planning global development

2.10. References

2.1 Aspects of Strategic Planning

Planning is critical both when beginning a new development programme and later in the design stage of each MRCT protocol. Refer to the E17 guideline, strategy-related issues section 2.1 and the figure below. (Figure 2.1)

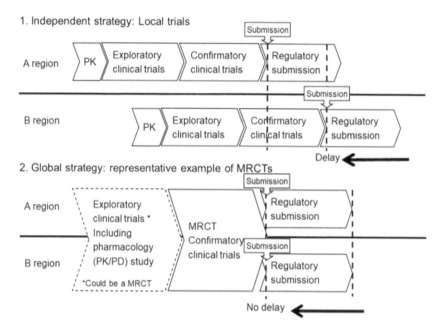

FIGURE 2.1
Figure 1 of ICH E17 section 2.1. Strategy-related issues. Illustrations of clinical drug development workflow across regions for drug submission and regulatory review in independent and global strategies. *: Marketing Authorisation Application/New Drug Application. **: Could be parallel single region trials or MRCTs.

When developing new treatments, the planning activities are usually initiated before the start-up of phase I. The aim of the development programme is to generate data which can support marketing authorisation in all relevant geographic areas, i.e., where the people in need live and may potentially benefit from the new treatment. Therefore, the development programme should include populations which represent all the geographic areas, where the treatment is planned to be authorised and marketed. The complexity needs to be understood to the widest extent possible. Many aspects need to be considered early in the planning phase and preceding any clinical development. Some of these aspects are:

- Identifying populations, globally, suffering from the disease or condition in question, i.e., that potentially may benefit from treatment with the investigational drug
- Prospects of global marketing, aiming at geographic areas where the product is planned to be authorised
- Ethical aspects related to the targeted population(s) and marketing prospects

- Pharmacological effects of the investigational drug
- Epidemiological information for the relevant geographic areas
- Including information about how an underlying disease is diagnosed across areas
- Standard of care, including current treatments and any concomitant treatments and other cultural aspects
- Professional society treatment guidelines
- Real-world information as applicable and available for each geographic area
- Laws and requirements for product authorisations in concerned geographic areas and regulatory guidelines
- Sponsor and local resources, e.g., qualified investigators.

2.2 Pre-considerations of Regional Variability

Global development is a time-consuming, complex, and challenging process. It involves extensive planning including research about the disease and/or condition, which may exist in most parts of the world. Differences among regions are not unusual, and these differences need not be barriers against the conduct of MRCTs. Not only finding differences, but also identifying differences, which affect treatment effect, is of paramount importance. Most importantly, is then how to manage these differences in MRCTs.

It is important that clinical trial participants represent the populations most likely to use the potential drug or treatment, no matter where they live. Sponsors can apply the E17 principles to confront global health care disparities, and make sure that clinical trials for drugs are more inclusive of various populations. FDA (U.S. Food and Drug Administration) issued a guideline in November 2020 underlining the importance of including populations with different demographic characteristics, like sex, race, ethnicities, age, and other demographic characteristics like people with organ dysfunctions, comorbid conditions, disabilities, extreme body weights; and populations with diseases or conditions with low prevalence (FDA, Enhancing the Diversity of Clinical Trial Populations—Eligibility Criteria, Enrolment Practices, and Trial Designs Guidance for Industry 2020). This guideline is also applicable to MRCTs, and by doing global studies, we may learn more about how drugs work in populations, which used to be underrepresented in clinical studies, e.g., populations from remote areas and low-income communities. So, the planning needs to address variabilities in disease symptoms, demographic characteristics, functional status among populations/subjects, and geography (see also below section 2.6).

When recruiting people from different parts of the world, it is expected that the population to be targeted is more diverse compared to development, that is limited to one part of the world, e.g., Europe and North America. Including more heterogeneous populations in MRCTs may necessitate larger subject enrolments than traditionally anticipated, which used to be based on experience from regional development. Each MRCT protocol is also expected to include considerations related to pre-planned subgroups or subpopulation analysis, based on subject and disease characteristics, still with the overall objective as the basis for powering each MRCT (Refer to Chapter 5). Planned subgroup- or subpopulation analyses are usually based on factors that a priori are known to vary among regions, and are hypothesised to be prognostic or predictive.

Regional development strategies may include fewer subjects in each protocol; however, when using global MRCTs the intention is that the total number of study participants will not increase (Refer to Chapter 5 on sample size considerations). When recruiting broadly for each MRCT, the diversity will increase with inclusion of minorities from remote places, low-income communities, and old people, who are often underrepresented in studies. Having global studies that include diverse populations may provide new insights into how drugs work in different populations.

2.3 The Targeted Population and Definitions

The disease and the targeted population must be defined for the overall development programme as well as for each protocol. Clarity of such definitions is crucial for a global development programme and particularly when the programme is using the ICH E17 principles in the development programme and planned clinical studies. The complexity involved with these definitions becomes more critical in global programmes vs. local/part of the world programmes, due to the expected increased inherent differences between multiple parts of the world. The differences may be due to heterogeneity among the populations. Culture, language, educational attainments are also examples of factors that need to be identified in the planning phase of a new global development programme.

The ICH E17 promotes simultaneous drug development and can potentially include subjects from all over the world, e.g., from developed, middle, and low-income countries into the same programme and MRCTs, and thereby supports simultaneous marketing authorisations. This approach is very appealing and is expected to reduce the delay of access to new drugs to some areas of the world, that usually get new treatments late compared to other countries (refer to discussions on intrinsic and extrinsic factors in Chapter 3).

2.4 Global Drug Development and Business Perspectives

When a sponsor prepares a clinical development plan, it is also important, at the early planning phase, to consider the strategy for where to launch the product. It is also important to keep this strategy updated during the development to ensure that areas participating in clinical trials are also ready to authorise and market the drug, once the development has been completed. The simultaneous global development is attractive as it may bring new treatments faster to all subjects in need. This requires that sponsors are ready with resources to support marketing in areas that contributed to the development. Not all countries may necessarily join the MRCTs but may still have populations that can benefit from the new drug. The data from the global programme should also be assessable by authorities in areas that did not contribute during the development phases. All subjects in need, no matter where they live, may have access to the new treatment, when the global programme is conducted under the E17 principles.

There are, however, still hurdles that need to be considered carefully to ensure resource-efficient drug-development programme. Regulatory requirements for local data not based on scientific rationales may still exist, especially in areas that are not so familiar with or have not yet fully implemented the E17 guideline. Timely regulatory approvals of clinical trial applications may prevent timely recruitment which may also lead to a lack of participants from some areas. When MRCTs turn out to be impractical to include all relevant populations and regions, it may be necessary to conduct local or regional studies in order to reach out to all relevant areas of the world, see also below section 2.5.

2.5 Identify Influential Ethnic Factors (Effect Modifiers) and Mitigation Strategies

Information which should be pre-considered in the early planning phase includes, but is not limited to, local epidemiological and real-world information including prevalence and severity of the disease, cultural aspects, standard of care, and specific genetic information e.g., prevalence of genetic polymorphisms. It is important that as many details as possible are collected and analysed in the planning phases.

The treatment effects, efficacy as well as safety, may be influenced by ethnic factors, so the need for pharmacological studies in the early phases of the drug development programme is determined based on the initial research of epidemiological information, race, culture, real-world data, etc. as well as the exploratory and pharmacological properties of the investigational drug. As an example, many of the chemical entities are metabolised and transported via hepatic enzyme systems, and it is well known that populations display genetic variants in hepatic metabolic enzymes. The need for pharmacogenetic testing of the targeted populations may therefore also consider the metabolic pathways for the investigational drug. Hence, in the case of a hepatically metabolised investigational drug, it is recommended to explore the detailed metabolic pathways for the drug and consider identifying subgroups of the populations with certain genetic variants, or phenotypes, e.g., poor or extensive metabolizers. Both *in-vitro* and *in-vivo* studies, as well as studies in healthy subjects and/or diseased subjects, may be needed depending on the pharmacological properties of the drug and the level of know-how about the effects of the drug. Variants among human genes for hepatic enzymes are categorised as intrinsic factors according to the ICH E5 guideline. There is more discussion on "ethnic factors" in Chapter 3.

There are other ethnic factors that may matter in relation to global development, like the prevalence of specific diseases or conditions within a geographical area. This kind of information may be collected as epidemiological information, e.g., differences in the prevalence of specific diseases across areas of the world. Some differences could be due to population adaptation to special environmental conditions, or due to existing genetic factors. This kind of information may become valuable in the design phase of the global MRCTs. For some biologicals, "ethnic sensitivity" as mentioned in ICH E5 is less critical to the development programme, because the metabolic pathway of the investigational drug may be rather simple and not utilising complex metabolic pathways. Finally, the development programme may have a different focus, if the treatment depends on identification of biomarkers and/or biogenomics relevant for a specific group of people, e.g., treatment of some oncology conditions like in non-small cell lung cancer states, where mapping of the extrinsic factors is not so important to the development programme (see below Case Example 3 and also ICH E17 training Module 2, Example 2). When initiating a new treatment all these research activities are highly valuable. Usually much more information is collected and analysed, and only some are included in the overall demographic information in the study protocols. This information has sometimes been valuable, as history has shown that such data could explain surprising results and contributed to new knowledge. One example is the PLATO study (Wallentin et al. 2009), ICH E17 trainidesign of the confirmatory global MRCTs.ng Module 6, discussed in Chapter 6, and below is an example with the treatment of non-small cell lung cancer.

Zhou et al. (2021) describe the planning of a confirmatory MRCT investigating the effects of pevonedistat in three oncological indications. The study is global including both Western and Asian regions. The East Asian region is a pooled region consisting of subjects from the Republic of Korea,

Japan, and China. The pooling of the East Asian subjects was based on scientific considerations of commonality of intrinsic and extrinsic factors and statistical evaluations to define the number of East Asian subjects needed to evaluate consistency with the overall study data. The study sample size was estimated to be 450 subjects and the number of subjects in the East Asian region to 30 subjects. (Study ID U1111–1189-8055). The study completed recruitment in 2020 and included a broad targeted population with all states of diseases and comorbidities.

2.5.1 Developing strategies

It is recommended to support the design of MRCTs by planning for global development from the early development phases, and thereby optimising the design of the confirmatory global MRCTs. It is however also possible to do the global MRCTs even if the early studies might have been performed locally with a less global focus. The MRCT design may include some pharmacology data and, if needed, some supplementary exploratory studies and/or bridging aspects. It is always recommendable to maximise the use of existing data from early development, i.e., through simulation models, in order to have the best possible planning information for the MRCTs. Additional studies may be included in the confirmatory MRCT protocol or conducted simultaneously with the MRCT to ensure the global applicability of the overall development programme.

Once the global target population has been identified, and appropriate information about ethnic factors has been collected and analysed, the development plan for pharmacology studies is made (see also Case Example 4, below).

The end of the exploratory phase and planning of the confirmatory phase is the critical parts for getting MRCT designs right. The defined targeted population to be investigated in MRCTs is key to the design of MRCTs and should be agreed upon across different parts of the world and with concerned regulatory authorities. While the aspiration would be to get consistent agreement on the study design, it may not always be possible in every detail, see below in section 2.6.

In addition to generating early clinical pharmacology and exploratory data across broad patient groups and ethnicities, there are other aspects that need to be considered as part of the development strategy. When designing MRCTs, the calculation of sample-size must consider using some of the principles defined in Chapter 5. The variability and distribution of the subjects among participating regions should be considered at this stage. Other design aspects, such as the selection of endpoints that are acceptable broadly by regulators across the world, should be considered. The question of concomitant medications, and how they vary within different regions should also be considered. As discussed in the ICH E17 guideline, to ensure the robust quality of the clinical data, GCP principles as defined in ICH E6 should be followed. Thus for MRCT, global harmonisation and alignments across all participating sites require thorough planning, standardisation, training, and control—something that may be less critical in the case of local development.

2.6 Consultation with Regulatory Authorities

ICH guidelines do usually not provide disease-specific requirements. There are several regulatory scientific guidelines that cover different therapeutic areas and describe the requirements for the development of a new drug for a specific disease and/or condition within a specific jurisdiction. These guidelines are issued by different regulatory bodies and may address the development requirements in their jurisdictions in different ways. The guidelines do often not agree on all development aspects and required criteria. Thus, having one development programme and single MRCT protocols covering all relevant regions will in most cases require a harmonised approach to each development programme across various regulatory authorities. It may not always be possible to comply with all parts of the guidelines issued by local regulatory bodies, thus necessitating consultation with authorities to reach study design compromises for the overall development programme and MRCTs, applying the E17 principles. Some of the key questions could be MRCT pooling strategies, agreements on primary and secondary endpoints, inclusion- and exclusion criteria, acceptance of concomitant treatments, and, last but not least the control treatment(s). A common example of discussions between regulatory bodies in various jurisdictions and sponsors is the use of non-inferiority margins. The inconsistencies among the regulatory scientific guidelines are not likely to be harmonised in a near foreseeable timeframe. This makes these consultations with authorities key to all global development programmes, in order to support successful global marketing authorisations. In the future, international collaborations among authorities and within organisations, like ICH, may support the development of international master protocols, including advice on topics like design options, adaptive platforms, primary endpoints, and characteristics of study populations. This may be some of the discussions in the ICH guideline development projects.

For the success of a global development programme, it is crucial that sponsors consult with regulatory authorities from the early planning stage to ensure that the advice from multiple authorities is informed and taken into consideration as much as possible. It is likely that several discussions and follow-up activities with authorities are needed to reach regulatory concurrence prior to a new global development programme and prior to each MRCT. In recent years, regulators have collaborated across countries on access to medicines. This has led to major benefits, not only for populations' access to new medicines, but also for authorities' learning from each other, by sharing discussions and assessment of data. The success of this kind of collaboration encourages other countries to work together to secure sustainable access to medicines.

Various work-sharing initiatives (e.g., ACCESS, ORBIS) are being put together by regulatory bodies, which may in time allow for a simultaneous consultation process for MRCTs and marketing authorisation applications. While currently, there are very few options for sponsors having parallel advice with multiple authorities on specific development programmes, it is encouraging to see the growth of international collaboration, e.g., ICMRA (International Coalition of Medicines Regulatory Authorities). These were very important when guidelines for the development of treatments and vaccines for the COVID-19 diseases were urgently needed. The COVID-19 crisis has changed much of the clinical trial world. However, the need for experts and professionals from sponsors and authorities, to come together and discuss how to successfully assess and manage clinical studies and processes, and to understand the need for data and evidence, remains the same.

It is expected for sponsors to tailor the submission of marketing authorisation applications to the needs of and agreed with respective regulatory authorities. The clinical data sets from the studies submitted, include usually several MRCTs. Post hoc analyses are summarised and include analyses within and across MRCTs, with a focus on the needs and requirements from respective authorities. In addition to the overall and regional outcomes reported for each MRCT, and summaries across studies, there are specific ad hoc analyses of data provided by sponsors based on requests from individual authorities. Even if the same set of clinical data are submitted to regulatory authorities, it is acknowledged that the need for information about efficacy and safety data may be different depending on different regulations, health care systems, cultures, traditions, etc. in the areas where the drug is going to be used.

A development programme conducted according to the ICH E17 principles is using pooling strategies in MRCTs. Populations sharing ethnic factors that may impact the effects of the drug are pooled into regions, which may be up to five in each MRCT. It is not expected that each MRCT can provide statistical conclusions for any subgroup or region included in the MRCT. The sample size in MRCTs is based on the overall objective of the trials, and allocation of subjects to regions are equally balanced (e.g., method 1 and 2 in the E17 guideline) with no specific defined sample size per region. Geography is often used when defining the regions as surrogates for ethnicities of the pooled populations. Each global MRCT includes typically about 30–40 counties representing the global targeted populations in almost 200 countries. A global development programme includes often more than one MRCT, whereby different topics like standard treatments/ controls and targeted populations are investigated further. Each MRCT may not always be representative for all targeted populations. It is the total sample size of the global development programme that ensures a global representative population demonstrating efficacy and safety for the targeted populations. Authorities from different jurisdictions/countries may have different interests and approaches to assessment of the overall clinical dataset. Several post hoc analyses may be required within and across studies by different jurisdictions/countries for each authority to assess the benefits and risk relevant to their targeted population. The overall assessment by international authorities may be very similar, also including important learnings about how the drug performs in diverse populations. The benefit-risk assessments by different authorities may differ due to differences in population characteristics in each jurisdiction/country. The decision outcomes made by these authorities may therefore vary.

2.7 Overcoming Regional Variabilities

The sample size should not increase, when the ICH E17 principles are used in a global development programme. The pooling principle is key to ensure this, when the populations targeted in the clinical development programme become increasingly diverse. The reason for pooling populations into regions in an MRCT is the sharing of ethnic factors within each pooled population. Geography as such is not important and is merely a surrogate for pooling of populations. It is important to provide a scientific rationale for the pooling strategies and definition of regions in the protocol (see Chapter 4). The protocol should present the background for the defined ethnic factors that potentially may impact the effects of the investigational drug (effect modifiers) and how these factors are shared among the subjects pooled into one region. Pooling is only simple in the case where there are no effect modifiers due to ethnic differences. It is important, that the clinical data from pooled populations is shown to be representative for each country, where the data are submitted to support marketing authorisation.

Both the recruiting of increasingly diverse populations in global development and MRCTs (see section 2.2 above) and the handling of these more heterogeneous populations in MRCTs can be challenging. Some of the variabilities across regions may be difficult to harmonise, like different control treatments and disease diagnoses, but this may be overcomed by tailoring parts of the study design to regional needs. Molecular biology and master protocols, which include several sub-clinical studies, are well known in the area of oncology. This is a useful approach that can be applied to other disease areas. Global development and MRCTs include diverse target populations and conducting phase I–III according to each subpopulation may be unrealistic. In some diverse disease areas, it may make sense to make sub-investigations within the MRCT protocol, including populations with different subtypes of the disease in different subgroups or subpopulations.

Another important recent learning is the use of virtual trial methodologies, including methods like telemedicine and virtual visits as vital tools to support safety of patients enrolled in clinical trials. These tools have steadily and gradually been adopted and advanced, especially during the COVID-19 crisis, where mobile devices are used to supplant or supplement traditional visits at the clinic or sites. These virtual methods are important tools for MRCTs, as both recruitment and retainment of global patients are greatly facilitated. For example, decentralised clinical trial platform can be operated from a mobile device, and thereby enable and coordinate study-related procedures and assessments that used to take place at a hospital. Authorities developed guidelines in 2020 during the COVID-19 crisis (e.g., FDA Guidance on Conduct of Clinical Trials of Medical Products during COVID-19 2020; EMA-HMA, Guidance on the Management of Clinical Trials during the COVID-19 2020), to support these virtual approaches and vital tools, as the pandemic transformed how sponsors and regulators need to think about the executions of clinical studies. The virtual tools were logical tools mitigating some of the risks associated with the COVID-19 disease. These learnings helped reduce the burden on personnel and systems, not only in the extraordinarily difficult circumstances due to the COVID-19 crisis but also because reducing obstacles like traveling may improve the retainment of subjects and facilitate recruitment of subjects in remote areas and "low-income" communities. These new approaches are useful in facilitating the conduct of MRCTs, where some populations are living in remote areas or cannot easily travel to hospitals for visits. The development of these virtual solutions may also ease the collection of real-world data as part of drug development. Real-world data may further inform trial designs and provide new insights on the global development journey. Global MRCTs may eventually minimize the current differences in the access to data and to innovative treatments among regions.

The phase of collecting ethnic factors is very important in the planning of the development programme, see ICH E17, Training Module 2. Realising the value of collecting a broad, diverse, and global set of intrinsic and extrinsic factor information, is critical for successful planning of the development programme, leading to an effective and lean clinical programme. The collection of ethnic information should never be focused on the "need to know." It is recommended to collect information and data with an open mindset, accepting that it may not be all collected information that is needed in the first place, but the information may be useful later in development, in post-marketing phases, or for other projects.

The use of digital approaches, such as and wearables, may open opportunities for evaluating new study endpoints and participants' experiences. For example, digital tools allow participants to enter information immediately. These new tools support the usual questionnaires and dairies and may change the way sponsors can increase the value of MRCTs, especially bringing value to dispersed sites participating in MRCTs. Subjects far from university hospitals, populations that are usually not elected for clinical studies, may now become included, due to the remote visit options offered by the digital study tools.

The intrinsic factors like occurrence of different genes measure vital signs or are used to diagnose, e.g., metabolising systems, biomarkers, and races are collected. Importantly is also the collection of extrinsic factors, like concomitant medicines and standard of care in the different areas. The diversity of health care systems among regions has always been a concern for the conduct of global MRCTs. MRCTs may be one of the tools that will improve the knowledge about diverse healthcare systems and lead to further global harmonisation of the systems. Tools like digital wearables, that can measure vital signs or are used to diagnose subjects, will need to be validated, and standards across regions should be developed. However, the increased harmonisation and global cooperation between sponsors and authorities has already demonstrated, even with a great diversity of populations, that global MRCTs can be very successful and can support global marketing authorisation. In addition to the patient-reported outcomes (PRO) new subjects' experience data has emerged and provided a platform for understanding effects observed directly by study participants, online, and more real in the participant's own environment. These new endpoints, and generally the use of digital measures in MRCTs, may provide new insights in future studies.

2.8 Concluding Remarks

MRCTs conducted in accordance with the ICH E17 guideline, will improve the know-how and understanding of both similarities and differences in how the new treatment performs in different regions. It is therefore important for the planning of a global development programme and MRCTs to identify differences and similarities in intrinsic and extrinsic factors. Prespecified pooling of regions and/or subpopulations may help provide flexibility in sample size allocation to regions, facilitate the evaluation of consistency in treatment effects across regions, and support regulatory decision-making. The pooling strategy should be justified based on the distribution of the intrinsic and extrinsic factors expected to affect the treatment response, the disease under investigation, and similarity of those factors across regions. Differences among regions are not unusual and these differences should not be a barrier against the conduct of MRCTs in most cases. It is of paramount importance to find and identify differences, which affect treatment effect, early before start of MRCTs. Important is then how to manage such differences, in order to conduct and participate in MRCTs.

It is important for the planning of a global development programme to get the best possible overview of the different situations regarding the ethnic factors in the different areas. This know-how may also be valuable, when surprising results may occur and need to be assessed. Last, but not least, it supports global marketing and access to drugs. Sponsors have one global development plan and one set of data generated by the clinical studies, and all the different questions from different authorities must be answered using that same dataset. Therefore, it is important to ensure that each population within an area, is represented in the dataset, for the relevant authority to be able to assess the risks and benefits for that population.

2.9 Case Examples

Case Example 1: Diabetes outcome studies provided some early experience with the MRCT concepts. The investigation of the cardiovascular risk involved with the treatment of diabetic type 2 patients with liraglutide (the LEADER study) was a global study involving 32 countries, grouped in four defined regions, see below Figure 2.2. to represent all diabetic type 2 subjects in the world the allocation of subjects was balanced to make up four regions. From the presentation of data, it looks as if the participating subjects from North America may have a higher risk of CV events compared to the other regions. The results showed that the overall treatment effect based on all subjects was statistically superior to the control; however, the point estimate of treatment effect in patients from USA was numerically inferior (Marso et al. 2016).

The results were investigated in detail, and different sets of sub-analyses were performed. It was not obvious why the subjects from the USA seemed to behave differently, and the overall study conclusions were accepted by all involved authorities. FDA in the USA also approved that there was no increased risk to diabetic CV patients regarding their CV disease and that treatment with liraglutide was superior to placebo, thereby protecting diabetic patients towards deterioration of their CV disease. This kind of apparent difference in treatment effect has also been seen in other MRCTs, e.g., the PLATO study. New knowledge was learned about the effect of the drug, like in the PLATO study, where baseline characteristics were the reason for a difference between the subjects from the USA vs. all subjects in the study, see also Chapter 6. Back in history, researchers learned that African-Americans have reduced blood pressure responses to monotherapy

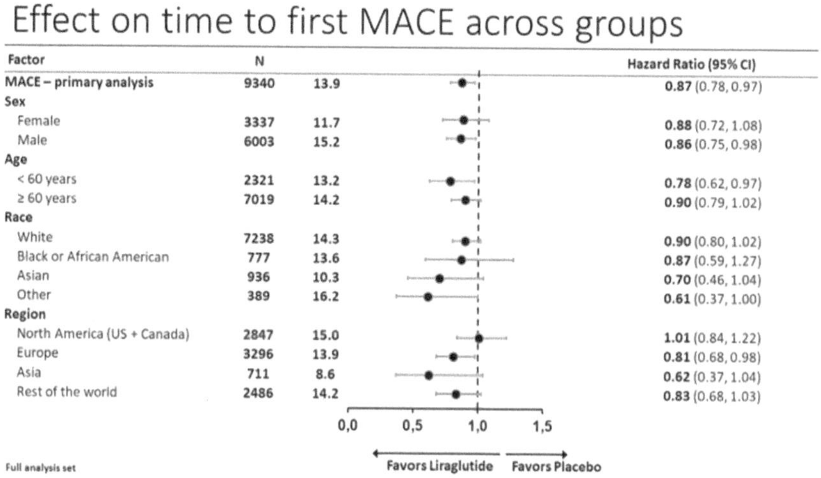

Effect on time to first MACE across groups

Factor	N			Hazard Ratio (95% CI)
MACE – primary analysis	9340	13.9		0.87 (0.78, 0.97)
Sex				
Female	3337	11.7		0.88 (0.72, 1.08)
Male	6003	15.2		0.86 (0.75, 0.98)
Age				
< 60 years	2321	13.2		0.78 (0.62, 0.97)
≥ 60 years	7019	14.2		0.90 (0.79, 1.02)
Race				
White	7238	14.3		0.90 (0.80, 1.02)
Black or African American	777	13.6		0.87 (0.59, 1.27)
Asian	936	10.3		0.70 (0.46, 1.04)
Other	389	16.2		0.61 (0.37, 1.00)
Region				
North America (US + Canada)	2847	15.0		1.01 (0.84, 1.22)
Europe	3296	13.9		0.81 (0.68, 0.98)
Asia	711	8.6		0.62 (0.37, 1.04)
Rest of the world	2486	14.2		0.83 (0.68, 1.03)

0,0   0,5   1,0   1,5

Full analysis set

← Favors Liraglutide   Favors Placebo →

FIGURE 2.2
Effects on time to first MACE across subgroups and regions.

with beta-blocker, and this has also been shown with ACE inhibitors, or ARBs, when compared to diuretics or calcium channel blockers (Brewster and Seedat 2013). Examples like these may be captured early during the conduct of global MRCTs with new investigational drugs, because different populations are investigated in parallel in the same study.

Case Example 2: In the training material, Module 2, is an example of a development programme for a new long-acting basal insulin product, i.e., an insulin product with long time between injections. It is critical for diabetic persons to keep their blood sugar within normal levels to limit the risk of diabetic complications as much as possible. Long-acting insulin products, provide a stable blood concentration, not varying too much over time, and are needed to treat the basal glucose metabolism in the body. Diabetes occurs all over the world, so the development plan is targeting diabetic subjects globally. The treatment needs to cope with many different lifestyles, age groups, concomitant diseases, disease severity, cultures, and many more extrinsic as well as intrinsic factors, where Body Mass Index is one of the key effect modifiers when deciding the initial dosing regimen. Both intrinsic factors and extrinsic factors are important for development of the disease, and disease risk factors include both kinds of ethnic factors. There are for example different, prevalence of several complications among diabetic populations across regions (Kenealy et al. 2012). Risk factors due to lifestyle for type 2 diabetes mellitus (DM) are the factors that matter the most for the increasing worldwide prevalence, that has been observed for the disease, especially in Asia. The meals in Asia have usually a high content of carbohydrates, whereas Americans take meals with a high fat and protein content relative to the Asian populations. Also, lifestyles, like daily exercise, are risk factors for the disease and vary between populations. There are also different treatment traditions across regions, which need to be informed and addressed in the planning of the development programme and each MRCT. The epidemiological data, disease information, and treatment guidelines from regions are collected in the planning phase. Based on these data, the know-how about the PK-PD properties of the in-vestigational drug and experience from other development programmes, are the ethnic factors that potentially may influence the effect of the drug defined (See Chapter 6 and Effect modifiers, ICH E8, R1). See medicines' sensitivity to ethnic factors, ICH E5, and refer to Chapter 3.

As discussed in Chapter 4 on pooling strategies, populations sharing common effect modifiers can be pooled together into one region. As an example, regions defined in a confirmatory MRCT investigating treatment in type 2 DM populations are based on commonalities in eating habits (note also period of fasting in some cultures) and daily exercise. The planning of an MRCT needs to consider the possibility to evaluate the consistency of the effects across regions. So, even if the number of subjects to be included in the MRCT must be calculated based on the overall trial objective, it is also important to balance the number of subjects per region (see ICH training module 4). It is recommended to keep the number of regions low, e.g., up to five regions in one MRCT, to make it possible to compare results across regions (see also Chapter 6). In a global trial, like this example, the Asian populations are pooled, the European-Eurasian populations are pooled, and the Americas can be pooled as one region. A region including the remaining populations is often defined to make up the last region, the so-called "Rest of the World" region. The "ROW" region includes more diverse popula-tions compared to the other regions, in order to allow inclusion of some low- and middle-income areas/countries and "new" university hospitals. These are areas where the know-how about ethnic factors is more scarce and will therefore also introduce more uncertainties. It is expected that the number of subjects to be included in global MRCTs may increase, compared to regional studies, in order to handle these more diverse populations. Some MRCTs may therefore turn out to be "overpowered," because the risk of having included very variable populations and uncertainties is considered when the sample size is decided. Ultimately it is always a balance of how much uncertainty can be allowed. For example, for a disease such as dia-betes type 2, which is extensively studied, it may be alright to have a broadly variable population. However, for less known diseases, this may be difficult or not recommended.

Case Example 3: Included in the training material module 2, is another example of important knowledge learned from global development. That is a treatment of non-small cell lung cancer (NSCLC) with gefitinib (Yang 2008; Vansteenkiste and Wauters 2018). Gefitinib is a small molecule, which inhibits EGFR tyrosine kinase. At the time of development, not much was understood about the predictive marker, i.e., mutated EGFR. The phase II programme included two studies with populations from the USA and Japan, and the results were different in these two regions. The response showed significant improvements in the Asian population, while the results of the study in the USA were disappointing and did not demonstrate the same efficacy as was seen in early exploratory studies and in the Asian population. Hence, it was speculated why the Asian subjects responded much better to treatment compared to the subjects from America. Upon further analysis, it turned out that the incidence of mutated EGFR was much higher in Asia vs. America, and overall the incidence of the mutated EFFR is down to 20–30% of patients with NSCLC. Had it not been for the remarkable effect in the Asian subjects, the company may have relied on the low level of efficacy in other populations and never discovered this re-markable effect in NSCLC patients with mutated EGFR and thereby es-tablishment of the first-line treatment of NSCLC. With today's improved tools to study genomics, it may be possible to identify genetic differences and identify predictive biomarkers early in drug development when de-signing MRCTs.

Case Example 4: In the figure below is an overview of sponsor planning phases based on the E17 principles and the considerations described in this chapter. The first part is the collection of information phase, where the sponsor collects the internationally available information about the targeted disease, knowledge from international societies, data from pre-clinical re-search, and any other relevant information regarding similar research projects. This general information is summarised and provided to regional experts, who then add information about regional conditions, epidemiolo-gical data, know-how about the disease, and cultural aspects to the overall background information. All this collected input is then evaluated and analysed to summarise the information about the ethnic factors from where the factors that may potentially influence the effects of the investigational drug are to be defined (effect modifiers). Questions asked may include:

- What is known about the biology of the disease?
- Where does the disease occur and how (prevalence, severity) does it occur?
- What are the investigational drug characteristics (mode of action, pharmacology)?
- What are the intrinsic and extrinsic factors where the disease occurs?

Based on the answers to these questions, including information from the pre-clinical research and the international and regional experts, the intrinsic

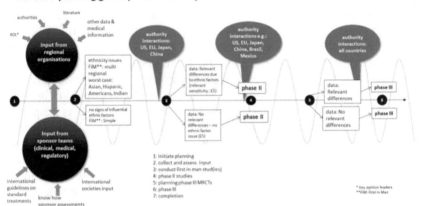

FIGURE 2.3
Planning global product development.

and extrinsic factors, that potentially may influence the effect of the drug, are defined (effect modifiers). The planning of the first studies in man, i.e., pharmacological and exploratory studies, phase I–II, is then completed. If the investigational drug is expected to be highly sensitive to intrinsic and extrinsic factors (see ICH E 5), i.e., that these factors are expected to have an influence on the efficacy of the drug, then this is the "worst case," where the sponsor should consider including different populations in the early studies to collect and compare PK and PD data between the different populations. (Figure 2.3)

Before entering phase II, it is imperative to engage with international regulatory authorities to discuss the sufficiency of the programme for development and marketing authorisations. The outcome of phase II studies supported by the collected information about influential ethnic factors should inform the design of each confirmatory MRCT. Meetings with involved regulatory authorities are recommended to discuss the sufficiency of each MRCT protocol for marketing authorisation.

The defined influential factors, effect modifiers, are key to the definition of regions for each MRCT. Each region should consist of populations sharing influential factors/effect modifiers. Ethnic factors may influence both efficacy and safety endpoints, and the whole picture may not be fully understood in the design phase of the confirmatory studies. It is the planning of the overall programme and how the MRTCs are designed that are key to the success of the development. This also includes how the planned studies can support each other to eventually provide a dataset that is sufficient for the planned marketing authorisations. Throughout the development, it is important to adjust the programme to ensure that all relevant populations are represented by the programme.

References

Brewster LM and Seedat YK. Why do hypertensive patients of African ancestry respond better to calcium blockers and diuretics than to ACE inhibitors and β-adrenergic blockers? A systematic review. *BMC Med*. 2013; 11: 141. https://www.ncbi.nlm.nih.gov/pmc/articles/PMC3681568/

EMA-HMA: Guidance on the Management of Clinical Trials during the COVID-19 (coronavirus) Pandemic Version 3 28/04/2020. https://ec.europa.eu/health/sites/health/files/files/eudralex/vol-10/guidanceclinicaltrials_covid19_en.pdf

FDA. Enhancing the Diversity of Clinical Trial Populations—Eligibility Criteria, Enrolment Practices, and Trial Designs Guidance for Industry, November 2020. https://www.fda.gov/regulatory-information/search-fda-guidance-documents/enhancing-diversity-clinical-trial-populations-eligibility-criteria-enrollment-practices-and-trial

FDA. Guidance on Conduct of Clinical Trials of Medical Products during COVID-19 Public Health Emergency Guidance for Industry, Investigators, and Institutional Review Boards, March 2020. https://www.fda.gov/news-events/press-announcements/coronavirus-covid-19-update-fda-issues-guidance-conducting-clinical-trials

FDA. The Orbis project by FDA 09/17/2019. https://www.fda.gov/about-fda/oncology-center-excellence/project-orbis and Project Orbis: Strengthening International Collaboration for Oncology Product Reviews, Faster Patient Access to Innovative Therapies | FDA.

FDA. Drug trials snapshots 2015–2019 Five-Year Summary and Analysis of Clinical Trial Participation and Demographics, November 2020. https://www.fda.gov/media/143592/download

Kenealy T, Elley CR, Collins JF, Moyes SA, Metcalf PA and Drury PL. Increased prevalence of albuminuria among non-European peoples with type 2 diabetes. Nephrol Dial Transplant. 2012; 27:1840–1846.

Kim ES, Bruinooge SS, Roberts S, et al. Broadening eligibility criteria to make clinical trials more representative: American Society of Clinical Oncology and Friends of Cancer Research Joint research statement. *J Clin Oncol*. 2017; 35: 3737–3744.

Marso SP, Daniels GH, Brown-Frandsen K, Kristensen P, Mann JFE, Nauck MA, Nissen SE, Pocock S, Poulter NR, Ravn LS, Steinberg WM, Stockner M, Zinman B, Bergenstal RM, and Buse JB. Liraglutide and cardiovascular outcomes in type 2 diabetes, the LEADER study. *N Engl J Med*. 2016; 375: 311–322.

Nielsen HK, DeChairo S and Goldman B. Evaluation of consistency of treatment response across regions. The LEADER trial. 2021. Pending publication.

The Access Consortium by Australia-Canada-Singapore-Switzerland-United Kingdom: https://www.tga.gov.au/australia-canada-singapore-switzerland-united-kingdom-access-consortium

Vansteenkiste J and Wauters E. Ann Oncol. 2018; 29: Supplement 1. https://www.annalsofoncology.org/article/S0923-7534(19)31673-4/fulltext.

Wallentin L, Becker RC, Budaj A, Cannon CP, Emanuelsson H, Held C, Horrow J, Husted S, James S, Katus H, Mahaffey KW, and Scirica BM. Ticagrelor versus clopidogrel in patients with acute coronary syndromes. *N Engl J Med*. 2009; 361:1045–1057.

Yang CH. EGFR tyrosine kinase inhibitors for the treatment of NSCLC in East Asia: Present and future. *Lung Cancer*. 2008; 60(Suppl. 2):S23–S30.

Zhou X, Friedlander S, Kupperman E, Sedarati F Kuroda S, Hua Z, Yuan Y, Yamamoto Y, Faller DV, Haikawa K, Nakai K, Bowen S, Dai Y, Venkatakrishnan K. Asia-inclusive global development of pevonedistat: Clinical pharmacology and translational research enabling a phase III multi-regional clinical trial. *Clin Transl Sci*. 2021; 00:1–13.

3

Consideration of "Ethnic Factors" in Design and Conduct of Multiregional Clinical Trials (MRCT)

Rominder Singh and Vibeke Bjerregaard

3.1 Introduction

The International Council for Harmonisation of Technical Requirements for Pharmaceuticals for Human Use (ICH) E5 guidelines were developed in 1998 and have since then undergone series of revisions. Many terms used in the E5 guidelines are over two decades old and warrant revisiting given that the science has evolved and so has our knowledge of how to conduct global clinical trials. The terms such as "ethnic factors" may mean different things in the context of race and ethnicity. Terms like "genetic" were originally meant to be a catch-all term for all things related to the inherited genes and epigenomics lumped under the umbrella of "intrinsic factors" but may have broader implications in drug development. Finally, the definition of the region, the "R" in MRCT, has also evolved under the E17 guidelines. This chapter will provide a historic perspective of how the terminology used in E5 and E17 guidelines are best interpreted and applied for the conduct of multiregional clinical trials (MRCT).

Content:

1. History of ICH E5

2. Definition of intrinsic and extrinsic "ethnic factors"

3. "Ethnic Sensitivity" as described in ICH E5

4. Interpretation and Application of ICH E5—Challenges and Gaps

    a. Definition of Race and Ethnicity in Drug Development Needs to Be Revisited

    b. What are Foreign Clinical Data?

    c. Intrinsic Factors

DOI: 10.1201/9781003109785-3

3.2 History of ICH E5

The concept of MRCTs is not new. In the past, however, clinical trials of a new medicine were often performed separately in different regulatory regions to fulfill the regulatory requirements of each region or specific country. This resulted in a great deal of repetition and extra expense. In addition, because it was difficult to conduct many trials simultaneously, some countries would have to wait for studies to be conducted in their region or country resulting in delays to drug approvals.

To improve the efficiency of drug development globally, ICH released the E5 guidelines entitled "Ethnic Factors in the Acceptability of Foreign Clinical Data." The ICH E5 guidelines, first released in 1998, provides a general framework for evaluating the potential impact of ethnic factors on the acceptability of foreign clinical data, with the underlying objective of minimizing duplication or repetition of clinical studies. ICH E5 also describes the concept of bridging studies for the extrapolation of foreign clinical data to a new region. In other words, ICH E5 provides guidance for how to justify the use of data from other countries for registration, based on common characteristics such as genetic factors, diet, and disease patterns to reduce, or avoid, the need to conduct separate studies in every country.

Despite the intent of the E5 guidelines, questions remained about how best to plan and perform individual clinical studies that were intended for registration in many countries, and drug developers often continued to conduct standalone clinical trials in individual countries, which resulted in continued high costs and delays to regulatory submission and access in some countries and regions.

To address this continuing challenge, beginning in 2014, the ICH commissioned an expert working group consisting of various regulatory agencies in partnership with pharmaceutical industry groups to develop a new guideline devoted to the planning and conduct of MRCTs. These new guidelines are now referred to as ICH E17 ("E17 General Principles For Planning And Design Of Multiregional…" 2017). More details on the evolution of E17 guidelines are presented in Chapter 1.

3.3 Definition of Intrinsic and Extrinsic "Ethnic Factors"

As per the ICH E5 guidelines, defines intrinsic and extrinsic factors as:

- *Extrinsic ethnic factors are factors associated with the environment and culture in which a person resides. Extrinsic factors tend to be less genetically and more culturally and behaviorally determined. Examples of extrinsic factors include the social and cultural aspects of a region such as medical practice, diet, use of tobacco, use of alcohol, exposure to pollution and sunshine, socio-economic status, compliance with prescribed medications, and, particularly important to the reliance on studies from a different region, practices in clinical trial design and conduct. "*

- *On the other hand, intrinsic ethnic factors are defined as factors that help to define and identify a sub-population and may influence the ability to extrapolate clinical data between regions. Examples of intrinsic factors include genetic polymorphism, age, gender, height, weight, lean body mass, body composition, and organ dysfunction."*

As shown in Figure 3.1, there are factors that are interdependent on each other such as smoking, food, stress, etc., that are represented in between the intrinsic and extrinsic factors.

INTRINSIC		EXTRINSIC
Genetic	Physiological and pathological conditions	Environmental
Gender	Age (children - elderly)	Climate
		Sunlight
	Height	Pollution
	Bodyweight	
	Liver	**Culture**
	Kidney	Socio-economic factors
	Cardiovascular functions	Educational status
	ADME	Language
	Receptor sensitivity	
Race		Medical practice
		Disease definition/Diagnostic
Genetic polymorphism		Therapeutic approach
of the drug metabolism	Smoking	Drug compliance
	Alcohol	
	Food habits	
	Stress	
Genetic disease	Diseases	
		Regulatory practice/GCP
		Methodology/Endpoints

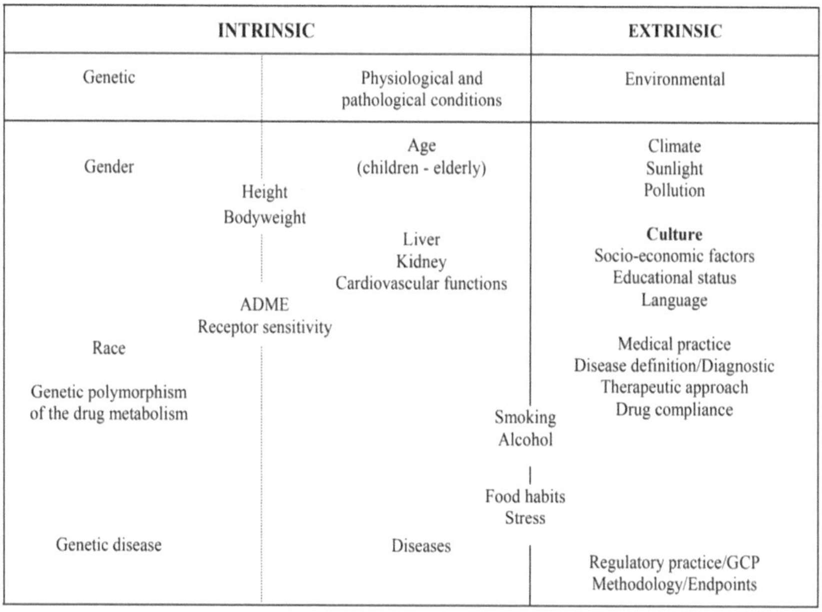

FIGURE 3.1
Classification of intrinsic and extrinsic factors as described in Appendix A of the ICH E5 guidelines.

As discussed in Chapter 1, the ICH E17 is captured in the seven principles described in the document. Principles 2 and 3 specifically reference how intrinsic and extrinsic factors are relevant in the design and conduct of MRCTs. For example, Principle 2 states that *"The intrinsic and extrinsic factors important to the drug development program, should be identified early. The potential impact of these factors could be examined in the exploratory phases before the design of confirmatory MRCTs. Information about them should also be collected during the confirmatory trial for evaluation of their impact on treatment effects."* And Principle 3 states that *"MRCTs are planned under the assumption that the treatment effect applies to the entire target population, particularly to the regions included in the trial. Strategic allocation of the sample size to regions allows an evaluation of the extent to which this assumption holds."* Thus, it is critical that early evaluation of "intrinsic and extrinsic" factors be conducted.

3.4 "Ethnic Sensitivity" as Described in ICH E5

As per the ICH E5 guidelines, *"characterization of a medicine as 'ethnically insensitive', i.e., unlikely to behave differently in different populations, would usually make it easier to extrapolate data from one region to another and needless bridging data."*

This led to many agencies reference the E5 guidelines as the rationale for local clinical studies which were used to "bridge" to the broader global clinical data. It was not uncommon that local clinical studies were conducted again in multiple countries instead of truly leveraging the guiding principle of E5 which states *"This guidance is based on the premise that it is not necessary to repeat the entire clinical drug development program in the new region and is intended to recommend strategies for accepting foreign clinical data as full or partial support for approval of an application in a new region."*

To request a clinical trial waiver, the sponsors need to submit the Ethnic Sensitivity Waiver Request (ESWR) based on E5 Appendix D. With it came a set of questions, and the evaluation by the agencies was not always consistent or predictable. While the generation of pharmacokinetics (PK) data was usually the starting point but not necessarily the end to show that *"characterization of a medicine as 'ethnically insensitive', i.e., unlikely to behave differently in different populations, would usually make it easier to extrapolate data from one region to another and need less bridging data."*

Moreover, the bridging studies did not always work as intended; the results were prone to varying degrees of interpretation. This resulted in an increased number of local clinical studies, which at times included large patient numbers (e.g., 300 patients from China or 15% of the total study population in Japan). There was little consistency in what the various agencies required for bridging based on what was highlighted in ICH E5 *"a bridging study is defined as a study performed in the new region to provide pharmacodynamic or clinical data on efficacy, safety, dosage and dose regimen in the new region that will allow extrapolation of the foreign clinical data to the population in the new region."* Thus, intrinsic and/or extrinsic ethnic factors mentioned in the context of E5 which are listed in Figure 3.1 are generally considered to be "broad" factors. For example, gender, race, and genetics are composites of many other facets which need to be addressed in the context of a drug development program.

3.5 Interpretation and Application of ICH E5—Challenges and Gaps

3.5.1 Definition of Race and Ethnicity in Drug Development Needs to Be Revisited

The concept of race is largely considered a social construct and with only a small difference in the genetic between races (Boris 1994). As per the American Anthropological Association (AAA), *"Evidence from the analysis of genetics (e.g., DNA) indicates that most physical variation, about 94%, lies within so-called racial groups. Conventional geographic 'racial' groupings differ from one another only in about 6% of their genes. There is greater variation within 'racial' groups than between them"* ("American Anthropological Association Draft Official Statement On "Race"" 1997). Race is a better predictor of physical traits (e.g., the color of the skin or shape of the eyes) rather than a comprehensive prognosticator of biological characteristics. Over generations, because of migration and interbreeding, the human phenotypes have been diluted and it is almost impossible to have a singular race category. Even having a regional classification of East Asians classified as a specific race or ethnicity in drug development based on phenotypic traits seems arbitrary at best.

The US Food and Drug Administration (FDA) recently issued guidelines on the collection of race and ethnicity data in clinical trials (2019 FDA). The driver behind these guidelines is to have a standardized terminology based on the Office of Management and Budget (OMB) definitions. OMB defines "Asians" as people having origins in any of the original peoples of the Far East, Southeast Asia, or the Indian subcontinent including, for example, Cambodia, China, India, Japan, Korea, Malaysia, Pakistan, the Philippine Islands, Thailand, and Vietnam ("Office Of Management And Budget (OMB) Standards | Office Of Research On Women's Health" 2021). For drug development and clinical trials, there is no scientific basis for this clarification, and collecting the "Asian" data could lead to false results. Yusuf and Wittes (2016) in their analysis have concluded that most variations in results among countries are probably due to chance, variations can occasionally reflect important differences among countries in either the true benefits of an intervention or its true harms. While there is a need to be a representation of the minority population in clinical trials, and race and/ or ethnicity characteristics could impact the treatment outcome, there needs to be a more consistent definition, and validation, of race and ethnicity in drug development.

3.5.2 What Are Foreign Clinical Data?

The ICH E5 guidelines reference "foreign clinical data." What is "foreign"? How much is "foreign"? Why is it "foreign"? "Foreign" to whom? Historically, clinical data were first generated in the "West" (e.g., US/EU) and then bridged to the other regions ("foreign"). This is an outdated concept. It is not uncommon to have most, if not all, clinical data be generated in countries other than where it is being used for registration. For example, data generated exclusively in China could be used for registration in the US—so in this case which is the "foreign country"? The ICH E17 was designed to help address some of these archaic concepts. In the interconnected world of drug development and medicine, the concept of "foreign" data is no longer be applicable.

3.5.3 Intrinsic Factors

3.5.3.1 Gender

The term gender refers to a complex interrelation and integration of sex, as a biological and functional determinant, and psychological and cultural behavior due to ethnical, social, or religious background (Buoncervello et al. 2017). Gender, in the context of E5 was intended to study the disparities between females and males and the related biological mechanisms as well as human physiology, pathophysiology, and clinical outcomes common to women and men. Over the years since the publication of E5 guidelines in the late 1990s, the field of gender-medicine has become an important transversal dimension in the practice of medicine and in the design of clinical trials. These describe the differences within the same disease of symptoms, clinical evolution, and the treatment effect between men and women—all of which need to be considered in drug development (Gemmati et al. 2019). Thus, understanding the gender differences, and enrolling representative gender populations in MRCTs will allow for better interpretability of results.

3.5.3.2 Race and Ethnicity

When conducting a literature search on race and ethnicity in medicine or drug development, these terms appear to be used interchangeably. The ICH

E5 guidelines say that *"three major racial groups most relevant to the ICH regions (Asian, Black, and Caucasian) is critical to the registration of medicines in the ICH regions."* The question is who is Asian? Who is Black? How does one define race and/or ethnicity?

Race and ethnicity, by themselves, are poor surrogates to measure the meaningful clinical effects and should be used with caution in drug development (Collins 2004). Other approaches are needed to define a population other than race or ethnicity or their belonging to the geographic region or a country. Ethnicity and race are social constructs that are self-reported and introduce varying degrees of subjectivity. Instead, influencing factors that are prognostic or have predictive biomarkers responsible for disease causation and treatment should be identified early in the drug development process. These influencing factors may, or may not, be related to race, ethnicity, or a geographic region.

Thus, the concept of using ethnicity and race in drug development needs to be revisited. In a country there are multiple ethnicities and races, the ethnic factors can be intrinsic or extrinsic. Thus, grouping populations based on self-reported race or ethnicity does not accurately predict the genotype or drug response of the patient (Bonham et al. 2016). Self-reporting of race and ethnicity has its pitfalls (Magaña López et al. 2016) and at best is a poor surrogate to determine the drug response in patients. Thus, other ways are needed to define a population other than race or ethnicity for efficient assessment and promoting drug development.

3.5.3.3 Genetics

Likewise, the other broad intrinsic factor—genetics—is a catch-all for all things hereditary. It does not consider epigenetics which is influenced by the environment (and is listed as an extrinsic factor). In drug development, the genetic polymorphism of CYP450 has been widely studied in various populations and regions (Zanger and Schwab 2013). To understand the genetic polymorphism, over the last decade multiple studies and analysis were conducted to evaluate the difference (and similarities) in PK in East Asia (Japan, China, Korea). These studies focused on evaluating the inter- and intra-regional differences (e.g. East-Asian vs. Caucasians) (Asano, Uyama and Tohkin 2017). The results were at times contradictory but directionally suggesting that the difference may be restricted to drugs that are metabolized by CYP450 enzymes that have known polymorphism. In these studies, the premise was that the East-Asian have a similar genetic background based on ethnicity and race and thus could be combined as a group and compared to another "ethnic group," the Caucasians.

Furthermore, in the late 1990s when the ICH E5 guidelines were issued, the majority of the new drugs were small molecules or new chemical entities (NCE). These NCEs were susceptible to intra-population variabilities related to the ADME of the drug (Wilson et al. 2001). The ICH E5 guidelines focus extensively on the various intrinsic factors (e.g., drug-metabolizing enzyme polymorphism) that can cause differences in drug metabolism and dispositions in various populations (or regions). Today, biologics make up a majority of new therapeutics and these new medicines are generally not as susceptible to the drug disposition differences between populations.

3.5.4 Extrinsic Factors

Over the years, as our knowledge of genetics and biology of diseases has improved, the pharmaceutical industry and academia have become adept in taking into account the E5 intrinsic factors. However, there has been a lag in taking into account the extrinsic factors (Figure 3.1). The recent call for diversity in clinical trials has its roots in better understanding and addressing, the "extrinsic factors." Extrinsic factors related to socio-economic factors, education status, access to preventive medical care can be addressed through the inclusion of diverse patient populations in MRCTs. Thus, identifying the extrinsic factors which are rather subjective, has been difficult to incorporate into the study design, especially in MRCTs.

As per the Centers for Disease Control and Prevention (CDC) guidelines, health outcome is influenced by many factors, and it may generally be organized into five broad categories known as the determinants of health: genetics, behavior, environmental and physical influences, medical care, and social factors ("Social Determinants Of Health | CDC" 2021"Social Determinants Of Health | CDC" 2021). These five categories broadly capture the extrinsic factors (as defined in E5) and could be considered when designing MRCTs.

Furthermore, a recent report (NEJM 2017), highlights 12 social determinants of health. Notable examples of social determinants of health include income level, education, gender, race, physical environment, access to healthy food and safe water, etc. If one looks at these determinants through the E5 lens, these cover the various "intrinsic and extrinsic factors" as originally conceived in the E5 guidelines. Thus, ideally, a broad inclusion representative of the target patient population should be developed early during the design of MRCT taking into ICH E5 factors as a guide. After all, clinical trials (especially randomized clinical trials) are controlled studies that are meant to represent real-life future applications in broader populations in their native settings. The social determinants of health provide a much broader aperture through which one could design the MRCTs using the principles of E5 and E17.

3.5.5 Definition of "Region"

Over the last two decades, since the ICH E5 guidelines were issued, the definition of the "region" in MRCT has also evolved. While ICH E5 guidelines extensively reference the "ICH Region," "New Region," and "Foreign Region"—the definition of "region" has been redefined in the new ICH E17 guidelines.

During the new drug registration process, some regulatory agencies in Asia (e.g., Japan, China, Korea, Taiwan, India) frequently require that additional safety and efficacy data should be generated in "Asians" or "global" clinical data be "bridged" to "East Asians." This raises the fundamental question: who is an Asian? The use of a single ethnic label of "Asians" or "East Asian" in drug development underestimates the genetic diversity in the vast continent yet could overstate its impact on variability to drug response. Geographic location, race, and ethnicity by themselves have been shown to be poor surrogates to determine meaningful clinical effects. Findings reported in a recent publication in Clinical Pharmacology and Therapeutics (Singh and Teo 2019) shed further light on this argument.

The recently released guidelines of ICH E17 on MRCTs introduce a new concept and context for defining the region as a **Region**. Under the ICHE17 guidelines, there are three types of regions—**Geographical Region, Regulatory Region,** and **Pooled Region.**

The *Regulatory Region* has a common set of regulatory requirements applied to drug approval. For example, the EU, with a harmonized set of guidelines, is a region. Traditionally, the *Geographical Region* is where the countries are in physical proximity, e.g., East Asia, which at times all of Asia has been lumped into this category of "Asian." Finally, the *Pooled Region* is made up of countries or population that has common intrinsic factors (ICH E5). A region is, according to ICH E 17, generated by pooling populations that share key ethnic factors. So, each region in an MRCT consists of populations that are pooled together because they share common "ethnic factors," which potentially may influence the effect of the investigational drug.

3.6 New Concepts in ICH E17 of Pooling and Subpopulations

As previously described, the *Regulatory Region* has a common set of regulatory requirements applied to drug approval. However, with E17 guidelines, the *Pooled Region* has more scientific classification that allows to pool data from countries or populations that have commonalities in ethnic factors (Figure 3.1). Thus, one can consider pooling data from East Asian countries (e.g., Japan, China, Korea) that consist of a subset of the subjects from this region with similarly defined subsets from other regions to form a pooled subpopulation whose members share one or more intrinsic or extrinsic factors important for the drug development program. If the intrinsic factors such as gender, body weight, genetic polymorphism, kidney function, concomitant diseases are of interest, the pooling of the population may not only be restricted to a geographical region but can also involve the pooling of populations across continents. For example, patients of Japanese origin having common genetic factors in disease causation can be pooled from across Japan, the US, or Latin America. More details on pooling strategies are discussed in Chapter 5.

3.7 Can Asia Be a "Pooled Region"? Mapping Human Genetic Diversity in Asia

Genome-wide patterns of variations across individuals provide an important source of information on similarities, or differences, of races. With the recent availability of powerful molecular biologics analytical techniques, analysis using data from single-nucleotide polymorphism (SNP) couple with powerful biostatistics tools has yielded important information on the genetic diversity of populations. Based on the Maximum Likelihood Tree and analysis of haplotype diversity, haplotype sharing, and population phylogeny relationships can be established between Asians (South East Asians, East Asians).

The drug development paradigm over the last few years has focused on conducting pivotal clinical studies in the West (US/EU) and then those data are used to extrapolate the results to other regions (e.g., Asia) which were considered to be different. Regulators from major countries such as China, Japan, Korea, Taiwan, and India require "local" patient data in their own population that is exposed to local medical practice, and find it trustworthy for making a regulatory decision. As part of getting a waiver for those local studies, "ethnic sensitivity analysis" is conducted using the ICH E5 guidelines to "bridge" the local data or the "Asian data" to the global data. Asia is a diverse continent spanning 30% of the world's landmass and over 60% of the world's population. Thus, the question always remained, who is Asian? Geographic location, race, and ethnicity by themselves are poor surrogates to determine the meaningful clinical effect. A single ethnic label of "Asian" may not represent the broad diversity between collections of people in Asia. Thus, the "Asian" phenotype underestimates the genetic diversity of Asia yet potentially overstates its impact on the variability in drug disposition and pharmacodynamics.

3.8 How to Apply the Intrinsic and Extrinsic Factors in Context of ICH E17 Guidelines

To investigate the causes of regional differences, E17 introduces a "structured exploration of regional differences." We should take care of both prognostic factors of the disease and predictive factors of the treatment response.

The first step is a pre-planned analysis for known influential factors—the intrinsic and extrinsic factors described earlier in this chapter.

The second step is an ad hoc analysis for possible factors based on the accumulated data in the MRCT, first focusing on prognostic factors of the disease and then investigating predictive factors of the treatment response.

The third step is further ad hoc investigation, through usual subgroup analyses. Checking internal or external consistency may be conducted in this step.

We should investigate these general factors first. If we find some factors affecting treatment responses, we would need to investigate further. Each factor could be a gateway to further investigate the explainable factors. Over the years the drug developers have become apt in collecting intrinsic data—the genetic information, enzyme polymorphism, or disease state have standard measures. However, identifying, and collecting, the extrinsic factors is not that easy. For example, the food effect or the standard of medical care has been difficult to collect and standardize. Thus, early knowledge of the intrinsic and extrinsic factors as part of pre-consideration and mitigation of large differences across regions can support adequate interpretability of the results of MRCT in different regions.

In response to the globalization of drug development with MRCTs, a different approach is needed to assure a benefit or risk of a drug in a local population. E17 provides a few different ways how to efficiently accumulate clinical data which are useful for different regulatory agencies for making such a decision. If all ethnic factors important to drug response are well understood and absolutely insensitive to drug response, local population data may not be required. However, in reality, such clear situations are not always true. In a process of drug development, there is continuous learning based on accumulated evidence. Therefore, the inclusion of a local population in an MRCT could be a practical and acceptable approach. As scientific data and regulatory experiences accumulate, approaches can be more flexible.

As discussed in Chapter 2, the inclusion of diverse demographics should be part of the design of MRCT to establish diversity as a key scientific variable across the research portfolio. The US FDA has instituted policies to better understand the barriers for, and increase participation among, more diverse participants. Recently, the US FDA has issued guidance documents on *enhancing the Diversity of Clinical Trial Populations— Eligibility Criteria, Enrollment Practices, and Trial Designs Guidance for Industry* (FDA 2020).

The plan to address broad inclusion representative of the target patient population should be developed early during the design of MRCT taking the ICH E5 factors into account. After all, these factors are indicative of treatment response.

3.9 Determining Intrinsic and Extrinsic Factors—Closing Thoughts

The concept of using ethnicity and race in drug development is a poor surrogate to determine the drug response in patients. Race or ethnicity as a determinant of response may be an indicator of population-based differences in exposure response that occur in greater frequency but not exclusivity in certain populations. It is equally important to understand various other determinants early enough to justify a pooling strategy across geographical regions. Influencing factors (intrinsic and extrinsic) responsible for disease causation and treatment should be identified early in the drug development process. These influencing factors may, or may not, be related to race, ethnicity, or a geographical region.

There are bound to be intrinsic and extrinsic differences—identifying those differences early and managing these differences which affect the treatment effect will determine the success of MRCT. Thus, understanding the pre-considerations of regional variability is important in the design of MRCT because intrinsic and extrinsic factors may affect the treatment effect and the interpretation of the trial. A stepwise approach to identify these factors and some mitigation and design strategies could use the "collect, examine, decide" strategy as defined in E17 guidelines.

It is important to recognize that science and regulatory science has advanced considerably to allow drug developer and regulators to better understand and predict sources and amount of intrinsic variability in dose-exposure-response relationships (e.g., metabolism and receptor polymorphisms). External sources of variability remain and comprise a long list including medical practice, the standard of care (SOC), and endpoint performance due to cultural and linguistic differences.

Considering the broadly defined intrinsic and extrinsic factors in E5 while designing MRCT is like casting a wide net hoping to capture a large patient pool that would be representative of the broader population. This approach lacks the selectivity and specificity of the selection of a targeted population. In order to be selective of the intended target population, various biological, genetic or epigenetic, social, cultural, environmental factors, and other determinants of health that impact medical practice differences need to be understood. The intrinsic and extrinsic factors as described in the ICH E5 guidelines should be used as a rough guide and not the end-all and be-all for the design and conduct of MRCT. As part of E17 guidelines, pre-consideration of regional variability should be reflected in the trial design to lead to a successful MRCT.

As a concluding thought, one must "follow the science" and apply the "learn/confirm model" that is highlighted in the ICH E17 guidelines. That is the only we can move away from the nonscientific, inconsistent, and, at times, arbitrary requirements for local studies, which are largely based on traditions and politics.

References

"American Anthropological Association Draft Official Statement on "Race"". 1997. *Anthropology News* 38 (6): 27. 10.1111/an.1997.38.6.27.1.

Asano, Kunihito, Yoshiaki Uyama, and Masahiro Tohkin. 2017. "Factors Affecting Drug-Development Strategies in Asian Global Clinical Trials for Drug Approval in Japan". *Clinical and Translational Science* 11 (2): 182–188. 10.1111/cts.12520.

Bonham, Vence L., Shawneequa L. Callier, and Charmaine D. Royal. 2016. "Will Precision Medicine Move Us Beyond Race?". *New England Journal of Medicine* 374 (21): 2003–2005. 10.1056/nejmp1511294.

Boris, Eileen. 1994. "Gender, Race, and Rights: Listening to Critical Race Theory". *Journal of Women's History* 6 (2): 111–124. 10.1353/jowh.2010.0349.

Buoncervello, Maria, Matteo Marconi, Alessandra Carè, Paola Piscopo, Walter Malorni, and Paola Matarrese. 2017. "Preclinical Models in the Study of Sex Differences". *Clinical Science* 131 (6): 449–469. 10.1042/cs20160847.

Cavalli-Sforza, L. Luca, and Marcus W. Feldman. 2003. "The Application of Molecular Genetic Approaches to the Study of Human Evolution". *Nature Genetics* 33 (S3): 266–275. 10.1038/ng1113.

Collins, Francis S. 2004. "What We Do and Don't Know about 'Race', 'Ethnicity', Genetics and Health at the Dawn of The Genome Era". *Nature Genetics* 36 (S11): S13–S15. 10.1038/ng1436.

"E17 General Principles For Planning And Design Of Multiregional...". 2021. *U.S. Food And Drug Administration.* https://www.fda.gov/regulatory-information/search-fda-guidance-documents/e17-general-principles-planning-and-design-multi-regional-clinical-trials.

FDA Guidance: Enhancing the Diversity of Clinical Trial Populations — Eligibility Criteria, Enrollment Practices, and Trial Designs Guidance for Industry November 2020.

Fda.Gov. https://www.fda.gov/media/75453/download.

Gemmati, Donato, Katia Varani, Barbara Bramanti, Roberta Piva, Gloria Bonaccorsi, Alessandro Trentini, Maria Cristina Manfrinato, Veronica Tisato, Alessandra Carè, and Tiziana Bellini. 2019. ""Bridging The Gap" Everything that Could Have Been Avoided if We Had Applied Gender Medicine, Pharmacogenetics and Personalized Medicine in the Gender-Omics and Sex-Omics Era". *International Journal of Molecular Sciences* 21 (1): 296. 10.3390/ijms21010296.

Hasunuma, Tomoko, Masahiro Tohkin, Nahoko Kaniwa, In-Jin Jang, Cui Yimin, Masaru Kaneko, and Yoshiro Saito et al. 2016. "Absence of Ethnic Differences in the Pharmacokinetics of Moxifloxacin, Simvastatin, and Meloxicam among Three East Asian Populations and Caucasians". *British Journal of Clinical Pharmacology* 81 (6): 1078–1090. 10.1111/bcp.12884.

"ICH Official Website: ICH". 2021. *Ich.Org.* https://www.ich.org/products/guidelines.html.

Jakobsson, Mattias, Sonja W. Scholz, Paul Scheet, J. Raphael Gibbs, Jenna M. VanLiere, Hon-Chung Fung, and Zachary A. Szpiech et al. 2008. "Genotype, Haplotype and Copy-Number Variation in Worldwide Human Populations". *Nature* 451 (7181): 998–1003. 10.1038/nature06742.

Kurose, Kouichi, Emiko Sugiyama, and Yoshiro Saito. 2012. "Population Differences in Major Functional Polymorphisms of Pharmacokinetics/Pharmacodynamics-Related Genes in Eastern Asians and Europeans: Implications in the Clinical Trials for Novel Drug Development". *Drug Metabolism and Pharmacokinetics* 27 (1): 9–54. 10.2133/dmpk.dmpk-11-rv-111.

Liu, Xuanyao, Dongsheng Lu, Woei-Yuh Saw, Philip J. Shaw, Pongsakorn Wangkumhang, Chumpol Ngamphiw, and Suthat Fucharoen et al. 2017. "Characterising Private and Shared Signatures of Positive Selection in 37 Asian Populations". *European Journal of Human Genetics* 25 (4): 499–508. 10.1038/ejhg.2016.181.

Magaña López, Miriam, Margaret Bevans, Leslie Wehrlen, Li Yang, and Gwenyth R. Wallen. 2016. "Discrepancies in Race and Ethnicity Documentation: A Potential Barrier in Identifying Racial and Ethnic Disparities". *Journal of Racial and Ethnic Health Disparities* 4 (5): 812–818. 10.1007/s40615-016-0283-3.

Miyazaki, Koichi, Yasunori Sato, Hideki Hanaoka, and Yoshiaki Uyama. 2017. "Current Status and Open Issues Concerning Global Clinical Trials (Gcts) in Japan And East Asia". *Clinical and Translational Science* 10 (6): 503–508. 10.1111/cts.12485.

Nakashima, Kae, Mamoru Narukaw, Yoshiko Kanazu, and Masahiro Takeuchi. 2011. "Differences between Japan and the United States in Dosages of Drugs Recently Approved in Japan". *The Journal Of Clinical Pharmacology* 51 (4): 549–560. 10.1177/0091270010375958.

N Catalyst–NEJM Catalyst, 2017–catalyst.nejm.org

Normile, Dennis 2009. "SNP Study Supports Southern Migration Route to Asia". *Science* 326 (5959): 1470. 10.1126/science.326.5959.1470.

"Office Of Management and Budget (OMB) Standards | Office Of Research On Women's Health". 2021. *Orwh.Od.Nih.Gov*. https://orwh.od.nih.gov/toolkit/other-relevant-federal-policies/OMB-standards.

Singh, Rominder, and Yik Ying Teo. 2019. ""Asian" Phenotype Underestimates the Genetic Diversity of Asia yet Overstates its Impact on Variability in Drug Disposition and Pharmacodynamics". *Clinical Pharmacology & Therapeutics* 105 (4): 802–805. 10.1002/cpt.1329.

"Social Determinants Of Health | CDC". 2021. *Cdc.Gov*. https://www.cdc.gov/socialdeterminants/index.htm.

Wilson, James F., Michael E. Weale, Alice C. Smith, Fiona Gratrix, Benjamin Fletcher, Mark G. Thomas, Neil Bradman, and David B. Goldstein. 2001. "Population Genetic Structure of Variable Drug Response". *Nature Genetics* 29 (3): 265–269. 10.1038/ng761.

Yi, SoJeong, Hyungmi An, Howard Lee, Sangin Lee, Ichiro Ieiri, Youngjo Lee, and Joo-Youn Cho et al. 2014. "Korean, Japanese, and Chinese Populations Featured Similar Genes Encoding Drug-Metabolizing Enzymes and Transporters". *Pharmacogenetics and Genomics* 24 (10): 477–485. 10.1097/fpc.0000000000000075.

Yusuf, Salim, and Janet Wittes. 2016. "Interpreting Geographic Variations in Results of Randomized, Controlled Trials". *New England Journal of Medicine* 375 (23): 2263–2271. 10.1056/nejmra1510065.

Zanger, Ulrich M., and Matthias Schwab. 2013. "Cytochrome P450 Enzymes in Drug Metabolism: Regulation of Gene Expression, Enzyme Activities, and Impact of Genetic Variation". *Pharmacology & Therapeutics* 138 (1): 103–141. 10.1016/j.pharmthera.2012.12.007.

4

Pooling Strategies

Osamu Komiyama, Shintaro Hiro, Nobushige Matsuoka, and
Hideharu Yamamoto

4.1 Introduction

The pooling strategy is one of the concepts introduced by the E17 guideline
of the International Council for Harmonisation of Technical Requirements
for Pharmaceuticals for Human Use (ICH). That is related to the following
sentence in section 1.2 of the guideline that describes the benefits of multi-
regional clinical trials (MRCTs);

> ... In addition, MRCTs conducted according to the present guideline
> may enhance scientific knowledge about how treatment effects vary
> across regions and populations under the umbrella of a single study
> protocol, and how this variation may be explained by intrinsic and ex-
> trinsic factors....

When regional differences are observed in the MRCT, the pooling strategy
may provide further insight into the exploration of the causes. The E17
guideline also states the value of pre-specification of pooling strategy in
sections 1.4 and 2.2.5;

> Pre-specified pooling of regions or subpopulations may help provide
> flexibility in sample size allocation to regions, facilitate the assessment of
> consistency in treatment effects across regions, and support regulatory
> decision-making.

This guideline recommends pooling strategies to be defined and described
in the protocol. By prespecifying the pooling strategies, the allocation of a
sample size to regions can be planned so that consistency among regions
can be evaluated appropriately. We have sometimes experienced a strong
dependence on the speed of enrollment, resulting in an exceptionally high

DOI: 10.1201/9781003109785-4

or low number of subjects in some regions. In order to prevent this, it is important to define the pooling strategies in advance. As the ICH E17 Training Material module five suggested, the use case of the pooling strategy is not limited to the planning of the MRCT but includes unplanned exploratory analyses after the MRCT completes as well.

4.2 What Are Pooling Strategies?

The E17 guideline introduced two types of pooling strategies, i.e., pooled regions and pooled subpopulations. The definitions, given in the glossary in the E17, are as follows.

> Pooled regions: Pooling some geographical regions, countries or regulatory regions at the planning stage, if subjects in those regions are thought to be similar enough with respect to intrinsic and/or extrinsic factors relevant to the disease and/or drug under study.

> Pooled subpopulations: Pooling a subset of the subjects from a particular region with similarly defined subsets from other regions whose members share one or more intrinsic or extrinsic factors important for the drug development programme at the planning stage. Pooled subpopulations are assumed as ethnicity-related subgroups and are particularly important in the MRCT setting.

Both pooling strategies are defined based on *commonality* in intrinsic and/or extrinsic ethnic factors known to potentially influence the treatment effect, which can be also called *effect modifiers*. As will be discussed later, the concept of effect modifiers is broader than ethnic factors and can be applied to more than just MRCT.

Suppose that the severity of the disease is an effect modifier, and its distribution is different among regions. Such a situation is illustrated in Figure 2a in the E17 guideline. In this case, if we consider commonality at the country level or geographical region level, every participating country or region has its own distribution of the severity, and we may pool countries or regions with similar distributions of the severity. This is an example of a pooled region. On the other hand, if we consider commonality at the subject level, each participating subject has his or her own disease severity, and we may pool subjects with similar disease severity. This is an example of a pooled subpopulation (see Figure 4.1).

If the disease severity is an important effect modifier, as in this example, and its distribution varies from region to region, then the average values of the treatment response from these regions will be different. This is a

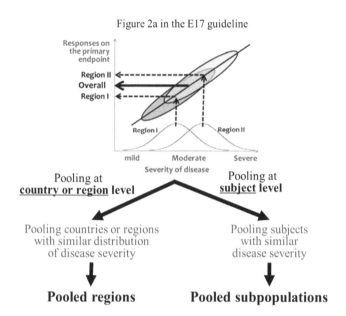

Figure 2a in the E17 guideline

FIGURE 4.1
Pooled regions and pooled subpopulations.

difference that is bound to happen, and it is a difference between regions that can be explained.

To maximize the ability to detect regional differences when they exist, equalizing the number of subjects across regions is the statistically correct choice. In practice, however, the number of patients may vary greatly among defined regions, and it may be difficult to enroll an equal number of subjects across regions within a reasonable time frame. The balanced approach recommended by the E17 guideline for sample size allocation to regions is to consider the extremes of reality and the statistical ideal and to balance them so that neither is significantly compromised.

In order to define pooled regions at the planning stage of the MRCT, the following conditions would be necessary.

  i. The severity of the disease is known to be an effect modifier and can be agreed upon with the regulatory authorities.
  ii. The distribution of the disease severity in the countries and regions participating in the MRCT should be available from earlier trials or epidemiological information.

Therefore, it will be important to collect data and/or gather information on effect modifiers from the early stages of development and to get to know effect modifiers.

4.3 Knowing Effect Modification

Regulatory agencies, who review and approve the drugs for use in their countries, would like to know the efficacy and safety of the drugs in the populations in their countries or regulatory regions. How do they know it? A simple and traditional approach would be to check the data for the target population in the country or region of interest. However, as is often the case in MRCTs, the smaller the data, the more likely the point estimate will deviate from the true value and the less accurate the estimation will be. These may be brought about just by chance, which clouds the truth. Knowledge of *effect modification* would improve this situation.

A biological phenomenon in which exposure has a different impact in different circumstances is called effect modification. In general, effect modification occurs when the magnitude of the effect of the exposure on an outcome (i.e., the association) differs depending on the level of a third variable (effect modifier). (Figure 4.2)

If we know the effect modifiers or those likely candidates and if data from countries or regions with similar effect modifiers, or with similar distributions of effect modifiers are available, we do not need to base our estimates of treatment effects in a country solely on data actually collected in that country; we can apply our estimates for the pooled region to that country. Further, pooling regions can also improve the precision of estimates of the treatment effects.

We should note that effect modifiers for efficacy endpoints may be different from effect modifiers for safety variables (e.g., clinically significant adverse events). In such a case, it is not reasonable to use pooled regions composed of effect modifiers in efficacy evaluation for safety evaluation.

4.4 Hierarchy of Factors Leading to Different Treatment Effects

To detect regional differences and to explore effect modifiers that can plausibly explain the regional differences, we conduct many stratified

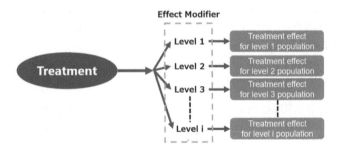

FIGURE 4.2
Effect modification.

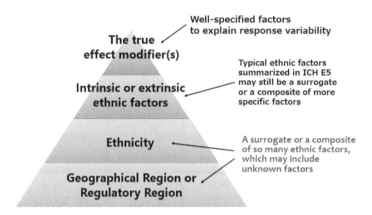

FIGURE 4.3
Hierarchy of factors leading to different treatment effects.

analyses, subgroup analyses, and/or model-based analyses. In such analyses, we use various factors, e.g., geographical regions, countries, culture, lifestyles, ethnicities, race, gender, or other ethnic factors. Figure 4.3 illustrates the hierarchy of these factors based on the granularity of information that these factors have.

Geographical region or regulatory region is a mixture of so many ethnic factors and may be a surrogate or a composite of true effect modifiers, which may include unknown factors. In other words, the treatment effect difference across regions can be a surrogate of the difference caused by the distributional difference in effect modifiers (known or unknown) across regions. If we would try to explain the different responses among people around the world only by geographical region, without further considering effect modifiers, different responses observed in a certain geographical region would not inform well the other geographical regions. Ethnicity gives further aspects beyond geography but still may be a surrogate or a composite of true effect modifiers. Intrinsic and extrinsic ethnic factors summarized in the ICH E5 guideline look more specific but still may be a surrogate or a composite of further specific factor(s). For example, we may regard a body weight (intrinsic ethnic factor) as an effect modifier. The true effect modifiers may be some genetic background, volume of distribution, diet, or some complications, and body weight may just be recognized as a phenotype of these factors. At the top of the hierarchy is a specific factor(s), the true effect modifier(s) that would explain well different treatment responses. A good example of the true effect modifier is the EGFR mutation in gefitinib for non-small cell lung cancer that explained well the different treatment effects in the patient population. This example is shown in the E17 Training Material module 2. The true effect modifier was not known at the beginning of its development program. There were no specific candidates of effect modifiers identified at the early stage. But in the phase II trial, race, gender, disease, and smoking history took the spotlight. Good responses in non-smoking Asian females were observed in adenocarcinoma. At last, it was shown that shown that a mutation in the Epidermal Growth Factor Receptor (EGFR) is the true effect modifier. This was an excellent story to tell about the learning process of effect modifiers. And the other lesson learned was that the inclusion of a broad global population in the development program was helpful for exploring effect modifiers. If Asian subjects had not been included in the phase II trial, identification of effect modifiers might be delayed.

The learning process of effect modifiers will proceed through a development program. At the early stage of drug development, we may have insufficient or no information of effect modifiers and we may consider different responses at geographical region level or ethnicity level. But as knowledge is accumulated, we may be able to approach the true effect modifiers.

4.5 What We Can Do at the Planning Stage Depends on Our Knowledge of Effect Modifier

The E17 guideline states the value of the pre-specification of the pooling strategy. If we can do that, we can allocate the overall sample size to each region taking the pooling into consideration. However, it is not so easy. We need to know effect modifiers with convincing evidences to form pooled regions or subpopulations when we are planning MRCTs, and we need to agree with the regulatory authorities on the identification of effect modifiers and the appropriateness of the pooling strategy using these effect modifiers. Without pre-specification of the pooling strategies, can we no longer use the pooling strategies? The answer is no. There are potential applications of pooling strategies, especially for exploratory purposes, e.g., sensitivity analyses, further exploration of effect modifiers, etc.

The extent to which effect modifiers are understood may vary from situation to situation. In some cases, we may have no idea of effect modifiers. In the other cases, we may just have candidates of effect modifiers and insufficient evidence available, or we may know that factor a is definitely an effect modifier, but factor b and factor c may just likely be effect modifiers. Therefore, depending on our knowledge of effect modifiers, what we can do at the planning stage of MRCTs and at the analysis of study results may be different.

Figure 4.4 illustrates what we can do in each case. The more information about effect modifiers is known at the planning stage of the MRCT, more analyses can be planned using effect modifiers and more findings from the MRCT could provide strong evidence.

Knowledge of effect modifier (EM)	Case 1	Case 2	Case 3	Case 4
Definitely EM	none	none	none	factor a
Likely EM	none	none	factor a	factor b, c
Just candidates of EM	none	factor a	factor b, c, ...	factor d, e, ...
Pooling strategy and analysis planning				
Known Known	cannot prespecify	cannot prespecify	plan analyses of factor a	plan analyses of factor a,b,c
Known Unknown	cannot prespecify	plan analyses of factor a	plan analyses of factor b, c, ...	plan analyses of factor a,b,c, d,e, ...
Unknown Unknown	*post hoc* analyses to investigate EMs based on actually collected data			

FIGURE 4.4
Knowledge of effect modifier and what can be done at the planning stage.

4.6 How to Pool

The first step for pooling is identifying effect modifiers from early trials or existing data. Candidates may be found in prognostic factors of the disease and/or predictive factors of the treatment. The second step is considering the extent to which these factors may explain the anticipated variability among regions or subpopulations. The third step is defining pooled regions and/or subpopulations based on similar distribution of the identified effect modifiers. The process to determine effect modifiers for pooling is similar to the process to determine stratification factors or covariates in the primary analysis in clinical trials, in general.

As shown in Chapter 4.2, pooling regions based on just one effect modifier is not so difficult. However, in cases where we should take more than one effect modifier into consideration, we will face technical difficulties. The following section is trying to give some ideas about possible approaches to such cases.

4.6.1 Statistical Methods

Cluster analysis is a powerful tool to pool regions. Key components of applying cluster analysis are (1) measuring a distance between regions, (2) grouping regions based on the distance matrix among regions. In each component, many approaches have been developed and the results of pooling depend on the applied approach. In this section, one of the approaches is introduced.

4.6.1.1 How to Measure a Distance Between Regions

A simple way to measure a distance between regions is to let a region have a representative value in each candidate parameter of effect modifier and plot regions on the parameter space. The basic methods for distance measures are Euclidean and Manhattan distances. In many cases, standardization of each parameter which is the transformation of the data into the standard normal distribution of $N(0,1)$ is needed to measure a difference between regions with the common scale across parameters. Various distance measures such as Pearson correlation distance, Eisen cosine correlation distance, and Spearman correlation distance[1] have been also proposed. The selection of distance measure is one of the key decisions; however, the most important point is considering correlation relationships between the parameters and response endpoint(s). In case that there are ten candidate parameters of the effect modifier, some parameters have a strong relationship with the response endpoint (effect modifier), and some parameters have no influence on the response (not effect modifier). In this situation, it is not a good choice to measure a distance with the same scale on a ten-dimension space. We should measure a distance with some weighting scale for parameters. It means that a difference in strong effect modifier should be handled as long-distance and a difference in parameters of not effect modifier should be handled as short distance. The simple idea of determination of weights for parameters is using some regression model of the response endpoint with candidate parameters of effect modifier. If Lasso regression model is applied, the weight of parameters not impacted on the response would be estimated as zero, and the difference of the parameters would be ignored in clustering analysis.

4.6.1.2 How to Pool Regions Based on the Distance Matrix Across Regions

In case of applying the cluster analysis to pool regions, samples are regions and clusters are pooled regions. There are various types of clustering such as hierarchical clustering, k-means clustering, distribution-based clustering, density-based clustering, etc. Because the basic approach is hierarchical clustering, we will focus on it here. This method provides a dendrogram with regions and we can select a level of hierarchy in considering the number of clusters (pooled regions). K-means clustering is also a basic

---

[1] DATANOVIA. "Clustering Distance Measures." Accessed April 23, 2021.
    https://www.datanovia.com/en/lessons/clustering-distance-measures/#:~:text=35%20mins-,Data%20Clustering%20Basics,a%20dissimilarity%20or%20distance%20matrix.

approach. As the difference from the hierarchical clustering, a pre-setting of the number of clusters is needed before the analysis. In case the number of pooled regions can be pre-defined (see section 4.6.1.3) then this method works efficiently.

4.6.1.3 How to Determine the Number of Pooled Regions

The number of pooled regions should be carefully considered because of the impact on the interpretation of findings from investigating the consistency of treatment effects across pooled regions and regulatory decision-making.

In cluster analysis, there are many approaches to determine the number of clusters. These discussions would be helpful to determine the number of pooled regions. In addition to the approaches, we can also determine them from the precision of statistical inference in subgroups in a clinical trial. Alosh et al. provided a comprehensive statistical consideration on subgroup analysis.[2] They investigated the probability that a negative subgroup effect is observed by chance assuming the underlying treatment effect is a positive and truly homogenous across subgroups. In their investigations, the probability of observing at least one subgroup with a negative treatment effect increases with the number of subgroups that are a major factor in this regard. For example, there would be more than 26% probability of obtaining a negative treatment effect in at least one subgroup in case more than or equal to five subgroups in the assumption of a study powered at 90% with the same treatment effect size of 0.25 among subgroups. Quan et al. also provided similar findings that more than four defined regions may impact the ability to demonstrate the consistency of treatment effect across regions.[3] Less than or equal to four pooled regions would be recommended from this point.

4.6.1.4 How to Interpret the Results of Pooled Regions or Pooled Subpopulations

Subgroup analysis stratified by pooled regions is one of the subgroup analyses stratified by candidate effect modifiers (e.g., sex, age, BMI, pre-treatments, medical history, etc.). But there might be a large difference in the meaning of the subcategory. As mentioned in section 4.6.1.1, pooled regions would be determined with the adjusted distance on the parameters of the effect modifier by a relationship with the response endpoint. Therefore, subgroup analysis by the pooled regions provides the results stratified by

---

[2] Mohamed Alosh, Mohammad F. Huque, Frank Bretz, Ralph B. D'Agostino Sr. "Tutorial on statistical considerations on subgroup analysis in confirmatory clinical trials." Statistics in Medicine 36(2017): 1334–1360.

[3] Hui Quan, et.al. "Assessment of consistency of treatment effects in multiregional clinical trials." Drug Information Journal 44(2010): 617–632.

clusters of regions based on distances in a space composed of candidate effect modifiers. For example, if there are two factors (e.g., gender and age) that impacted the treatment response, we can classify all regions into four pooled regions (male and younger, male and elder, female and younger, or female and elder).

Subgroup analysis with the four pooled regions provides investigation by a mixed factor of gender and age. Please note that this classification is considered as the distribution of the patient population in a region. In case that the proportion of male patients and that of younger patients are similar, then these regions can be pooled.

On the other hand, subgroup analyses by candidate effect modifiers support the investigation of the response difference by a single parameter. We should look into the response difference by a single parameter first, and then we can interpret the response difference by pooled regions as the response in regions with a similar subject background of effect modifiers.

One question arise here; Can we equate point estimates of treatment effect(s) for a certain pooled region to those for individual country or region included in the pooled region? Regulatory authorities are sometimes interested in risk-benefit balance in their own region. The above question comes up to evaluate the magnitude of drug efficacy in the own region. There is not a simple answer, but we should not focus on the point estimate of the pooled region or a region only. We should evaluate the magnitude of the impact of the effect modifiers including the pooled regions and interpret if these differences are clinically meaningful or not.

4.7 Concluding Remarks

Evaluation of consistency in treatment effects across regions and/or subpopulations is one of the most important elements of the ICH E17 guidelines and should always be considered in the design of MRCTs and in the interpretation of results.

Understanding effect modifiers and characterizing each population of interest by effect modifiers can be helpful in evaluating the consistency or inconsistency of treatment effects across populations. If effect modifiers that have a significant impact on treatment effect can be identified and agreed upon with regulatory authorities during the planning stage of an MRCT, we can construct pooled regions and allocate the overall sample size to these pooled regions. The discussion may be improved by pooled subpopulations with common effect modifiers rather than countries or regions. If there is insufficient information on effect modifiers at the planning stage of MRCTs, we will have to rely on post-hoc analyses, but efforts should continue to try to explain the consistency or inconsistency of treatment effects by effect modifiers.

A small number of effect modifiers with strong explanatory ability could be very useful in evaluating consistency across regions and subpopulations, as well as in estimating treatment effects in any given patient population or individual patient. There will be a long learning process in each drug development to become familiar with such effect modifiers. This learning process can begin early in the research and development of a drug. The pooling strategies based on effect modifiers can guide such a learning process and may even serve as a gateway.

5

Overall Sample Size and Allocation to Regions

Aloka Chakravarty[1], Xin Zeng[2], and William Wang[3]
[1]*US FDA*
[2]*China NMPA*
[3]*Merck & Co., Inc., Kenilworth, NJ, USA*

5.1 Introduction

In multi-regional clinical trials (MRCTs), sample size calculation, and allocation to participating regions need additional planning. Compared to a study that is conducted solely in a single region, the overall sample size is expected to increase primarily due to the added variability in a more heterogeneous population. Based on the combined data across all enrolled regions, there are two guiding principles:

1. The primary hypothesis to be tested is the focus of sample size planning.
2. The regional allocation is to be done such that (i) clinically meaningful treatment effect differences and (ii) variability of primary outcomes can be evaluated without a substantial increase to the sample size.

The sample size, adequate to address these two guiding principles, is calculated based on the anticipated overall treatment effect (OTE) that is:

- clinically meaningful to an entire target population
- relevant to all regions, disease process, mechanism of action of the drug
- incorporates prior knowledge on ethnic factors
- factors in the potential impact of ethnic factors on drug response in each region

DOI: 10.1201/9781003109785-5

- includes any data available from early exploratory trials with the new drug.

Prior information about intrinsic and/or extrinsic factors beyond ethnicity contributing to the heterogeneity of the enrolling population is important in planning MRCTs and should be discussed with regulatory authorities. In particular, the acceptability of the trial should be discussed if recruitment is expected to be heavily skewed towards select prevalent regions, as this may limit the ability to characterize regional differences in safety and efficacy. The use of pooled regions and pooled subpopulations may be pragmatic tools to maintain the total sample size while allowing the descriptions of treatment effect in its regional context. This will be discussed in detail later. In certain situations, such as rare diseases, or in response to an unmet medical need, sample size allocation in regions could generally be allowed more flexibility.

The ICH E9 discusses general principles and gives a detailed description of factors to be noted in determining sample sizes of clinical trials. As stated in E9, the overall sample size is determined by the primary objective of the trial in terms of study endpoints and specific hypotheses to be tested. In the planning for the hypotheses testing, the anticipated size of the treatment effect to be detected, background prevalence rate or control group event rates as well as the variability of the primary outcome need to be considered. Careful planning on the choice of appropriate test statistics, handling of missing data, multiplicity, and overall control of Type I error should be undertaken.

In planning MRCTs, additional factors may be pertinent. Different regions may have different regulatory requirements regarding endpoints or subgroup analysis requirements. Every attempt must be made to resolve to avoid this possibility by an early discussion with the relevant regulatory authorities.

   a. A single primary endpoint ensures that the overall sample size and power can be determined based on the overall population. If well-justified scientific or regulatory reasons preclude reaching an agreement on a primary endpoint, a single protocol should be developed with endpoint-related sub-sections tailored to meet the respective requirements of the regulatory authorities. In this case, because regulatory approvals are based on different primary endpoints by different authorities, no multiplicity adjustment is needed.
   b. Where the primary objective of an MRCT is to assess the equivalence of two drugs, the non-inferiority margin is a critical factor in determining the overall sample size and should be pre-specified in the study protocol. Ideally, the same margin would be acceptable to

all regulatory authorities. If different margins are required for different regulatory regions, the protocol should clearly specify the rationale and region specific margins. The sample size calculation should take into consideration the most stringent margin.

Only if the regional variation is known or suspected *a prior*to be of such a high degree that the treatment effect will be difficult to interpret; in that situation, conducting separate trials in at least some of the regions may be a more appropriate drug development strategy.

5.2 Pooled Regions and Pooled Subpopulations

While not new to practicing statisticians, pooling concepts are powerful tools in planning an MRCT. Science-based strategic pooling can bring efficiency and knowledge to regulatory decision-making. In ICH E17, they are defined as:

- Pooled Regions: Data obtained by pooling some of the enrolled regions, if subjects in those regions are thought to be similar with respect to intrinsic and/or extrinsic factors which are relevant to the disease area and/or the drug under study. Examples of pooled regions include East Asia, Europe, or North America.
- Pooled Subpopulations: Data obtained by pooling a subset of the subjects from a region with similarly defined subsets from other regions whose members share one or more intrinsic or extrinsic factors relevant to the disease area and/or the drug under study. Examples of pooled subpopulations include Hispanics living in North and South America or Caucasians living in Europe and North America.

As an example of a pooled subpopulation, in Figure 5.1b, an ethnic group B can either be enrolled from the region I, or alternatively, be enrolled globally (e.g., Regions I and II) to evaluate the impact of ethnic factors and regulatory decision-making. The allocation should also provide sufficient information to support the assessment of consistency in treatment effects in the regions.

The use of pooled regions and pooled subpopulations should be prespecified and described in the study protocol, along with its rationale. It should also be discussed at the planning stage how the analyses of *pooled regions and/or pooled subpopulations* may provide a basis for regulatory decision-making. The use of pooled subpopulation can further support the evaluation of consistency.

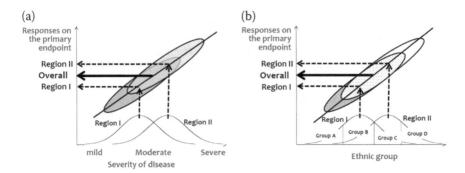

FIGURE 5.1
Illustration of primary endpoint responses modulated by intrinsic and extrinsic factors across regions (a) by the severity of disease, (b) by ethnic group.

Value of pooling strategies as statistical design elements are multifold and should not be considered only as analysis strategies. There are four major reasons for considering the use of pooled regions and pooled subpopulations.

1. Prioritize: To identify and understand intrinsic and/or extrinsic factors known to potentially affect the treatment effect.
2. Pool: To connect and leverage scientific information and resources beyond a single geographical boundary.
3. Plan: To allocate sample size and collect information efficiently to answer the key questions of interest.
4. Promote: To engage in early scientific discussion and agreement with regulatory agencies.

The above considerations for sample size planning to assess regional variation apply to assessing the consistency of treatment effect with respect to other intrinsic and/or extrinsic factors. It may be possible to pool regions or subpopulations in these assessments in order to increase the ability to evaluate consistency.

5.3 Sample Size Allocation to Regions

As drug development moves from the exploratory to confirmatory stage, knowledge of intrinsic and extrinsic factors accumulates. However, the region is always a valuable indicator for population differences in intrinsic and/or extrinsic factors. Figure 5.1 illustrates that the primary endpoint may be modulated by known factors such as disease severity (Figure 5.1a) or ethnicity (Figure 5.1b) across regions. Consequently, the treatment effect of the primary endpoint may be affected by those known factors, along with other potential unknown factors across regions. When these factors have different distributions across the regions, some variation in treatment effect among regions may be expected. Thus, careful planning for sample size allocation to the region is needed in order to describe the treatment effect in the multi-regional setting.

To understand the treatment effect in the multi-regional setting, MRCTs are usually stratified by region to reflect the similarity of patients within a region regarding genetics, medical practice, and other intrinsic and extrinsic factors. The sample size allocation to regions should be determined such that clinically meaningful differences in treatment effects estimated in different regions can be described. (Figure 5.2)

There are several approaches that have been practiced for regional allocation. Each of these approaches has its own pros and cons, thus careful understanding of the case in hand is needed during planning.

1. Proportional Allocation: In this strategy, subjects are allocated to regions proportional to the size of the enrolling region and disease prevalence in each region. The advantages of this approach are that

   a. It focuses on the regions of occurrence of the disease and is likely to get the best characterization of it.

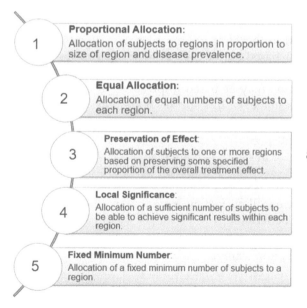

FIGURE 5.2
Five strategies for sample size allocation to regions.

    b. Recruitment is feasible and can be completed in a timely manner.

    c. It may provide adequate information to provide regional context to the drug evaluation.
However, there are a few disadvantages as well.

    a. A single region or a cluster of regions may dominate the allocation and drive the overall results.

    b. Adequate safety information may not be available in the global context a single region or cluster of regions primarily provide the information.

2. Equal Allocation: In this strategy, equal number of subjects are allocated to each enrolling region. The advantages of this approach are that

    a. It is intuitive and easily understood.

    b. It maximizes the power to examine the consistency and increases the likelihood to see similar trends in regions.

The disadvantages are that

  a. If disease prevalence varies widely among the regions, it will affect recruitment in the study.

  b. The recruitment may not be feasible or completed timely.

3. Preservation of Effect: In this strategy, the allocation of subjects to one or more regions is based on the preservation of a pre-specified proportion of the OTE. For example, if the planned OTE is 10%, the allocation in each region may be based to preserve 50% of that effect, i.e., 5%. The advantages of this approach are that

    a. There is an assurance that in each region, a certain minimal treatment effect is maintained.
The disadvantages of this approach are that

    a. The choice of a percent to be preserved may be subjective.

    b. If too many of the enrolling regions have this requirement, this strategy may not be feasible.

    c. This strategy is essentially similar to a formal test of heterogeneity with all its implications.

4. Local Significance: In this strategy, the allocation of subjects to each enrolling region must be sufficient to achieve statistically significant results in each region. The advantages of this approach are that

    a. This provides the most persuasive result for each enrolling region.

    b. There is assurance that significance is achieved in each enrolling region.

    The disadvantages of this approach are that

    a. This does not take the efficiency of MRCT into effect and, essentially, a collection of local trials.

    b. It may increase the sample size of the trial to the extent that it is too large to be feasible.

5. Fixed Minimum Number: In this strategy, a fixed minimum number of subjects are enrolled in each region. For example, at least 200 subjects are enrolled in each region. The advantages of this approach are that

    a. A minimal number of subjects are assured in each enrolling region.

    b. Adequate safety information is available in each region, providing local context.
    The disadvantages of this approach are that

    a. There may not be a scientific justification for this requirement. Any local safety requirement for a minimum number of subjects to be exposed to the drug is generally a program-level consideration and should not be a key determinant of the regional sample size in MRCTs.

    b. It may increase the sample size of the trial to the extent that it is too large to be feasible.

There is no uniformly acceptable strategy for regional sample size allocation. A balanced approach is needed to ensure that the trial is not only feasible but it also provides sufficient information to evaluate the drug in its regional context. Therefore, sample size allocation should take into consideration the size of the regions, common intrinsic and extrinsic factors, disease prevalence, and other logistical considerations to ensure timely recruitment.

5.4 Implementation and Methodological Considerations

In practical implementation, sample size allocation deliberations will reflect both scientific and logistical considerations. Figure 5.3 below illustrates some stepwise considerations:

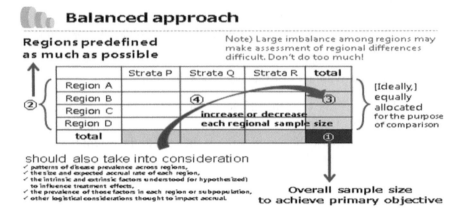

FIGURE 5.3
Practical implementation of sample size allocation

- Step 1: Overall sample size should be calculated to ensure sufficient power to achieve overall study success.
- Step 2: Pooled regions and subpopulations should be defined according to scientific knowledge.
- Step 3: An initial allocation may be determined that targets the population affected by the disease, taking disease prevalence and regional size into account. This initial allocation should ensure that the overall sample size can be achieved.
- Step 4: The allocation would then be modified to reduce any large imbalances in regional sample sizes and to support an evaluation of the consistency of treatment effects across regions. This modification could entail pooling some regions (as described in Section 4.2) to provide flexibility in sample size allocation. Minimum regional sample size targets that are scientifically justified could also be taken into consideration at this step.
- Step 5: The above steps may be iterated to achieve balance in its practical feasibility and scientific validity.

There are a few situations where minimum sample size can be specified based on specific scientific and regulatory considerations:

> In some cases, the minimal sample size required for specific regions will be justified to support the consistency assessment based on descriptive summaries, e.g., a minimum sample size to describe a regional effect with sufficient accuracy and precision (e.g., forest plot). In most cases, homogeneous treatment effects are anticipated, but if meaningful differences are observed (surprise!), the sample sizes within the regions where the differences are observed should be adequate to allow an

investigation of the factors that may be influencing the observed differences. In these cases, pre-specifying some minimum sample size needed for this exploratory analysis will help guide recruitment to ensure that the exploratory analyses can in fact be conducted. Minimum regional sample size could be specified based on the preservation of a prespecified proportion of the OTE, in other words, calculating the minimum regional sample size with an appropriate proportion then use Proportional Allocation and Equal Allocation to allocate the remaining sample size.

As pointed out in the ICH E17, the five approaches are not exhaustive. New approaches for sample size allocation in MRCTs can be developed based on the specific situations. Here are a few statistical and methodological points for further consideration:

- To ensure efficient sample size allocation and consistency evaluation, the number of regions should be limited. No more than 5 regions are recommended as a practical guide (Hung et al. 2010; Quan et al. 2010)

- With the number of regions limited to four or five, it is possible to adapt the PMDA method 1 and method 2 (2007) in a multi-regional setting. For example, with 5 regions, one can set π to be $1/5$, and the prob (treatment effect in each region> π*overall treatment effect) to be greater than 50%. This can be used to calculate the minimum sample size per region.

- The approaches previously discussed for sample size allocation can also be applied in the non-inferiority situation. In that case, instead of using 0 as a reference point for method 1 and method 2, the non-inferiority margin should be used to replace the reference point.

- These sample size allocation approaches can also be applied in consideration of primary and secondary endpoints, clinical endpoints, and surrogate endpoints. For the outcome trials with relatively rare endpoints, sample size allocation may be determined based on surrogate markers.

5.5 Case Example

Ultibro (indacaterol/glycopyrronium) is a combination drug indicated for the relief of symptoms secondary to airway obstructive disorder in chronic obstructive pulmonary disease (chronic bronchitis, emphysema) when a combination treatment of an inhaled long-acting anticholinergic and a long-acting beta-2 agonist is needed.

The Japanese sample size was determined to detect consistency between the overall result and the Japanese result with a probability of 80% and more. The primary efficacy endpoint was forced expiratory volume (FEV1). FEV1 is the amount of air one can force from their lungs in one second.

Since the primary purpose of the study was to verify the superiority of indacaterol/glycopyrronium over indacaterol and glycopyrronium respectively, the criterion for consistency was assumed that the trough FEV1 after 26 weeks in each treatment group was shown to be (1) indacaterol/glycopyrronium superior to glycopyrronium, (2) indacaterol/glycopyrronium superior to glycopyrronium, and (3) indacaterol/glycopyrronium superior to placebo.

In calculating the sample size, the assumptions were

- The difference between indacaterol/glycopyrronium and placebo, glycopyrronium and placebo, and indacaterol and placebo were 210 mL, 120 mL, and 150 mL, respectively.
- The standard deviation was 245 mL.
- The dropout rate was 20%.

Based on the following assumption, the required number of Japanese subjects was calculated to be 185.

5.6 Concluding Remarks

The overall sample size calculation and allocation to regions is based on Principles 3 and 4 of the Seven Principles ICH E17 highlighted. Evaluation of the overall treatment effect (OTE) based on data from all regions is the primary hypothesis of interest. The overall sample size and its allocation to regions should be carefully determined so that treatment effect in the regional context can also be evaluated. This should be done without substantially increasing the total sample size. To do so, pooling strategies can be utilized to increase the efficiency of an MRCT.

It should further be pointed out that the goal for MRCT design is that the resulting data can be used for each country or jurisdiction for assessment of the benefit-risk, but this does not mean that there is minimum sample size for each country or jurisdiction, nor that there are subjects included from all countries that the product is going to be used in. The E17 principles allow for the pooling of populations that share commonalities in ethnic factors, so that MRCTs using the E 17 principles can represent the global target populations, no matter how each region is defined. The pooled region is an important concept in the ICH E17 for the MRCT design. To be practically

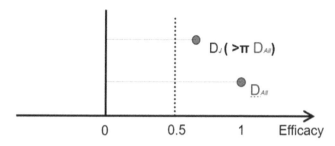

FIGURE 5.4
An illustration of Method 1 in the 2007 PMDA guideline.

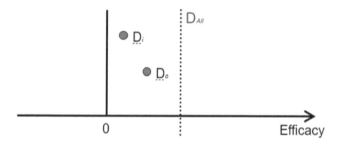

FIGURE 5.5
An illustration of Method 2 in the 2007 PMDA guideline.

useful, consider limiting the number of pooled regions in the trial design for stratification and for sample size allocation. (Figure 5.4 and 5.5)

References

Hung HMJ, Wang SJ, O'Neill RT. Consideration of regional difference in design and analysis of multi-regional trials. Pharm Stat. 2010;9:173–178

Ministry-of-Health-Labour-and-Welfare. Basic principles on global clinical trials (0928010 Evaluation and Licensing Division, Pharmaceuticals and Food Safety Bureau). 2007. Available from: http://www.pmda.go.jp/files/000157900.pdf (accessed April 11, 2021).

Quan H, Zhao PL, Zhang J, Roessner M, Aizawa K. Sample size considerations for Japanese patients in a multi-regional trial based on MHLW guidance. Pharm Stat. 2010;9:100–112.

Ultibro new drug application to Pharmaceuticals and Medical Devices Agency, Japan. https://www.pmda.go.jp/drugs/2013/P201300135/index.html (accessed April 11, 2021).

6

Consistency Evaluation in MRCTs

William Wang, Armin Koch, and Osamu Komiyama

6.1 Introduction

One of seven key principles in the ICH E17 guideline promotes structured exploration to examine the consistency of treatment effects across regions and subpopulations. In this chapter, we will first introduce the definition of consistency and explain why the consistency evaluation in confirmatory multi-regional clinical trials (MRCTs) is necessary (Section 6.1). We will introduce the structured approach for consistency evaluation and discuss the holistic evaluation in consistency assessment in Section 6.2. A summary of various statistical approaches for consistency evaluation is provided in Section 6.3. This section will also discuss the linkage between the regional consistency evaluation and subgroup analyses. The Platelet Inhibition and Patient Outcomes (PLATO) trial will be used as a case study in Section 6.4 to illustrate key concepts. An expanded discussion will be provided in Section 6.5 to link the ICH E17 MRCT consistency evaluation with the new concepts in the recent revision of the ICH E9 and E8 as well as other key principles in the ICH E17. The concepts in this Chapter are largely based on the ICH E17 training model VI (https://www.ich.org/page/efficacy-guidelines).

According to the ICH E17 guideline, MRCTs, if properly designed and executed, can facilitate more efficient drug development and increase the possibility of submitting marketing authorization applications simultaneously to regulatory authorities in different regions. They can enhance scientific knowledge about how treatment effects vary across regions and across populations under a single study protocol. A single primary analysis approach for hypothesis testing and estimation of the overall treatment effect should be planned so that it is acceptable to all concerned regulatory authorities. In addition, a structured exploration to examine the consistency of treatment effects across regions and subpopulations should be planned. The targeted disease condition determines the clinical context, targeted study population, treatment regimen, the primary and other key endpoints. An ideal clinical trial

DOI: 10.1201/9781003109785-6

endpoint is one that is clinically relevant, accepted in medical practice (e.g., by regulatory guidance or professional society guidelines) and sufficiently sensitive and specific to detect the anticipated effects of the treatment.

6.1.1 Definition of Consistency of Treatment Effect

Evaluation of consistency examines the extent to which the overall treatment effect applies to the breadth of the trial population. In the ICH E17, the consistency of treatment effect is simply defined as "A lack of clinically relevant differences between treatment effects in different regions or subpopulations of an MRCT." In this definition, "clinically relevant difference" depends on the condition or indication under investigation, the primary or secondary endpoints, and, to some extent, the anticipated treatment effect. The anticipated treatment effect will also depend on the estimand strategy for the treatment effect (ICH E9 R1), including the handling of intercurrent events and the metrics to measure the treatment effect (e.g., risk ratio or risk difference).

Regional differences that go beyond the variabilities and are clinically relevant should be the focus of consistency evaluation. Non-inferiority margins for quantification of what should constitute an irrelevant difference between treatment groups have successfully been established in many therapeutic contexts. For example, a non-inferiority margin of 0.3% for HbA1c has typically been used for Type 2 diabetes drugs. These margins can be used as a reference and may provide some guiding principles for such a discussion at the planning stage of an MRCT.

MRCTs are planned under the assumption that one true treatment effect exists that can be observed in all regions. MRCTs offer a unique opportunity to evaluate the extent to which this assumption holds. If clinically relevant differences are observed, there should be further exploration to determine if these differences can be attributed to differences in intrinsic and/or extrinsic factors. That evaluation should help the benefit-risk assessment across regions globally or in a particular region. Where this assumption is considered not plausible, the MRCT may have limited value for the full benefit-risk evaluation across regions.

As emphasized in the ICH E17 and shown in Figure 6.1 below, the foundation of the MRCT consistency evaluation is the primary analysis

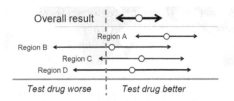

FIGURE 6.1
Illustration of overall treatment effect and its realization in MRCT.

approach for the estimation and hypothesis testing of the overall treatment effect. The primary analysis strategy should carefully consider (1) the target population, (2) the endpoints or variables of primary interest, (3) the known or potential intrinsic and extrinsic factors in the multi-regional, multi-subpopulation context, and (4) the population level summary of data required to describe the treatment effect. For MRCTs, the primary analysis will correspond to a test of the hypothesis about the treatment effect and the estimation of that effect, considering data from all regions and subpopulations included in the trial.

In those cases where the outcome in regions is consistent without major differences, this provides strong support that the treatment effect is little, or not affected by regional differences in co-medication or the concomitant setting that may exist despite a careful description of study procedures in the study protocol. On the contrary, a consistency evaluation in an MRCT, especially with an expected and/or unexpected inconsistency finding, offers an opportunity to perform a structured and holistic evaluation of how treatment effect can be modified by intrinsic or extrinsic factors across regions. After the evaluation, if the inconsistency can be explained by the distributional difference of those effect modifiers across regions, then the treatment effect can be considered consistent across regions by the level of effect modifiers.

Using Figure 2 of the ICH E17 as an example, if the regional difference of treatment effect is found to be caused by the distributional difference of disease severity across regions, the treatment effect is actually consistent across regions by disease severity, an informed discussion about the efficacy of the experimental treatment depending on disease severity can take place and inform the benefit or risk decision making overall. A similar phenomenon happens often in multiregional oncology drug development where drug may depend on biomarker status (eg biomarker positive or biomarker negative) . Consequently, the treatment effect is still consistent across regions for subjects with the same biomarker status. Such findings in an MRCT offers insight on how drugs work across different subpopulation and different regions, despite potential observed regional difference. To achieve this objective, a consistency evaluation should be planned to the extent possible to assure that the treatment effect applies particularly to the regions included in the MRCT.

6.2 General Approaches to Consistency Evaluation

As stated in multiple sections of the ICH E17, consistency of treatment effects across regions should be planned and evaluated in a structured way. The structured evaluation of regional differences, and how these differences link to intrinsic and/or extrinsic factors, requires a sufficient amount of information in each of the regions. The needs of this information should be

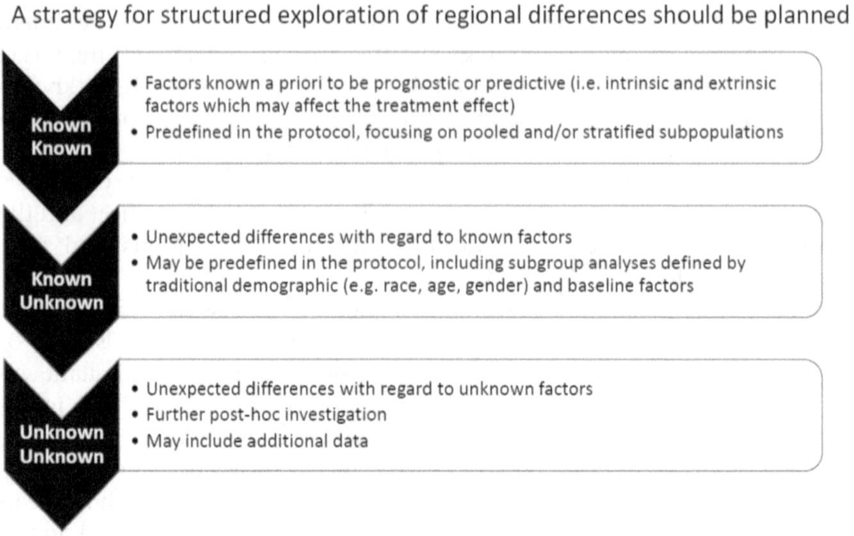

A strategy for structured exploration of regional differences should be planned

Known Known
- Factors known a priori to be prognostic or predictive (i.e. intrinsic and extrinsic factors which may affect the treatment effect)
- Predefined in the protocol, focusing on pooled and/or stratified subpopulations

Known Unknown
- Unexpected differences with regard to known factors
- May be predefined in the protocol, including subgroup analyses defined by traditional demographic (e.g. race, age, gender) and baseline factors

Unknown Unknown
- Unexpected differences with regard to unknown factors
- Further post-hoc investigation
- May include additional data

FIGURE 6.2
Structured exploration of regional difference.

Source: ICH E17 training module 6

carefully considered in the overall design of the MRCT, either in sample size allocation, in intrinsic or extrinsic factor collection, or in the statistical analysis planning.

A structured exploration of these differences should be planned. Figure 6.2 illustrates such a structured approach. It constitutes the following steps:

- Based on the pre-consideration of regional variability and its potential impact on primary endpoints, factors known a priori to vary among regions and hypothesized to be prognostic or predictive should be planned for and evaluated in the analysis model. Examples of intrinsic and/or extrinsic factors likely to be prognostic include disease severity, race, specific subject characteristics, medical practice/therapeutic approach, or genetic factors (e.g., polymorphisms in drug-metabolizing enzymes). Examples of subject characteristics include smoking status, body mass index. Medical practices include different background therapies and their different doses across regions. These factors should be based on well-established evidence from literature and early stage of investigation. How to better understand these factors should be an essential part of drug development planning. More discussions were provided in Chapters 2 and 4.

- In addition to those prognostic factors that are often referred to as effect modifiers (see Chapter 4 and ICH E8 R1), there are subject characteristics that can potentially contribute to regional variability in responses in either treatment or control groups. Even though these factors do not always need to be included in the primary analysis model, traditional factors that reflect subject characteristics such as age, gender, race, and disease status should be examined. These known factors may provide further explanations for consistency or inconsistency across regions.

- Regional differences not explained by examination of known factors may require further post-hoc investigation to either identify plausible reasons for the differences or to better understand the observed heterogeneity. Searching for unknown factors that may explain the unexpected regional difference (referred to as unknown/unknown in Figure 6.2 requires a holistic approach in exploration. In some cases, additional data, including data from other clinical trials (e.g., in earlier phases), or supportive evidence from other sources, may be needed to understand the regional differences observed. An example of unknown or unknown exploration is the effect of high-dose Aspirin in the PLATO trial when used in combination with Ticagrelor (see the case study in Section 6.4).

Figure 6.3 further illustrates the holistic ways of consistency evaluation. The holistic evaluation is aiming to gather as much evidence as required to

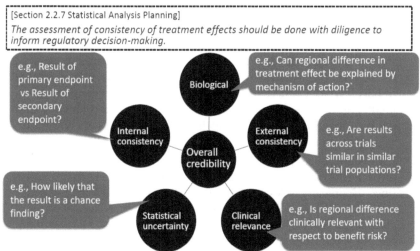

FIGURE 6.3
Holistic evaluation of consistency evaluation.

Source: ICH E17 training module 6

explain the potential reasons for the differences across regions. There are multiple dimensions in this evaluation process

- **Biological plausibility** is a concept describing the extent to which a particular effect might be predicted, or might have been expected, based on clinical, pharmacological, and mechanistic considerations. In this evaluation, one tries to evaluate whether the difference between regions and subgroups is plausible due to clinical and pharmacological judgment. Unless this is considered at the planning stage, this is usually not directly quantifiable or measurable based on post-hoc findings.

- **Internal consistency** refers to whether an impact on treatment effect by a particular factor is seen across multiple settings within the trial. In an MRCT, we typically examine treatment effects, across regions, across subpopulations, and across subgroups within the trials. We also evaluate treatment effects across various study endpoints such as primary and secondary endpoints. Internal consistency is supported if the estimates of treatment effects are quantitatively similar across these subgroups. Internal consistency is strengthened if the internal consistency is shown for various study endpoints (e.g., primary, secondary, and other supportive endpoints).

- **External consistency** refers to whether an impact on treatment effect by a particular factor is seen in multiple data sources: specifically, whether an inconsistency in one confirmatory clinical trial is also seen in independent clinical trial data (another phase III trial, phase II exploratory trial). Sometimes, we also examine trial results from outside the development program. Before examining external consistency across different experimental conditions, it is important to check whether the experimental conditions are similar in treatment regimens, study populations, endpoint measurements, and their summary metrics as well as the intercurrent events and multi-regional context (ref ICH E9 R1 and ICH E17).

- **Clinical relevance** indicates whether the results of a study are meaningful or not for several stakeholders. In the regulatory setting, a clinically relevant intervention is the one whose efficacy outweighs the risk. In a multi-regional context, a large difference across regions or subgroups may deem as quantitively large but not clinically relevant, or vice versa. These will take the targeted population, burden of disease, study endpoint, medical practice into consideration. Clinical relevance also depends on the estimand of treatment effect, including the metrics to summarize the treatment effect (e.g., risk ratio or risk difference).

- **Statistical uncertainty** arises from the play of chance or random fluctuations in measurement across multi-regional experimental conditions. In an MRCT, when there are many regions, and other subgroups, the play of chance can result in inconsistency of treatment estimates, especially when the sample size is small in and across regions. Obviously also the reverse is true: even though inconsistent effects may exist in subgroups, these effects may go undetected due to unequal distribution of subgroup sizes in different regions. For this reason, pooling regions based on a priori knowledge needs to be balanced against a loss in the opportunity to see consistency across regions. That's why we should try to balance the number of pooled regions (not too many) and the need to understand regional variabilities. It should be based on the pooling strategy in the ICH E17. See relevant considerations in Chapters 4 and 5.

It should also be noted that the learning of the intrinsic and/or extrinsic factors and potential effect modifiers is iterative throughout the drug development process. This should be planned at the overall program development level from exploratory clinical trials to confirmatory clinical trials and should extend to the postmarketing studies if needed. During the design of MRCTs, the ICH E17 emphasized that these eventualities of the trial outcome should be carefully considered at the planning stage. The eventuality is to "keep the end in mind," and to consider potential obstacles to the straightforward interpretation of the overall treatment effect in a multiregional context. Based on the principles in the ICH E17, here are a few practical points of design consideration in the preparation of these eventualities of consistency evaluation:

- The designers of MRCTs should search and examine the completed or ongoing studies for relevant evidence. Key intrinsic or extrinsic factors, especially those effect modifiers, should be listed with qualitative or quantitative evidence. These factors should be considered as stratification factors and possibly be built into the primary analysis model. See Chapters 1–4 for more discussion.

- These factors should also be used to define regions based on pooling principles. See Chapter 4 for more discussion on the pooling strategy. The pooled region should be considered as a stratification factor and should be part of the primary analysis model.

- To prepare for the consistency evaluation, not only the overall treatment estimand strategy should be well defined and the study should be sufficiently powered by the overall sample size, the total sample size should be properly allocated to these (pooled) regions. See Chapter 5 for various ways of sample size allocation. Sample size in the pooled region can be further allocated into countries or sub-regions according to clinical/regulatory/operational considerations

- In the protocol and SAP, overall study estimates, regional estimates, and their consistency evaluation should be spelled out. See Section 6.4 for various analytical approaches for consistency evaluation. This involves evaluation of the statistical likelihood of inconsistent findings due to chance.

- In reality, the design may go through multiple design scenarios and may compare or contrast multiple design assumptions. Design adaptation should also be planned if these assumptions change during the study execution.

Eventually, if any inconsistency among regions is observed, it's important to evaluate in the first place, whether this regional difference is clinically relevant in size and implication. Assessment of clinical relevance will take regional context into consideration and evaluate whether the drug has a positive benefit-risk balance in both regions, where the treatment effect is substantially different. Post-hoc and in-depth analyses are often needed for these. These potential activities should be part of an overall project and resource planning.

The total evidence from the aforementioned considerations will support the overall credibility of the study findings and the extent of consistency to which the overall treatment effect applies to the breadth of the trial population. It will further enhance the decision-making by the relevant regulatory authorities.

6.3 Statistical Approaches for Regional Consistency

The statistical analysis strategy should include the evaluation of the consistency of treatment effects across regions and subpopulations. Various analytical approaches to this evaluation, possibly used in combination, include but are not limited to (1) descriptive summaries, (2) graphical displays (e.g., forest plots), (3) model-based estimation including covariate-adjusted analysis, and (4) test of treatment-by-region interaction. There are strengths and limitations to any method (e.g., interaction tests often have very low power), and these should be carefully considered during analysis planning.

Descriptive summaries help describe and understand the features of a specific data set by giving short summaries about the sample and measures of the data. Descriptive statistics consists of two basic categories of measures: measures of central tendency and measures of variability (or spread): Measures of central tendency describe the center of a data set; measures of

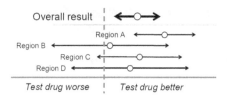

FIGURE 6.4
Graphical evaluation of regional consistency.

Source: ICH E17 training module 6

variability or spread describe the dispersion of data within the set. To evaluate the consistency of treatment effect across regions and subpopulations, sample size, min, max, mean, median, and their 95% confidence intervals are typically used to summarize by treatment group across regions, key subpopulations, and other subgroups. In addition, treatment effects and 95% confidence intervals are also calculated by adapting the analytical approaches for the overall population. These descriptive summaries, when planned properly, can give a good sense of robustness and consistency of treatment effects across regions and subpopulations.

Graphical displays, including visual analytical techniques that emerged in recent years, can be used to further examine the robustness and consistency of treatment effects across regions and subpopulations. It utilizes various types of graphs to visually display, analyze, clarify, and interpret quantitative evidence in multi-regional and multi-subpopulation settings. As an example, the consistency of the MRCT results can be evaluated visually using a forest plot (see Figure 6.4). Another commonly used graphical tool to assess treatment effects from regions is the so-called funnel plot. The observed treatment effects from individual regions are plotted against the sample sizes (or the number of events for time-to-event endpoint). The confidence interval around the overall treatment effect gets narrower when the sample size increases and forms funnel-shaped bounds around the overall treatment effect. This approach can take the sample size of the individual regions into consideration. An equivalent alternative of a funnel plot is the Galbraith plot, in which the observed treatment effect in each region is plotted against its inverse of the standard error (Carroll and Fleming, 2013, see PLATO case study below).

Model-based methods, including covariate-adjusted analyses and Bayesian-based Shrinkage estimates, could be utilized for a more comprehensive evaluation of treatment consistency across regions. In general, the choice of model should reflect an understanding of how intrinsic and/or extrinsic factors affect the regional estimates and be based on appropriate statistical methods. Sensitivity analyses should be planned that vary the assumptions required for any model if used. Covariate-adjusted analyses can be particularly useful if the intrinsic and/or extrinsic factors are not distributed evenly across regions or countries. If the population characteristics (e.g., age or baseline value) or the medical practice (e.g., background medication) are different across regions, one can take those as covariates to estimate the adjusted treatment effect so the consistency of treatment effect will be examined under a similar setting. One of the reasons that the ICH E17 promotes that stratification by region is to mitigate any imbalance of these intrinsic and/or extrinsic factors by treatment group at the regional level. If the sample size in a region is so small that the naïve estimates of treatment effect will likely be unreliable, the use of other methods should be considered, including the search for options for additional pooling of regions based on commonalities, or borrowing information from other regions or pooled regions. The model-based methods can also be used to predict the study outcome at the individual subject level based on the global model parameters and individual effect modifiers. By doing so, one can compare the predicted distribution of the study outcome to the observed distribution of the study outcome, as another way to evaluate the consistency of the regional results to global results. Please see Chapter 4 for more discussions on the use of effect modifiers and pooling strategies.

Methods using weighted averages of the overall effect estimate and the estimate using data from individual regions (shrinkage estimates) may be considered as post-hoc analysis, particularly when regional sample sizes turned out to be small and outlying values may be overly influential. The application of the shrinkage estimators in the analyses of the LEADER trial provides a good example of how it can be used for regulatory decision-making in consistency evaluation (Pennello and Rothmann, 2018).

The test of treatment-by-region interaction may also be used for the consistency evaluation of treatment effect across regions. It should be emphasized here that evaluation of regional consistency is NOT the confirmatory testing in an MRCT, but a supportive and descriptive investigation. Usually, the treatment-by-region interaction has lower power, and it should be carefully considered during analysis planning. Even if the interaction is statistically significant, it should be used as signal detection and a gateway for a more holistic evaluation.

Proactive use of subgroup or subpopulation analyses can be very helpful in the evaluation of regional consistency. In an MRCT, region as a special subgroup differs from other subgroups because a region often serves as a surrogate for disease incidence, prevalence, and severity as well as a surrogate for the standard of care across geographical locations. Subgroup analyses based on those factors can be used to not only evaluate the consistency of treatment effect across subgroups but also to deep dive into the reasons for the regional differences.

Usually, a forest plot that includes all relevant subgroups and shows consistency in the direction and magnitude of the treatment effect is generally accepted as adding validity to the overall conclusion that the outcome of the trial applies to the studied patient population. If multiple confirmatory trials are presented, a forest plot on a pooled dataset might be presented, in addition to assessing consistency between trials. Statistical tests for interaction can also be tried to explore the need to further investigate subgroups of the trial population. These subgroup analyses may lack the power due to limited sample size and can also be subject to the chance of error findings when the number of subgroups is large.

The aforementioned subgroup analyses, including region as a special subgroup, are usually planned and performed marginally. To prepare the eventuality that a regional difference may be observed, an in-depth analysis of subgroup by region can provide insight into the contributing factors for the difference across regions. These analyses can be particularly revealing if the subgroup is defined by an intrinsic and/or extrinsic effect modifier (see Chapter 4 for more description on effect modifier).

Examples of such effect modifiers can include disease severity in Figure 2 of the ICH E17 and the Aspirin dose level in the PLATO trial case study (see Figure 6.5 in Section 6.4). If the estimated treatment effects by subgroup (e.g., Aspirin dose) are observationally consistent across the region, and the regional difference may result from the distributional difference of the effect modifier across the region, one can argue that the mechanism and the magnitude of the treatment effect are still consistent across the region once we stratify the study population by those effect modifiers.

Therefore, we recommend that the following analyses should be planned in case regional difference is observed for primary endpoints: (1) summary of subject characteristic in terms of effect modifiers by region, (2) estimation of treatment effect by region and by effect modifier, and (3) estimation of

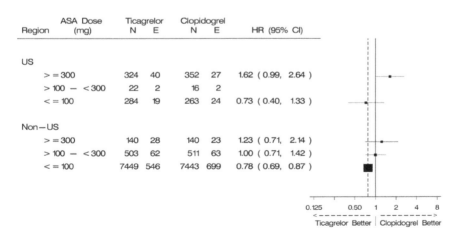

FIGURE 6.5
Estimate of treatment effect by region and ASA dose level.

Source: ICH E17 training module 6

treatment effect by each intersection of effect modifier and region. One cautionary note is the potential play of chance due to the small sample size and multiple analyses in many subgroups of intersections. This caution highlights the importance of pooling strategy and sample size allocation in case of observed regional differences. Other post-hoc analyses, such as model-based regression analyses or advanced machine learning methodologies, can also be considered to explore potential contributing factors. Sometimes, unplanned pooling using potential effect modifiers can also be used in the consistency evaluation. The following case study illustrates an interesting example for such exploration.

6.4 A MRCT Case Study: The PLATO Trial

We will use the PLATO trial as a case study to illustrate (1) a structured approach to better understand the observed regional heterogeneity, including the identification of intrinsic and extrinsic factors that could potentially explain regional differences and (2) various analytical approaches to evaluate consistency.

The PLATO trial compared ticagrelor with clopidogrel in patients with acute coronary syndrome (ACS). The primary endpoint was a composite of cardiovascular death, myocardial infarction (MI), and stroke. The PLATO trial was an MRCT that recruited 18,624 patients from 43 countries. The overall results showed a statistically significant benefit for ticagrelor, as the primary endpoint occurred in 9.8% of patients for ticagrelor and 11.7% for clopidogrel (HR 0.84; 95% CI: 0.77–0.92; $P < .001$) (Wallentin et al. 2009, James et al. 2009).

To evaluate the overall consistency of efficacy, extensive and structured analyses were planned and performed to evaluate the treatment effects across regions and across subgroups. A total of 31 pre-prespecified subgroup factors were evaluated. These factors included baseline disease characteristics such as clinical risk scores, diabetes mellitus, hypertension, previous stroke or transient ischemic attack (TIA), previous MI/revascularization history, prior antiplatelet therapy, concomitant IIb/IIIa inhibition, etc. It also included the traditional factors such as age, gender, race, and geographic region. Various statistical approaches were used to evaluate consistency. These included descriptive summaries graphical plots (e.g., forest, QQ plots), treatment-by-subgroup interaction.

Among 31 prespecified treatment-by-subgroup evaluations, most of the subgroup analyses show effects consistent with the overall results. However, a qualitatively different outcome by region was revealed. The pooled region was used to evaluate consistency across these pooled regions. Regions were prospectively defined and pooled across countries and

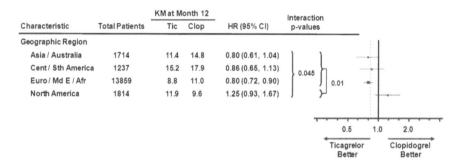

FIGURE 6.6
Treatment effect by region in the PLATO trial.

Source: ICH E17 training module 6

defined as (1) Europe, Middle East, and Africa (74.2%); (2) Asia and Australia (9.2%); (3) Central and South America (6.7%); and (4) North America (9.9%; 7.8%, n = 1,413 US patients) and the interaction between randomized treatment and region was $P = 0.045$ on 3 degrees of freedom. The data by region and the corresponding forest plots are displayed in Figure 6.6 (Figure 1 from Fleming's paper).

Holistic evaluations were performed to further examine the heterogeneity of treatment effect across regions and to understand the overall credibility of study findings. These include the examinations of study conduct, internal and external consistency, biological plausibility, and statistical uncertainty. Study conduct issues were carefully examined and ruled out as the cause for regional interaction. These included systematic issues in trial conduct, errors in drug delivery at US sites, site management issues at specific sites (including evaluation of large vs small sites), and regional differences in discounting treatment effect modifier and its distribution across regions, as well as the source of blinded trial monitoring.

The statistical uncertainty and the play of chance were evaluated extensively. As shown in Figure 6.6, treatment-by-region interaction has a P-value = 0.045. The estimated treatment effect focusing on US data had a hazard ratio of 1.27, with treatment by the US vs non-US interaction P-value = 0.0095. The treatment-by-region interaction should be interpreted with caution due to concerns of multiplicity and lack of statistical power in planned evaluation. Graphical methods such as Galbraith, QQ, and funnel plots can be used to see how unusual the US result is in the context of the multi-regional estimates and overall estimates. For example, the funnel plot (Figure 6.7) displays how the regional or country-specific estimates are relevant to the statistical error determined by the regional or country-specific sample size and assumed overall treatment effect. Although the US result is an outlier in the funnel plot, one should not completely rule out that this result could be due to a play of chance. More comprehensive evaluations

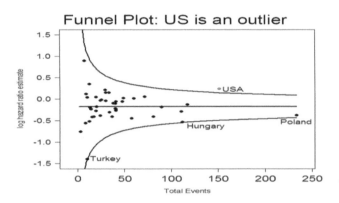

FIGURE 6.7
Funnel plot of treatment effect by sample size.

Source: ICH E17 training module 6

were needed to find potential factors that contribute to this regional heterogeneity.

A number of post-hoc analyses beyond those prespecified in the protocol, adjusting for both baseline and post-baseline characteristics, were performed to investigate whether there were any imbalances across regions that might account, at least in part, for the efficacy estimate in the US. These analyses revealed that the observed treatment-by-region interaction was little changed by the addition of any factors, with the sole and notable exception of maintenance aspirin dosage [ASA (acetylsalicylic acid) dose]. When included in analysis models, and depending on definition, median ASA dose was found to attenuate 80–100% of the observed interaction. This pattern is more clearly revealed if hazard ratio is displayed as a function of ASA dose as a continuous covariate (see Figure 6.7 in this Chapter and Figure 7 in Carroll and Fleming 2013). More detailed information about the PLATO trial can be found in the briefing documents for the FDA advisory commitee meeting (FDA 2010, Astra Zeneca 2010).

Based on the results from the PLATO trial and other supportive trials, Ticagrelor was approved by various regulatory authorities, including US FDA, EMA, Japan PMDA, and China NMPA, for patients with ACS to reduce the rate of thrombotic cardiovascular events. Special warning on aspirin dose was described in the Ticagrelor label in various regions. As an epilogue to the PLATO trial, the PEGASUS trial (Bonaca et al. 2015) was launched in 2010. Over 21,000 patients with prior MI were randomized to ticagrelor 90 mg twice daily, ticagrelor 60 mg twice daily, or placebo. All patients were to receive low-dose aspirin and were followed for a median of 33 months. The results supported the primary finding in the PLATO trial, with HR against placebo of 0.84 for both dose groups. In the framework of a holistic evaluation of consistency evaluation in the PLATO trial, the efficacy results from the PEGASUS trial can be viewed as evidence for external consistency.

There are a few points we can learn from the PLATO case study

- From the perspective of study design, there are some learning from the PLATO trial to consider at the design stage: Sample size should keep balanced across regions and pre-specified pooling of regions may help provide flexibility in sample size allocation to regions. Effect of ASA maintenance dose was not known. Had we known that the use of aspirin was potentially predictive, we should have stratified the trial by it or restricted it to low-dose aspirin.

- From the perspective of analysis planning, pre-specified extensive subgroup analyses were performed on 31 known factors (intrinsic and extrinsic). These analyses showed that the treatment was largely consistent across these factors, except regions. Descriptive summaries, graphical plots (e.g., Forest, QQ plots) and treatment-by-region interaction play a major role in detecting the unexpected finding regarding the effect of aspirin use.

- The subgroup analyses by aspirin dose across regions provide critical insight for the observed regional difference. The regional consistency and benefit-risk evaluation by regulatory authorities have been a holistic evaluation on the study conduct, internal consistency (e.g., the impact of ASA dose, across the US and non-US regions), biological plausibility, and statistical uncertainty (i.e., the play of chance).

6.5 Discussion

It has almost been a 20-year journey from the publication of the ICH E5 to that of the ICH E17. The ICH E5 introduced the concept of bridging evidence from one region to a new region. The main focus in this situation was usually the availability of data or evidence for a licensing decision in one region and the discussion about what would be needed to assure that sufficient information is available that the respective evidence is of relevance in another region, where licensing is under discussion. Even though the idea of planning this approach prospectively and discussing a sound basis for decision-making in more than one region is mentioned in the ICH-E5, it is the role of ICH E17 to expand the bridging concept to the idea of joint global evidence for decision-making, using one MRCT trial and the concept of consistency. The focus is on the provision of global and overall evidence from MRCTs and a thorough discussion of the applicability of the global evidence to the individual region(s). Compared with the bridging strategy in the ICH E5, MRCTs following the ICH E17 provide a fundamental change in drug-development strategy. Such a strategy also offers an efficient way to understand how a drug work in a global population, not only in the evaluation of its global treatment effect but also in a comprehensive examination of intrinsic or extrinsic factors or effect modifiers.

Since the finalization of the ICH E17 in 2017, there has been important progress in other regulatory guidance development that have important implications for the implementation of the ICH E17. One of this progress is the finalization of ICH E9 R1 (2019). The estimand framework in the E9 R1 provides additional ways of looking at regional consistency in MRCTs. In the estimand framework for the discussion of a treatment effect, one needs to examine and clarify the following key attributes: targeted study population, treatment regimen, endpoint definition, intercurrent events, and summary metrics for the treatment effect. While trivially the MRCTs should have overall estimand strategies for efficacy and key safety endpoints, the evaluation of regional consistency should also examine these key estimand attributes across the regions in should be part of this framework. From these points, the ICH E9 R1 offers an additional framework to consider consistentcy evaluation in an MRCT. The ICH E17 and the ICH E9 R1 should be considered together in their implementation.

Since 2017, the ICH has embarked on an effort to revise the ICH E6 and ICH E8. The draft of ICH E8 Revision 1 (reference ICH E8 R1)) introduced the concept of critical to quality factors for clinical development programs and clinical trial E9 R1esigns. The concept of critical to quality factors can readily be applied to the MRCT design and in particular to the consistency evaluation. In particular, Annex 3 of the ICH E8 (R1) has highlighted the key critical quality factors for MRCTs. These include eligibility criteria, randomization, types of controls, endpoint determination, study and site feasibilities, data monitoring, and management. All these factors will impact MRCTs quality and the consistency evaluation. The holistic evaluation of regional consistency should examine these critical quality factors at the end of the trial, but even more importantly, these quality factors should be monitored already during the trial execution. As the trial team monitors these factors across sites and across regions, problematic sites should quickly be given corrective instructions. An evaluation of the implication of emerging data trends may require considerations of many "what-if" scenarios and potential study adaptations.

Linking to other key principles in the ICH E17 and other chapters in this book, the planning of a structured consistency evaluation will require careful design considerations, including a careful choice of factors for stratification (Chapter 3), finding a good balance between sample size allocation (see Chapter 4), and pooling strategies for regions (see Chapter 5). This process should always start with proactively understanding intrinsic and extrinsic factors which may affect the treatment effect (also called effect modifiers) and should prioritize the importance of these factors for each specific drug development program. The study should power the primary hypotheses with proper planning of overall sample size also accounting for variabilities across regions and subpopulations. In terms of sample size allocation, proportional allocation to regions according to disease prevalence or capabilities of regions enables faster recruitment, while equal allocation optimizes the likelihood of detecting and learning about inconsistency; a balanced approach is needed to guarantee that a robust assessment of the importance of intrinsic and extrinsic effect modifiers. One such balance is to limit the number of pooled regions in stratification, for sample size allocation and in primary analyses. That's why the ICH E17 introduced the pooling strategy based on the commonality of intrinsic and extrinsic factors across regions.

Taken all these together, a good understanding of intrinsic or extrinsic factors especially those that are event modifiers and impact on the treatment effect can enable good pooling strategies. A good pooling strategy can guide proper stratification and sample size allocation. From these, not only the overall treatment effect can be estimated and tested scientifically, but a structured holistic consistency evaluation can also be planned and executed to characterize the drug effect globally. These can lead to an improved understanding of how medicines should be used in the multi-regional and multi-ethnic patient population with more comprehensive benefit-risk knowledge.

References

Astra Zeneca. 2010. "Briefing document for cardiovascular and renal drugs advisory committee meeting". Food and Drug Administration Cardiovascular and Renal Drugs Advisory Committee Meeting. Available at https://wayback. archive-it.org/7993/20170405212347/https://www.fda.gov/downloads/Advisory-Committees/CommitteesMeetingMaterials/Drugs/CardiovascularandRenalDrugs-AdvisoryCommittee/UCM220197.pdf (accessed on March 28, 2021).

Bonaca M.P., Bhatt D.L., Cohen M., et al. 2015. Long-term use of ticagrelor in patients with prior myocardial infarction. New England Journal of Medicine, 373(13), pp. 1271–1275. Available at https://www.nejm.org/doi/pdf/10.105 6/NEJMoa1500857?articleTools=true (accessed on March 28, 2021).

Carroll, K. and Fleming, T., 2013. Statistical evaluation and analysis of regional interactions: The PLATO trial case study. Statistics in Biopharmaceutical Research, 5(2), pp. 91–101.

European Medicines Agency, Guideline on the investigation of subgroups in confirmatory clinical trials, 2019. Available at https://www.ema.europa.eu/en/documents/scientific-guideline/guideline-investigation-subgroups-confirmatory-clinical-trials_en.pdf (accessed on March 28, 2021).

FDA, Center for Drug Evaluation and Research. FDA Briefing Information for Cardiovascular and Renal Drugs Advisory Committee Meeting, Food and Drug Administration Cardiovascular and Renal Drugs Advisory Committee Meeting, 2010. Available at https://wayback.archive-it.org/7993/2017040415 0613/https://www.fda.gov/AdvisoryCommittees/ CommitteesMeetingMaterials/Drugs/ CardiovascularandRenalDrugsAdvisoryCommittee/ucm220190.htm (accessed on March 28, 2021).

ICH E8 (R1). "General considerations for clinical studies", Available at https:// database.ich.org/sites/default/files/E8-R1_EWG_Draft_Guideline.pdf (accessed on March 28, 2021).

ICH E9 (R1). "Addendum on estimands and sensitivity analysis in clinical trials to the guideline on statistical principles for clinical trials", Available at https://database.ich.org/sites/default/files/E9-R1_Step4_Guideline_2019_12 03.pdf (accessed on March 28, 2021).

ICH E17. Training modules on the ICH E17: General principles for planning and design of multi-regional clinical trials https://www.ich.org/page/efficacy-guidelines (accessed on March 28, 2021).

James, S., Åkerblom, A., Cannon, C., Emanuelsson, H., Husted, S., Katus, H., Skene, A., Steg, P., Storey, R., Harrington, R., Becker, R. and Wallentin, L., 2009. Comparison of ticagrelor, the first reversible oral P2Y12 receptor antagonist, with clopidogrel in patients with acute coronary syndromes: Rationale, design, and baseline characteristics of the PLATelet inhibition and patient Outcomes (PLATO) trial. American Heart Journal, 157(4), pp. 599–605.

Pennello G. and Rothmann M., 2018. Bayesian subgroup analysis with hierarchical models. Karl E. Peace, Ding-Geng Chen, Sandeep Menon, Eds. Biopharmaceutical Applied Statistics Symposium Volume 2: Biostatistical Analysis of Clinical Trials. Springer.

Wallentin, L. et al. 2009. Ticagrelor versus clopidogrel in patients with acute coronary syndromes. New England Journal of Medicine, 361, pp. 1045–1057. Supplementary appendix available at http://www.nejm.org/doi/suppl/10.1 056/NEJMoa0904327/suppl_file/nejm_wallentin_1045sa1.pdf (accessed on March 28, 2021).

7

Implementation of the ICH E17 Guideline in Japan

Yoko Aoi, Shuji Kamada, Yasuto Otsubo, and Yoshiaki Uyama

7.1 Background

In 2007, before implementation of the ICH E17 guideline, a guideline entitled "Basic principles on global clinical trials" was published in Japan, followed by the publication of two related guidelines in 2012 ("Basic Principles on Global Clinical Trials (Reference Cases) (PFSB/ELD Administrative Notice)" 2012) and 2014 ("Basic Principles for Conducting Phase I Trials in the Japanese Population Prior to Global Clinical Trials (PFSB/ELD Administrative Notice)" 2014) as summarized in Table 7.1.

As shown in Figure 7.1, the number of clinical trial notifications on multi-regional clinical trials (MRCTs) has gradually increased since 2007 and more than 50% of clinical trials conducted in Japan were MRCTs in the fiscal year 2019.

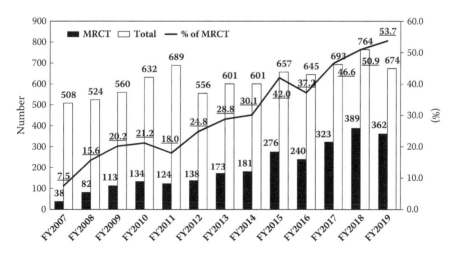

FIGURE 7.1
Trends in MRCT-related clinical trial notifications in Japan.

DOI: 10.1201/9781003109785-7

TABLE 7.1

Japanese guidelines on multi-regional clinical trial (MRCT)

Guideline	Issued year	Content
Basic principles on global clinical trials	2007	• Basic requirements to conduct an MRCT • Basic points to consider in designing an MRCT
Basic principles on global clinical trials (reference cases)	2012	• Points to consider for MRCTs in East Asia • General points to consider for MRCTs
Basic principles for conducting phase I trials in the Japanese population prior to global clinical trials	2014	• Reference cases regarding the necessity of conducting a phase I trial in the Japanese population

As listed below, the 2007 Japanese guideline "Basic principles on global clinical trials," the 2012 guideline "Basic principles on global clinical trials (reference cases)" and the 2014 guideline "Basic principles for conducting phase I trials in the Japanese population prior to global clinical trials" mentioned several items that are considered similar in the ICH E17 guideline:

- Compliance with good clinical practice (GCP)
- Importance of pharmacokinetic comparisons between regions (Japan and foreign)
- Assuring safety in regional (Japanese) population in an early phase clinical trial including Phase I trial prior to participation in MRCTs
- Development plan for dose-response studies
- Comprehensive evaluation of consistency in treatment effects between the overall population and regional (Japanese) population
- Points to consider when the active comparator is not approved in a specific region (Japan)
- Recommendation of consultation meetings with regulatory authorities from an early stage of MRCTs planning

Thus, even in the period before the implementation of the ICH E17 guideline in Japan, sponsors (pharmaceutical industries) were generally planning MRCTs including Japan taking these points into consideration but may have given less consideration to the items newly described in the ICH E17 guideline, such as specific measures to reduce regional variability and pre-specified pooling of regions or subpopulations (Asano et al. 2020).

7.2 Challenges in Implementing the ICH E17 Guideline in Japan

After the implementation of the ICH E17 guideline (general principles for planning and design of MRCTs) in Japan on June 12, 2018 (MHLW 2018), more active participation of Japan in global drug development is expected. Many discussions, including a public workshop ("The Public Workshop on the ICH E17 Guideline" 2019), have been held between the Pharmaceuticals and Medical Devices Agency (PMDA) and industries for the smooth implementation of the ICH E17 guideline in Japan. Below are some of the major topics that have been discussed.

1. Methods of consistency evaluation among regions and corresponding sample size allocation to Japan, aiming for submission of marketing authorization applications in Japan.

In this context, the 2007 Japanese guideline ("Basic Principles on Global Clinical Trials (PFSB/ELD Notification No. 0928010)" 2007) describes two practical methods of sample size allocation as an example supposing that no generally recommendable methods are established, whereas the ICH E17 guideline describes several approaches on sample size allocation to a region. In a practical situation like a scientific consultation meeting with the pharmaceutical industry, not only the sample size estimated based on the two methods described in the 2007 guideline but also the feasibility of subjects enrolment in Japan corresponding to the proportional allocation stated in the ICH E17 guideline have been taken into consideration to determine Japanese sample size in the MRCT planned by the industry even before the implementation of the ICH E17 guideline. Sample size allocation to the region will continue to be a major discussion point. All available methodologies should be put on the table and then we can discuss the approaches that are fit for the purpose of the study and the ones that are best to follow the principles of the ICH E17 guideline (see Chapter 5). Therefore, the approaches and methods described in both the ICH E17 guideline and the 2007 Japanese guideline can be used complementarily to determine the best method in light of the practicalities of the situation.

2. Practical application of the concept of pooled regions or subpopulations

The concept of pooled regions or subpopulations, which was newly described in the ICH E17 guideline, was not included in the 2007 Japanese guideline. Thus, the practical application of this concept is a challenge for Japan. Probably, there are no clear and uniform criteria to determine whether or not a pooling strategy is acceptable. It depends on how much information and data on ethnic factors are available to support the pooling of different regions or subpopulations into one region. In considering pooling for a particular drug, the target population, and disease, as well as the characteristics of the product, should be carefully evaluated in terms of the impact of ethnic factors on drug responses. Therefore, it is important to discuss, based on scientific data presented at the scientific consultation meeting between the pharmaceutical industry and the PMDA, intrinsic and extrinsic factors that may affect the treatment effect, the extent to which regional variability can be explained by intrinsic and extrinsic factors, the potential to influence the study results, and the strength of evidence.

From another viewpoint, the pooling concept may have an impact on the evaluation of data from an MRCT. Historically in Japan, the benefit and risk assessment of a drug was based on data from the Japanese population because owing to the impact of ethnic factors, drug responses may differ between Japanese and western populations, resulting in, for example, different pharmacokinetic parameters and/or different approved doses for some drugs (Myrand et al. 2008; Arnold, Kusama and Ono 2010; Nakashima et al. 2011). Before the early 1990s in Japan, clinical trials submitted for the regulatory approval of a drug usually included only Japanese subjects. Thus, the focus was on Japanese data during the review of that drug. However, after MRCTs became popular as a strategy for new drug development, it became difficult to evaluate the benefit and risk of a drug by focusing solely on Japanese data. Specifically, inconsistent results between the Japanese and overall populations have been sometimes observed, especially in cases where relatively fewer Japanese subjects participated in the MRCT (e.g.; "PMDA Review Report on Pertuzumab (Genetical Recombination) for Drug Approval" 2013). Such inconsistent results might be the outcome of a real ethnic difference or a chance finding due to the small sample size. In this regard, the pooling concept of the ICH E17 guideline may promote a more scientific approach on both consistency evaluation among populations and understanding of the impact of ethnic factors on drug responses because consistency evaluation can be based on the pooled regions or subpopulations that are expected to have a sufficient sample size for analysis. Thus, scientific considerations regarding the appropriateness of the pooling are important with respect to whether or not the Japanese population can be pooled with other regions, based on scientific information and data supporting sufficient similarity with respect to intrinsic and/or extrinsic factors relevant to the investigational product or the disease. For that purpose, it is encouraged to accumulate data that contribute to pre-considerations of regional variability leading to pooling regions by continuous participation of Japan in MRCTs from an early phase rather than participation only in confirmatory MRCTs.

3. Specific and detailed recommendations described in the ICH E17 guideline

The ICH E17 guideline provides specific measures to reduce regional variability in some items. Specifically, the ICH E17 guideline includes more specific and detailed recommendations than the 2007 Japanese guideline on the use of guidelines or guidance for disease definitions and primary endpoints, conduct of training and/or validation on subject selection and primary endpoint, standardization in efficacy and safety data. Such items may have been less considered in previous MRCTs that were started before the implementation of the ICH E17 guideline (Asano et al. 2020). Therefore, it is expected that MRCTs planned after the implementation of the ICH E17 guideline should consider more carefully those items that lead to the success of an MRCT and appropriate data interpretation.

As described above, better planning and design of MRCTs including Japanese subjects are expected after the implementation of the ICH E17 guideline in Japan. It should be noted that, although the series of Japanese guidelines on MRCTs ("Basic Principles on Global Clinical Trials (PFSB/ELD Notification No. 0928010)" 2007; "Basic Principles on Global Clinical Trials (Reference Cases) (PFSB/ELD Administrative Notice)" 2012; "Basic Principles for Conducting Phase I Trials in the Japanese Population Prior to Global Clinical Trials (PFSB/ELD Administrative Notice)" 2014) are still effective, the contents of those guidelines are basically consistent with the ICH E17 guideline. The use of these guidelines in a complementary manner will help to determine the best strategy for the development of a particular drug in Japan. Discussion with the PMDA at the scientific consultation meeting, including sharing scientific knowledge and discussing possible options acceptable for drug approval in Japan, will be important for the proper implementation of the ICH E17 guideline.

7.3 Impacts of the ICH E17 Guideline in Drug Development in Japan

7.3.1 The "SAKIGAKE" Designation System

It has been reported that global drug development with MRCTs can contribute to shortening the drug lag in Japan relative to local drug development (Ueno et al. 2014). To further promote research and development in Japan aimed at early practical patient access to innovative drugs and other medical products, the Ministry of Health, Labour, and Welfare (MHLW) announced the "SAKIGAKE" designation system in 2014, followed by the formal establishment via an amendment of the law in 2019 (Oye et al. 2016; Matsushita et al. 2019). A product designated SAKIGAKE must fulfill several requirements, including having highly significant effectiveness, meeting a large medical need, showing technological innovativeness, and in principle, being developed and submitted for application in Japan prior to other regions. The "SAKIGAKE" products are given special incentives, such as priority consultation, prior data assessment before submission of the marketing authorization application, and priority reviews with a reduction in the review time to as little as six months (which is half the standard review period). As of April 2020, eight SAKIGAKE pharmaceutical products have been approved in Japan ahead of other regions (Table 7.2). Of these, five were approved mainly based on data from MRCTs.

TABLE 7.2

Pharmaceuticals approved under SAKIGAKE designation

Generic name	Indication	Pivotal study	Approval
Baloxavir marboxil	Influenza A or B virus infections	Phase III MRCT including Japan	23 Feb 2018
Sirolimus	Skin lesions associated with tuberous sclerosis complex.	Phase III trial only in Japan (not MRCT)	23 Mar 2018
Gilteritinib fumarate	Relapsed or refractory FLT3 mutation-positive acute myeloid leukemia	Phase III MRCT including Japan	21 Sep 2019
Viltolarsen	Duchenne muscular dystrophy patients amenable to exon 53 skipping therapy	Phase I /II trial only in Japan (not MRCT) and phase II trial in US and Canada	25 Mar 2020
Borofalan [^{10}B]	Boron neutron capture therapy for the treatment of unresectable locally advanced or locally recurrent head and neck cancer	Phase II trial only in Japan (not MRCT)	25 Mar 2020
Tafamidis meglumine	Transthyretin cardiac amyloidosis (wild-type and hereditary)	Phase III MRCT including Japan	26 Mar 2019
Entrectinib	NTRK fusion gene-positive advanced or recurrent solid tumors	Phase II MRCT including Japan	18 Jun 2019
Tepotinib	Unresectable advanced or recurrent NSCLC with METex14 Skipping Alterations	Phase II MRCT including Japan	25 Mar 2020

Underlined: Approved mainly based on data from MRCTs.

7.3.2 Promoting the Accumulation of Better Scientific Evidence for Drug Approval

One of the important roles of MRCTs is to provide better scientific evidence in each region as described in the ICH E17 guideline (see also section 1.4 of

Chapter 1). Such an example has been realized in oncology drug development in Japan. For example, approval of docetaxel for the indication of oesophageal cancer in Japan in January 2004 was based on local clinical trials that included only Japanese patients and whose primary endpoint was response rate. In recent drug development (e.g., nivolumab and pembrolizumab) for the same indication (i.e., oesophageal cancer), data from MRCTs including Japanese patients were reviewed in the process for approval. The primary endpoint in the MRCT was overall survival, which is a true therapeutic goal and more objective than response rate. Currently, data on hard outcomes, such as overall survival, from MRCTs including the Japanese population have been usually submitted as a part of a data package for marketing authorization application, resulting in better availability of scientific evidence during regulatory review for drug approval.

As mentioned above, implementation of the ICH E17 guideline in Japan will further promote the design and conduct of MRCTs and marketing authorization in Japan; it is also expected to promote international harmonization in conducting MRCTs and contribute to the more efficient development of innovative drugs for patients.

7.4 Concluding Remarks

- To reduce drug lag, Japan has utilized MRCT data even before the implementation of the ICH E17 guideline through the issue of relevant Japanese guidelines. The concepts of these guidelines are basically consistent with the ICH E17 guideline.

- It is expected hereafter that drug development in Japan becomes more efficient by actively conducting MRCTs planned and designed based on the ICH E17 guideline with more attention to the newly described items (e.g., specific measures to reduce regional variability, pre-specified pooling of regions or subpopulations).

- From our past experiences, we have recognized the importance of data accumulation for considering the impact of ethnic factors on treatment effect in order to determine the best drug development strategy for approval in Japan.

- For better planning of MRCTs including the Japanese population, scientific knowledge and data for evaluating the impact of ethnic factors on treatment effect should be continuously accumulated. Lessons learned from actual cases of the MRCTs facilitate proper implementation of the ICH E17 guideline in Japan and promote continuous participation of Japan in MRCTs from an early stage as well as appropriate application of pooling strategy.

References

Arnold, FL, M Kusama, and S Ono. 2010. "Exploring Differences in Drug Doses between Japan and Western Countries". *Clinical Pharmacology & Therapeutics* 87 (6): 714–720. 10.1038/clpt.2010.31.

Asano, K, Y Aoi, S Kamada, Y Uyama, and M Tohkin. 2020. "Points to Consider for Implementation of the ICH E17 Guideline: Learning from Past Multiregional Clinical Trials in Japan". *Clinical Pharmacology & Therapeutics* 109 (6): 1555–1563. 10.1002/cpt.2121.

"Basic Principles on Global Clinical Trials (PFSB/ELD Notification No. 0928010)". 2007. *Ministry-of-Health-Labour-and-Welfare*. https://www.pmda.go.jp/files/000153265.pdf.

"Basic Principles on Global Clinical Trials (Reference Cases) (PFSB/ELD Administrative Notice)". 2012. *Ministry-of-Health-Labour-and-Welfare*. https://www.pmda.go.jp/files/000208185.pdf.

"Basic Principles for Conducting Phase I Trials in the Japanese Population Prior to Global Clinical Trials (PFSB/ELD Administrative Notice)". 2014. *Ministry-of-Health-Labour-and-Welfare*. https://www.pmda.go.jp/files/000157777.pdf.

"General Principles for Planning and Design of Multi-Regional Clinical Trials (PFSB/ELD Administrative Notice)". 2018. *Ministry of Health, Labour and Welfare*. https://www.pmda.go.jp/files/000224557.pdf.

Matsushita, S, K Tachibana, K Nakai, S Sanada, and M Kondoh. 2019. "A Review of the Regulatory Framework for Initiation and Acceleration of Patient Access to Innovative Medical Products in Japan". *Clinical Pharmacology & Therapeutics* 106 (3): 508–511. 10.1002/cpt.1383.

Myrand, SP, K Sekiguchi, MZ Man, X Lin, R-Y Tzeng, C-H Teng, and B Hee et al. 2008. "Pharmacokinetics/Genotype Associations for Major Cytochrome P450 Enzymes in Native and First- and Third-Generation Japanese Populations: Comparison with Korean, Chinese, and Caucasian Populations". *Clinical Pharmacology & Therapeutics* 84 (3): 347–361. 10.1038/sj.clpt.6100482.

Nakashima, K, M Narukawa, Y Kanazu, and M Takeuchi. 2011. "Differences between Japan and the United States in Dosages of Drugs Recently Approved in Japan". *The Journal of Clinical Pharmacology* 51 (4): 549–560. 10.1177/0091270010375958.

Oye, KA, HG Eichler, A Hoos, Y Mori, TM Mullin, and M Pearson. 2016. "Pharmaceuticals Licensing and Reimbursement in the European Union, United States, and Japan". *Clinical Pharmacology & Therapeutics* 100 (6): 626–632. 10.1002/cpt.505.

"PMDA Review Report On Pertuzumab (Genetical Recombination) For Drug Approval". 2013. *Pharmaceuticals and Medical Devices Agency*. https://www.pmda.go.jp/files/000153631.pdf.

"The Public Workshop On The ICH E17 Guideline". 2019. *Pharmaceuticals and Medical Devices Agency*. https://www.pmda.go.jp/review-services/symposia/0101.html.

Ueno, T, Y Asahina, A Tanaka, H Yamada, M Nakamura, and Y Uyama. 2014. "Significant Differences in Drug Lag in Clinical Development among Various Strategies Used for Regulatory Submissions in Japan". *Clinical Pharmacology & Therapeutics* 95 (5): 533–541. 10.1038/clpt.2013.223.

8

ICH E17 and MRCT: Implementation and Regulatory Perspective in China

Xin Zeng, Jun Wang, Zhaoyun Wang, Zhimin Yang, and Min Li

8.1 Introduction

The National Medical Products Administration of China (NMPA) has reformed the regulatory review and approval system for drugs and medical devices in the last five years. The reform aimed to meet the public's needs and to promote the technological innovation and competitiveness of the pharmaceutical and medical device industry. One noteworthy act is encouraging global simultaneous R&D and allowing the use of overseas data to support the new drug application (NDA) for the Chinese market.

One of the most important reforms is *The Proposals on Reforming the Review and Approval System for Drugs and Medical Devices*. It states that "for new drugs aboard that are not approved in China, manufactures are allowed to carry out clinical trials in China simultaneously. Domestic institutions are encouraged to participate in international multi-center clinical trials. Trial data that meets the requirements is acceptable for the registration application" (2015, State Council). *The Proposals on Deepening the Reform of Review and Approval System to Encourage Innovation in Drugs and Medical Devices* states that "Foreign enterprises and scientific research institutions are allowed to simultaneously carry out new drug trials in China under the Chinese law. Data obtained from multi-center trials abroad that meet the regulatory requirements of China's drug and medical device registration can be used for the registration application. To apply for regulatory approval of drugs or medical devices in the Chinese market, the sponsor should provide clinical trial data to evaluate the impact of ethnicity" (2017, State Council).

The globalization of drug development has become more and more common in recent years. More and more sponsors plan to register their products in China through MRCTs. The implementation and evaluation of

DOI: 10.1201/9781003109785-8

MRCT have drawn the Chinese regulatory agency's attention. In China, when sponsors discuss the design and analysis of MRCTs, several guidelines are referred to, including *ICH E5: Bridging Studies, ICH E5 Q&A, ICH E17: General Principles For Planning And Design Of Multi-Regional Clinical Trials, General Principles For Planning And Design Of Multi-Regional Clinical Trials (NMPA 2015), Technical Guidelines for Accepting Data from Overseas Clinical Trials of Drugs (NMPA 2018)*, and *Clinical Technical Requirements for Overseas Listed and Domestic Unlisted Drugs (NMPA, 2020)*. In particular, the release and implementation of the ICH E17 guideline and its training material have become the basis for promoting MRCTs in China.

This chapter provides the author's view on MRCTs, ICH E17 guideline, and their implementation in China.

8.2 MRCT and Related Concepts

8.2.1 Understanding of MRCT

In the ICH guideline, the concept of MRCT was initially taken from ICH E5. Initially, without the global MRCTs promoted in the ICH E17 guideline, if a sponsor plans to market drugs in more than one region, the clinical trials would be conducted in selected regions separately. Later, the sponsors would carry out the clinical trial in these regions (e.g., the United States (US) and the European Union (EU)) and then bridge to other regions (e.g., China and Japan). Recently, more sponsors choose to carry out the MRCT (E17) covering regions globally.

The original approach of MRCT is to refer to bridging research in ICH E5: "from region to the whole world," i.e., first focus on the regional treatment effect and then compare these regional results with global results. For a long time, this idea was the basis of designing and evaluating MRCTs in regulatory guidelines and research literature before the emergence of ICH E17 in 2017. The E17 guideline proposes a new idea, which is "from the whole world to the region." In other words, first focus on the overall global treatment effect, the relevant region afterward, and how the data from MRCTs representing a region.

From the perspective of the ICH E17, the design of MRCT should be considered in the overall R&D strategy at the compound level, not just in the trial-level design and analysis period. The sponsor should consider possible regional differences in advance, identify intrinsic and extrinsic factors, estimate the potential impact on the results, and then decide the suitability of MRCTs under the overall R&D context. Therefore, the MRCT strategy should be fully pre-considered, designed, executed, and analyzed following the E17 principles.

8.2.2 Pre-consideration for MRCTs and Totality of Evidence

The evaluation of MRCTs should be based on overall consideration, and the totality of evidence should be fully evaluated. This totality of evidence includes early research of the compound, external knowledge gathering, plus the design of MRCT. These pre-considerations and the MRCT sample size allocation, and consistency evaluation are all related and should not be considered separately. Adequate early research and reasonable sample size allocation and consistency evaluation method can improve the interpretability of results.

The pre-consideration of regional differences is the prerequisite for MRCT. Generally, early trials such as pharmacokinetics and pharmacodynamics studies can reflect or prompt the impact of these differences on efficacy and safety. Therefore, the relevant regions to be included in the MRCT should preferably provide certain clinical data. It is recommended that the industry consider early research as soon as possible. Early research is a prerequisite for follow-up MRCT and also valuable support for confirmatory MRCT research. Especially in the unknown innovation field, there are still many uncertainties. Early research data is needed to help understand the impact of drugs as soon as possible. There should be a comprehensive dataset, evaluation, and information to support the simultaneous global approval. Relevant guidelines are being drafted and discussed by various regulatory authorities. NMPA Center for Drug Evaluation (CDE) is developing related guidelines, including considerations for conducting phase I trials in China prior to an MRCT. The time point and requirements for conducting a phase I trial in China will be comprehensively evaluated based on human tolerance, ethnic differences, and clinical needs of drugs. This guideline can facilitate guiding the related work, and promote China to participate in global development as soon as possible.

8.2.3 Pooled Regions (or Subpopulations)

The pooled region or subpopulation is discussed in the ICH E17 guideline, and in Chapter 4 and Chapter 5 of this book. The pooling strategy depends on the understanding of the influence of intrinsic and extrinsic factors on the drug response. The pooling strategy should be justified based on the distribution of the intrinsic and extrinsic factors known to affect the treatment effect and the similarity of those factors across regions (effect modifiers). Therefore, if the sponsor plans to use the pooling strategy in MRCT, more sufficient early data, including epidemiological information, may be needed to support the justification of the pooling strategy. These put higher requirements on early research and pre-consideration of regional differences when conduction global MRCTs verse regional drug development.

8.2.4 Study with Local Enrollment Extension

Although MRCTs are encouraged by ICH E17, the trial progress may differ across regions. In the past, the enrollment and execution of some MRCTs were carried out in China later than in other regions. To mitigate the situation, some sponsors adopted the strategy of adding an extension study to the global MRCT. In other words, if the regional sample size requirements approved by the regulatory agency are not completed at the end of the global trial, an extension trial of a global MRCT will be added to ensure that the regional sample size meets the requirements.

For regulatory agencies, extension study is not an ideal R&D path. On one hand, this R&D strategy of MRCT with an extension is a mixture of MRCT and bridging research. MRCT and bridging research are actually different. Their design, implementation, and analysis requirements are different and hard to be considered together. On the other hand, the analysis and declaration of MRCT will have an immeasurable impact on the implementation and subsequent evaluation of extension study, including the bias caused by the publication of trial results to the follow-up extension trial, and the multiple problems caused by multiple evaluations.

Therefore, if the sponsor considers using the extension study, even if some measures are taken in advance to control the bias caused by multiple evaluations, the influence may not be completely eliminated. Extension study is not the R&D strategy recommended by regulators. On the contrary, the regulators suggest sponsors should consider taking measures in advance to avoid using this design when designing MRCTs.

8.3 Views and Challenges on Trial Design, Implementation, and Analysis

- Sample size allocation
  ICH E17 guideline lists five sample size allocation methods and proposes a balance between the proportional allocation method and the equal allocation method (see Chapter 4).
  When the sample size distribution among regions is considered from the perspective of E17, the basic idea is to consider the overall allocation protocol instead of considering the sample size requirements of a single region. Now, with the adoption of the ICH E17, the regulatory agencies should not only focus on whether the sample size of a single region is sufficient but should also consider whether the allocation plan is consistent with the basic principles in the E17 guide. The sample size allocation plan should be included

in the trial plan, including what regions will be included in the trial and the planned sample size allocation for each region.

However, the idea recommended in E17 guideline is relatively inoperable and lacks a clear and quantitative measurement scale. In order to increase the operability, the sample size can be allocated in combination with other methods, but the basic principle of considering the overall sample size allocation should not be violated.

- Consistency evaluation

  The assessment of efficacy data suggested by E17 pays more attention to the overall population and an efficacy evaluation from multiple perspectives is required (see Chapter 6). These perspectives include examination of consistency across regions, estimation of regional treatment effects, and subgroup analysis. The ICH E17 also emphasizes the structured exploration after discovering inconsistencies. In the planning stage, the issues related to consistency evaluation should be considered in advance as far as possible.

  The E17 guideline mentioned that there are strengths and limitations to any analytical methods, and these should be carefully considered during analysis planning. Because the sample size calculation is usually not calculated based on consistency evaluation in the trial design, it is difficult to clearly presuppose statistical inferences based on a certain method and to draw statistical conclusions based on a certain method. The ICH E17 and its training material emphasize that the consistency evaluation is not hypothesis testing driven, and should focus on descriptive estimation and overall evaluation. Therefore, there is no recommended method for consistency evaluation, sponsors are encouraged to use various methods to evaluate the consistency, including description and inference methods.

  In case of inconsistent effects among regions, it is necessary to conduct a structured exploration to find out the possible reasons for differences. The possibility of structured exploration should also be considered in the design stage. Sufficient data collection should also be considered in Case Report Form (CRF) design to ensure that structured exploration can be carried out later. When the evaluation results of consistency show that there may be clinically relevant differences in treatment effects among regions, the sponsor should submit detailed structured exploration results, and explain the possible reasons for the differences based on the actual trial data results, instead of simply attributing the results to opportunities. The credibility of results should take into consideration biological rationality, internal and external consistency, the strength of evidence, clinical relevance, and statistical uncertainty.

- Comparators in drug research
  MRCTs use the same research protocol across regions. In principle, the key design affecting the efficacy and safety of MRCTs should be consistent. The control drug used in MRCT may be approved with different indications and dosages in different regions. However, it is still suggested that the control drug in different regions should be consistent.

  If the indications and dosages of control drug used in an MRCT are different from the current situation approved in China, the sponsors should evaluate the impact of the current choice on the overall study and whether it could be applied to evaluate the risk-benefit of Chinese subjects and discuss this issue with regulators promptly. The regulators will consider whether the control in this MRCT could be acceptable after assessing the risk-benefit and its impact on the drug evaluation.

- Concomitant medications
  In MRCTs, concomitant medications in each region should be consistent with local clinical practice. Therefore, the regulators suggest that sponsors should consider the differences of concomitant medications that patients in each region may receive and evaluate the impact on a drug evaluation. When a possible impact on efficacy or safety evaluation may exist, the sponsors should carefully consider whether MRCT design needs to be adjusted, such as taking scientific and reasonable measures in the design of the screening period or introducing a washing-out period.

8.4 Concluding Remarks

In recent years, MRCT has become a trend of drug development. Strategic use of MRCTs, properly designed and executed following E17, can reduce redundant trials and costs, shorten the marketing time difference across regions, and increase the efficiency of drug development and the accessibility of patients. ICH E17 guideline provides detailed suggestions for the designing and implementation of MRCTs. At present, the ICH E17 guideline is the basis for NMPA to evaluate MRCT, and sponsors are encouraged to conduct MRCT under the ICH E17 guideline.

The evaluation of MRCT is facing many challenges. Data quality is one of the major focuses of the regulatory review process. With the implementation of E9(R1) in China soon, considerations of estimands in different regions may become another focus. Sponsors are encouraged to communicate the core issues of designing and analyzing their MRCTs with the regulators.

NMPA keeps an open attitude towards MRCT design and analysis under the framework and guidance of ICH E17.

To further promote the implementation of E17 in China, CDE plans to carry out a series of training, based on the E17 guideline and the supporting training materials provided by ICH. CDE also plans to conduct scientific discussions on core issues in the design, implementation, and analysis of MRCT to communicate more with the industry and the academic communities. We hope to form more consensus or practical implementation practices or guidelines to facilitate high-quality MRCTs in China.

References

State Council (2015) The Proposals on Reforming the Review and Approval System for Drugs and Medical Devices (in Chinese). http://www.gov.cn/xinwen/2015-08/18/content_2914901.htm (accessed on April 16, 2021).

State Council (2017) The Proposals on Deepening the Reform of Review and Approval System to Encourage Innovation in Drugs and Medical Devices (in Chinese). http://www.gov.cn/zhengce/2017-10/08/content_5230105.htm (accessed on April 16, 2021).

9

Lessons Learned from Actual Multi-Regional Clinical Trials with Signals of Treatment Effect Heterogeneity

Bruce Binkowitz, Gang Li, Hui Quan, Gordon Lan, Soo Peter Ouyang, Weining Robieson, William Wang, Sammy Yuan, Yoko Tanaka, Josh Chen, Lanju Zhang, and Paul Gallo

9.1 Introduction

Accurately assessing treatment effects across regions is a fundamental principle when conducting and interpreting the results of multiregional clinical trials (MRCTs). The ICH E17 guideline (ICH, International Council for Harmonization of Technical Requirement for Pharmaceuticals for Human Use, 2017) defines consistency among regions as "a lack of clinically relevant differences." Most MRCTs are designed in a conventional manner, powered to detect a treatment effect of importance in the full trial population, so it seems somewhat implicit that at the design stage effects were not expected to differ meaningfully across regions. If there were sound reasons to expect a region to show substantially different effects than others, e.g., due to factors relating to genetics, culture, or local medical practice, then it would often make sense to investigate such a region in a separate trial, or at the very least in an expanded trial, sized to allow stand-alone investigation of regions of particular focus. Trials should be conducted in a manner that will minimize the chance of regional heterogeneity; to the extent possible there should be a uniform implementation of inclusion-exclusion criteria, objectively defined and centrally assessed endpoints, identical background therapy, etc.

Nevertheless, regardless of sound design, at times there are true effect differences across regions for reasons that may not have been anticipated in advance, and MRCTs play an important role in identifying these. It must also be acknowledged that the smaller sample sizes in individual regions

DOI: 10.1201/9781003109785-9

can easily lead to striking signals of differences that could have arisen solely by chance. As with all subgroup results, it is important to distinguish between situations where the overall results can be reasonably interpreted as relevant across the subgroups, versus cases where heterogeneity reflects a potentially meaningful true difference. Due to regions being a subgroup directly related to regulatory decisions, this distinction is a fundamentally critical aspect of analysis and interpretation of regional effects in an MRCT's results.

This question has received much attention in the literature in recent years, and a number of different quantitative criteria to help judge regional consistency have been defined, e.g., MLHW (Quan et al., 2010; Chen et al., 2010; Tanaka et al., 2012; Li et al., 2013; MHLW, 2015). Their properties and behavior are affected by the number of regions being investigated, the region sample sizes, and the analytical approach used to determine the overall treatment effect across regions. However, in addition to post-trial evaluation of consistency, it is of interest to explore how trials may be planned and conducted in a manner that decreases the chance of obtaining inconsistent results.

Despite collaborative efforts to design and conduct trials in a manner that will enhance the homogeneity of treatment effects across regions, and to minimize the chance of obtaining false signals of differences, inconsistent results have been observed in a number of recent large MRCTs. Some of these have raised challenges for the proper interpretation of studies included in regulatory submissions. This includes recent trials investigating vaccines and therapeutics to prevent or treat COVID-19 patients. Understandably, it is critical for regulatory authorities to decide whether or not they believe an investigational drug will be beneficial to patients in their regions of responsibility. In this manuscript, we review several studies in which regional heterogeneity was suggested, describe how they were interpreted by regulators or the medical community, and whether subsequent experience substantiated the signal of inconsistency. We summarize lessons that can be learned from these cases and provide recommendations for proper design, monitoring, and interpretation based upon them. We also provide illustrations of a type of statistical adjustment procedure that sometimes can provide helpful perspectives in the presence of unexpected signals.

9.2 The COVID-19 Pandemic

At the time of the writing of this chapter, the coronavirus continues to spread rapidly around the world after new daily cases hit a peak in January 2021, despite the initial deployment of vaccines that could eventually halt the pandemic and the many preventive measures being taken worldwide. According to Johns Hopkins University (https://gisanddata.maps.arcgis.com/apps/opsdashboard/index.html#/bda7594740fd40299423467b48e9ecf6), well beyond 2 million people have died of COVID-19, the disease caused by the virus, since it first emerged in Wuhan, China. The true case counts are probably far higher than the confirmed tally, due to widespread limitations on testing. Over 3 million fatal cases have been reported. With COVID-19 representing a global pandemic, requiring the development of vaccines and therapeutics that can be distributed on a worldwide basis, the concepts around multiregional clinical trials are at the forefront of study designs. Further complicating these MRCTs is the emergence of virus mutations. These variants begin in a specific geographical area prior to spreading more broadly. For example, there has been the "UK" variant and the "South Africa" variant. Large vaccines trials are necessary, but where these trials are taking place is impacting the interpretation of the results and the ability to generalize the results. As discussed in Chen et al. (2011), one premise of MRCTs is the reasonably small region variation. This premise is usually supported by medical knowledge of the disease, the mechanism of action of the compound, and any available nonclinical, preclinical, and early-phase data. As an example, if an anti-HIV compound is shown in vitro to be active against HIV-1 virus but not against the HIV-2 virus, an MRCT including regions with predominant HIV-1 but excluding regions with the predominant HIV-2 type may be appropriate. The premise of MRCTs as applied to the HIV virus has also emerged for COVID-19. COVID-19 vaccine trials have demonstrated a dimension of MRCTs that is not only about the "where," but also about the "when." With a mutating virus, trials with sites in regions that are either free of the variant or done in the region prior to the emergence of the variant become subject to limitations of data interpretation. This means that if two identical trials are conducted in the same regions, but at different times that are in sync with viral mutations in some or all of the locations, "when" the trials were conducted may drive differences in results between otherwise identical trials, with accompanying difficulties in performing side by side interpretations of the results between two such identical trials.

The timing of medical information that may change over time is nothing new. It is an acknowledged concept in FDA Guidance for Industry "Non-Inferiority Clinical Trials to Establish Effectiveness" (https://www.fda.gov/media/78504/download) in what the guidance calls the "constancy assumption," defined as an assessment of the likelihood that the current effect of active control is similar to that observed in the past studies used to estimate the active control effect. ICH E17 (International Council for Harmonization of Technical Requirement for Pharmaceuticals for Human Use, 2017) addresses the need to understand differences among intrinsic and extrinsic factors at the planning stage of a trial because of the potential of regional variability to influence the study results.

The most current and relevant data should be used to understand the potential sources of regional variability (e.g., early trials, previous experience of the drug class). However, regarding COVID-19 vaccine trials in 2020, there are no previous trials, little epidemiology information, and by necessity, extremely short runways for the planning stage of these trials including those that are multiregional. ICH E17 notes there may be differences in medical practices across regions and that such differences may have an impact on the trial results and/or their interpretation. In an evolving situation such as the COVID-19 pandemic, regions could start a trial with similar medical practices but the local medical practices may evolve differently. In addition, there may be continually morphing differences in the underlying infections triggering a disease within very short time spans such that even common regions may not be subject to the same interpretation and have different trial results. The COVID-19 pandemic has brought us the greatest example of Multi-regional Multi-Temporal Clinical Trials, suggesting an amendment to the classic Appendix A from ICH E5:

COVID-19 has now emphasized the question about the intrinsic factor of disease that should always be asked: Is the disease under study the same disease in name only? An answer of yes leads to additional confounding interpretation issues, as also mentioned in the HIV example.

INTRINSIC		EXTRINSIC
Genetic	Physiological and pathological conditions	Environmental
Gender	Age (children - elderly)	Climate / Sunlight / Pollution
	Height / Bodyweight	
	Liver / Kidney / Cardiovascular functions	**Culture** / Socio-economic factors / Educational status / Language
Race	ADME / Receptor sensitivity	
Genetic polymorphism of the drug metabolism		Medical practice / Disease definition/Diagnostic / Therapeutic approach / Drug compliance
	Smoking / Alcohol	
	Food habits / Stress	
Genetic disease	Diseases — When?	Regulatory practice/GCP / Methodology/Endpoints

Appendix A from ICH E5: Adding "When?"

For the COVID-19 vaccine trials, the concept arises with trials being conducted at different times. The Pfizer and Moderna sponsored vaccine trials were completed before the Johnson and Johnson sponsored vaccine trial. The overall efficacy of the Pfizer/BioNTech vaccine and the Moderna vaccine was 95% and 94%, respectively. The J&J vaccine's overall efficacy was 66%. Initial interpretations were that, comparatively, the J&J vaccine is inferior. But quickly, caveats to that interpretation arose. Experts began pointing out that overall efficacy of the J&J vaccine varied a bit geographically, especially in South Africa, where a new variant may reduce the immunity resulting from COVID-19 vaccines, which were designed to target earlier strains of the SARS-CoV-2 virus. Interpretations comparing the vaccines are confounded by virus mutations, which are further confounded by the regions where the trials were conducted. Comparing efficacy in a single region, the United States (US), for the Pfizer/BioNTech vaccine and the Moderna vaccine yields efficacy estimates of 95% and 94%, respectively while the J&J vaccine US efficacy was 72%. However, was the underlying disease the same due to the differing time periods when the trials were conducted? Were the viral variants the same? The answers to these questions drive the ability to compare the results.

MRCT studies of therapeutics for treating COVID-19 are demonstrating the usual interpretation issues as discussed in ICH E17. For example, note the World Health Organization (WHO) study that found Gilead Sciences Inc's antiviral remdesivir failed to improve COVID-19 survival (WHO Solidarity Trial Consortium, 2021). The WHO subsequently declared that remdesivir should not be used for patients hospitalized with COVID-19. The trial, called Solidarity, looked at four drugs, across 405 hospitals in 30 countries representing all six WHO regions with 11,330 (22% from Europe and Canada, 17% from Latin America, and 61% from Asia and Africa) participants entered into the trial across four treatments and standard of care. Solidarity found no COVID-19 survival benefit from treatment with the HIV drug lopinavir, the immune booster interferon, or the malaria drug hydroxychloroquine. Solidarity's findings were counter to efficacious results seen previously using remdesivir, which was shown to shorten COVID-19 related hospital stays by five days compared with a placebo in a trial based in the US. At the time of this writing, US FDA has authorized remdesivir for COVID-19 patients who require hospitalization, and the drug is being used globally to treat COVID-19. So why would the WHO-run trial come up with a different result? Enter the usual MRCT examinations of potential confounding by region.

An editorial in the New England Journal of Medicine (https://www.nejm.org/doi/full/10.1056/NEJMe2034294?query=TOC) cites problems with the WHO-run trial in classic MRCT form. The issues included inconsistency in data collection among countries, as well as variation in the medical practice and standard of care, and even the measurement of how sick a patient was. Such differences can create the appearance of regional differences, even though the region is a surrogate for the actual extrinsic underlying differences. As the editorial states "The Solidarity trial averages over another source of heterogeneity not normally encountered in a more conventional design—variation within and between countries in the standard of care and in the burden of disease in patients who arrive at hospitals." These are standard MRCT factors that everyone designing an MRCT should take into account and whenever possible, address at the planning stage.

A final note regarding the reporting of the Solidarity trial. Noted previously is the regional distribution of the trial participants, as taken directly from Table 1 in the publication: 22% from Europe and Canada, 17% from Latin America, and 61% from Asia and Africa. This raises the immediate question of why the regions were grouped like this? Was there an underlying commonality among key intrinsic or extrinsic factors that, e.g., allowed pooling of countries from Asia and Africa to form what ICH E17 notes are more homogeneous subpopulations to better understand the regional results of such a large trial? The authors do not address this point in the NEJM article, but the use of these three region groupings doesn't stop with reporting the demographics. Subgroup analyses were conducted for all four active treatments versus their control, and the three regions were examined as subgroups for mortality results. These regional subgroups were consistent in that the Latin America subgroup had mortality rates often 10–20% higher than the other two region groupings. Hence, it appears to be important to ask whether these regional groupings were arbitrary, or actually based on important underlying intrinsic and/or extrinsic factors, and, if arbitrary, would the regional results change with a different, more factor-driven definition of region?

9.3 Trial Monitoring to Identify and Mitigate Potential Heterogeneity

We begin with an example illustrating how careful trial monitoring can assist in identifying regional heterogeneity, and potentially implementing remedial action.

The Treatment of Preserved Cardiac Function Heart Failure with an Aldosterone Antagonist (TOPCAT) trial sponsored by the US National Heart, Lung and Blood Institute (NHLBI) was a randomized double-blind study comparing spironolactone to placebo in patients with symptomatic heart failure and left ventricular ejection fraction >45%. The primary outcome was a composite of death from cardiovascular causes, aborted cardiac arrest, and hospitalization for management of heart failure (HF). The trial was conducted in countries in the Americas (US, Canada, Brazil, Argentina), and in Russia and Georgia (R/G). A Data Safety Monitoring Board (DSMB) was constituted to monitor overall enrollment, adverse events, outcome rates, and country-specific data.

The primary analysis suggested an advantage for spironolactone, but this was not statistically significant (HR = 0.84, $p = 0.14$; see Pitt et al., 2014). It was subsequently noted (Pfeffer et al., 2015) that the mean follow-up durations were different for the two regions (2.9 years for the Americas and 3.7 years for R/G), and the composite event rate per 100 patient-years for patients from the Americas was about five times (11.5% vs. 2.4%) that of patients from R/G, strikingly unusual regional variations for a study conducted under a common protocol. While a nominally significant effect was obtained in patients from the Americas (HR = 0.82, 95% CI: 0.69–0.98), spironolactone showed an observed numerically negative effect in R/G (HR = 1.10, 95% CI: 0.79–1.51). Post-hoc analysis also revealed regional differences in many important baseline variables, suggesting that clinical diagnostic criteria were not implemented uniformly.

The DSMB monitoring the trial had detected the potential regional heterogeneity. The recommendations provided to the Steering Committee (SC), and the workable solutions identified after taking operational challenges into account, were presented in Bristow et al., (2016), along with guidance for DSMB oversight of potential geographic disparities in future MRCTs. We describe below brief summaries of the efforts for proper disease diagnosis, attempts to limit enrollment from Eastern Europe, and how the initial recommendations were compromised by operational challenges.

Since biomarker assays were not universally available at the time of trial design, a separate stratum based on HF hospitalization within the year prior to randomization was also included. The hospitalization diagnosis relied heavily on investigator judgment and could be prone to regional variation. The DSMB made several recommendations to try to ensure that patients enrolled had evidence of HF symptoms. Short of a meaningful improvement, the DSMB later recommended including on the case record form documentation of physical evidence of fluid overload as well as HF symptoms in addition to dyspnea. However, implementation would have required collection of signs and symptoms from the record of index hospitalization, necessitating a protocol amendment. Furthermore, at that point, there were less than 60 patients remaining in Russia's enrollment target, and implementation would have increased the site burden and trial cost with very limited return. Thus, an alternative strategy of accelerating site monitoring to verify HF diagnoses was agreed to by all parties.

In addition to recommending intensified efforts to enroll HF patients, the DSMB also proposed the possibility of discontinuing enrollment in countries where the trends were not reversed. The trial leadership pointed out that stopping or limiting enrollment in some countries could have a negative impact on overall trial recruitment and on how the trial's results would be interpreted. Therefore enrollment continued without any limitation under general guidance to increase enrollment in the US and Canada. The two European countries nevertheless enrolled nearly half the total study population.

The record of this study indicates that the DSMB detected issues and provided useful recommendations to resolve them. However, the operational issues and the long lag time between recommendations and their implementation made the corrective efforts ineffective. In future MRCTs, some issues encountered in

TOPCAT could be avoided. First, the subjective criteria for HF diagnosis seemed to be a major source of the regional inconsistency. When a subjective measure is used, clear guidelines should be developed and communicated to sites to ensure these measures are implemented consistently. Second, evidence of disease should be included in the data collection because the retrospective collection is costly, time-consuming, and ineffective. Third, data quality issues need to be identified, and corrective actions implemented, expeditiously. Even within a well-founded trial design, unexpected circumstances can arise. Therefore, a system for early detection of unexpected issues is needed. A mutually acceptable way for the sponsor and site to change the site enrollment target, including stopping enrollment, should be established before the trial start. As the trial team monitors the data quality from each site, problematic sites should quickly be given corrective instructions or disallowed from enrolling more patients. Furthermore, the clinical team also should monitor for emerging problematic trends based on blinded data as recommended in ICH E6 R2 (2018), not relying only on the DSMB. An evaluation of the implication of emerging trends while blinded may require considerations of many "what-if" scenarios. A capable statistical team should work with the SC and the trial leadership to assess the potential impact and formulate workable corrective actions. It is essential to go through the assessment and deliberation with a sense of urgency so that corrective actions can be effectively implemented.

TOPCAT also illustrates how information may arise after a trial that adds to the interpretation of region differences. In a recent correspondence (de Denus et al., 2017), new results were brought to light. To further explore potential regional disparities in medication use, the authors measured concentrations of an active metabolite of spironolactone in a subset of 366 patients from TOPCAT (206 from the Americas and 160 from Russia) who had sufficient serum samples available. Among those assigned to receive spironolactone who reported at the 12-month visit that they were taking study drug (76 of 101 from the Americas and 66 of 70 from Russia), metabolite concentrations were undetectable in a higher percentage of participants from Russia than from the Americas (30% vs. 3%). The authors suggest that these regional discrepancies in the reported use and actual use of spironolactone raise concerns regarding study conduct at some sites in Russia and, by implication, Georgia, and may impact on the ability to assess the actual drug effects.

9.4 Analysis and Interpretation of Inconsistent Results

9.4.1 Studies with Negative Overall Results

We next review two drug development programs, gefitinib for non-small cell lung cancer (NSCLC) and BiDil® for heart failure, where the significant advantage of the test treatment was not observed in the overall patient population, but the stronger benefit was seen in a subgroup identified by post-hoc analysis and confirmed much later in subsequent studies (the latter example does not involve region, but rather a subgroup defined by a factor, race, that often is closely related to region, and the issues raised are structurally very similar to those arising in MRCTs). These drugs were for the treatment of life-threatening diseases, so there were important implications of accurately interpreting the equivocal study results for patients, sponsors, and regulators.

9.4.1.1 Example: Gefitinib for NSCLC

Two pivotal studies for gefitinib in NSCLC, INTACT1, and INTACT2 were completed in 2002. INTACT1 was conducted mainly (80%) in Europe, and INTACT2 in the US. The primary objective of both studies was to determine whether there was survival benefit for gefitinib compared to placebo, but neither trial showed a significant advantage in the overall patient population (Giaccone et al., 2004; Herbst et al., 2004). Post-hoc subgroup analysis suggested benefits in Asian patients, but "reasons for this remain obscure and require further preclinical testing" (Giaccone et al., 2004). Nevertheless, gefitinib was approved by the Japanese Ministry of Health, Labor and Welfare (MHLW) for treatment of NSCLC based on these studies (Hama and Sakaguchi, 2004); full details of the studies and the basis of approval could not be found in the public domain. A third large study, ISEL, was conducted, and in a planned subgroup analysis, a stronger benefit of gefitinib was again seen in Asian patients (Carroll, 2004; Thatcher et al., 2005). The third trial with a similar pattern begins to form a pattern of external consistency and even without plausible biological explanation does support the possibility of a true association. At the time, there remained no clear explanation for the lack of benefit in non-Asians. Several years later though a rationale emerged: (Maemondo et al., 2010) reported that gefitinib is efficacious mainly in NSCLC with mutated epidermal growth factor receptor (EGFR) which has a much higher prevalence among Asians than Caucasians (40% vs. 10%).

MHLW's approval for gefitinib was based on post-hoc subgroup interpretation from the INTACT studies, despite the lack of significance in the overall population. The decision did not seem consistent with typical regulatory practice (ICH International Council for Harmonization of Technical Requirement for Pharmaceuticals for Human Use, 1998), especially as Asians constituted a minority of the study population. In general, there is a tendency for observed effects in the most beneficial subgroups to be overestimates. The *drop-min* approach in Chen et al. (2017) may be used to account for this potential bias and produce adjusted inferences. Here, as an illustration, we apply the drop-min approach to the ISEL data and present the results.

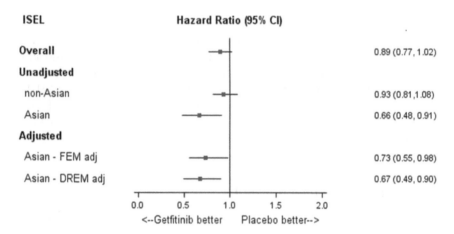

FIGURE 9.1
Hazard ratios for getfitinib vs placebo in the ISEL study – unadjusted and adjusted via FEM and DRM using the drop-min approach.

In ISEL, 1692 patients were randomized to gefitinib and placebo in a 2:1 ratio; Asian patients comprised 20% of the total. The overall HR was 0.89 (95% CI: 0.77–1.02, $p = 0.087$). Pre-planned subgroup analyses showed a much larger benefit for Asian patients (HR = 0.66, 95% CI: 0.48–0.91) than for non-Asians (HR = 0.93, 95% CI: 0.81–1.08). We applied the drop-min approach using two commonly-used models for MRCT data, a fixed-effect model (FEM) and a discrete random-effect model (DREM); these yielded adjusted HR estimates for the Asian population of 0.73 ($p = 0.035$) and 0.67 ($p = 0.008$), respectively. Figure 9.1 presents the unadjusted HRs for Asian and non-Asian patients in ISEL, and the adjusted HRs for Asian patients obtained using the drop min approach. Details of the calculations can be found in the supplement.

The MHLW interpretation of the evidence from the INTACT studies seems to have been given biological plausibility by the later results of ISEL, and perhaps validated by the genetic evidence presented some years later by Maemondo et al. (2010). Methods such as the drop-min approach can be helpful in such situations to provide more accurate inferences by adjusting for the bias associated with post-hoc subgroup identification.

9.4.1.2 Example: BiDil Studies (Subgroup Inconsistency)

MRCTs raise challenges because of the difficulties that may arise in interpreting results from subsets of trial data (i.e., regions) in trials that were mainly designed to address hypotheses in the full trial population. There are similarities with other settings where subgroup signals may be suggested. We now consider an example that does not involve an MRCT, but rather illustrates a subgroup issue quite similar to issues that may arise in MRCTs, because it involves a subgroup—race—that sometimes is highly confounded with region in MRCTs. Specifically, BiDil, a combination of isosorbide dinitrate and hydralazine, was approved by FDA in 2005 (FDA BiDil package insert, 2005) for the treatment of heart failure as an adjunct to standard therapy in self-identified *black patients* to improve survival, prolong time to hospitalization for heart failure, and improve patient-reported functional status. However, the clinical development of BiDil had been initiated decades earlier. More focused investigation of subgroup issues may have resulted in earlier availability.

The first clinical trial of BiDil, the Vasodilator-Heart Failure Trial I (V-HeFT I), was initiated in 1980 (Cohn et al., 1986). It randomly assigned 642 men receiving standard of care to additionally receive double-blind treatment with placebo, prazosin, or BiDil. Follow-up averaged 2.3 years. Mortality over the entire follow-up period was lower for BiDil than for placebo group, but did not reach statistical significance ($p = 0.053$). For two-year mortality, a major protocol-specified endpoint, cumulative rates were 34.3% for placebo and 25.6% for BiDil, a risk reduction of 34% ($p = 0.028$); at three years, mortality rates were 46.9% versus 36.2%, a risk reduction of 36%. Mortality in the prazosin group was similar to that of placebo.

Based on these promising results, the study was followed by V-HeFT II (Cohn et al., 1991), in which about 800 patients were randomly assigned to receive enalapril or BiDil. Two-year mortality was significantly lower for enalapril (18%) than for BiDil (25%) ($p = 0.016$; mortality reduction = 28.0%), and overall mortality trended lower but did not reach significance ($p = 0.08$).

A New Drug Application was prepared for BiDil on the basis of the V-HeFT trials. However, the FDA concluded the evidence of efficacy was insufficient and rejected the application. Carson et al. (1999) presented further analyses and identified a signal that BiDil appeared to work better in African-Americans. An additional study, A-HeFT (African-American Heart Failure Trial), was conducted and was stopped early based on a recommendation from its DMC due to overwhelming efficacy. On the basis of A-HeFT, the FDA approved BiDil in 2005 (Chen et al., 2017): "BiDil is indicated for the treatment of heart failure as an adjunct to standard therapy in self-identified black patients." In 2006, the Heart Failure Society of America included the use of BiDil as the standard of care for the treatment of heart failure in black patients.

The claim of a treatment benefit in a single self-identified racial group raised controversy. While advocates hailed the approval of BiDil as a breakthrough for African-Americans, critics (e.g., Roberts) argued that self-identification as an indicator for the race was not a sufficient categorization method because such self-identifications were socially constructed and have no biological connection to genomic data. Other relevant evidence supporting the effectiveness of BiDil on African-Americans was subsequently provided by Exner et al. (2001), suggesting that African-Americans with congestive heart failure (CHF) respond less effectively to conventional CHF treatments (particularly ACE inhibitors) than Caucasians, which may help provide a rationale for the racial interaction observed.

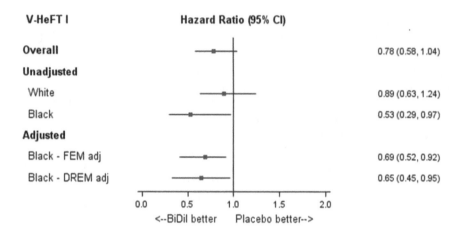

FIGURE 9.2
Hazard ratios for BiDil vs placebo in the V-HeFT I study – unadjusted and adjusted via FEM and DRM using the drop-min approach.

We now illustrate the application of the drop-min approach, shown in a previous example, to the V-HeFT data. The overall results from V-HeFT I (Cohn and Tognoni, 2001) suggested an advantage for BiDil over placebo that did not reach statistical significance (HR = 0.779, p = 0.093). For black patients, the HR of 0.532 was nominally significant (p = 0.041), while similar benefit for white patients was not seen (HR = 0.886, p = 0.48). Applying the drop-min approach to correct for the selection bias, adjusted HRs for FEM and DREM models were 0.61 (p = 0.018) and 0.55 (p = 0.035), respectively. Figure 9.2 presents the unadjusted HRs for white and black patients in V-HeFT I, and the adjusted HRs for black patients obtained using the drop min approach. As BiDil patients in both V-HeFT trials were similar, we also applied the drop-min approach using pooled BiDil data from the two studies. The initial nominal result in the black subgroup was HR = 0.62 (p = 0.03); the drop-min approach yielded HRs of 0.69 (p = 0.013) and 0.65 (p = 0.024) for the adjusted ones via FEM and DREM models, respectively.

Although gefitinib and BiDil failed to show benefits to the general population in the pivotal studies, the study results suggested that subgroups of the population could benefit from them, and further investigations seem to have borne this out. In the next several examples, we will review how inconsistency of regions may be addressed when overall results are positive.

9.4.2 Studies with Positive Overall Results

We next present five studies in which the overall results were positive, but with signals of region differences that raised concerns and engendered much follow-up investigation.

9.4.2.1 Example: The PLATO Study

The Platelet Inhibition and Patient Outcomes (PLATO) trial compared ticagrelor with clopidogrel in patients with acute coronary syndrome (ACS) (Wallentin et al., 2009). The primary endpoint was a composite of cardiovascular death, myocardial infarction (MI), and stroke. PLATO recruited 18624 patients from 43 countries; 7.6% of the trial population was enrolled in the US. The overall results showed a statistically significant benefit for ticagrelor, as the primary endpoint occurred in 9.8% of patients for ticagrelor and 11.7% for clopidogrel (HR = 0.84; 95% CI: 0.77–0.92; $p < 0.001$).

Among 31 pre-specified treatment-by-subgroup evaluations, a qualitatively different outcome by region was revealed. Among North American patients, the HR was 1.25 (95% CI: 0.93–1.67), suggesting a 25% greater risk with ticagrelor, clearly a signal of some concern. Extensive post-hoc exploratory analyses were performed to investigate the differences across regions. Examinations mainly focused on three possibilities: systematic issues in trial conduct in the US; differences between the US and non-US populations in important characteristics that could potentially explain the signal; and the play of chance.

Study conduct issues were carefully examined and ruled out as the cause for regional interaction. These included systematic issues in trial conduct, errors in drug delivery at US sites, site management issues at specific sites (including evaluation of large vs. small sites), and regional differences in discounting treatment effect modifier and its distribution across regions, as well as the source of blinded trial monitoring.

A number of post-hoc analyses, adjusting for both baseline and post-baseline characteristics, were performed to investigate whether there were any imbalances across regions that might account, at least in part, for the US observation. These revealed that the observed treatment-by-region interaction was little changed by the addition of any factor, with the sole and notable exception of maintenance aspirin dosage (ASA dose). When included in analysis models, and depending on definition, median ASA dose was found to attenuate 80–100% of the observed interaction. This pattern is more clearly revealed if HR is displayed as a function of ASA dose as a continuous covariate (see figure 8 in Carroll and Fleming, 2013). The credibility of an explanatory effect modifier is impacted by insights about biological plausibility. For the PLATO trial, there are some reasons for caution in interpreting these data regarding ASA dose, as there currently are not persuasive biological explanations for this interaction.

Based on the results from PLATO and other supportive trials, ticagrelor was approved by FDA (FDA Brilinta package insert, 2011) for patients with ACS to reduce the rate of thrombotic cardiovascular events. However, a "Boxed Warning" for ticagrelor warns about bleeding and the need to keep aspirin dose at or below 100 mg: "Maintenance doses of aspirin above 100 mg reduce the effectiveness... and should be avoided." Other agencies also approved the drug with similar label statements.

We note that in 2010, the PEGASUS trial was launched (Bonaca et al., 2015). Over 21,000 patients with prior MI were randomized to ticagrelor 90 mg twice daily, ticagrelor 60 mg twice daily, or placebo. All patients were to receive low-dose aspirin and were followed for a median of 33 months. The results supported the primary finding in PLATO, with HR against placebo of ~0.84 for both dose groups.

The next four examples also describe trials with positive results overall but showing weaker results in individual regions. After much investigation, it was, for the most part, considered that these signals likely arose largely due to chance (there are statistical tools available to calculate quantities such as the probabilities of a negative outcome in a region from the design perspective and based on the study results, as described in the supplement of this manuscript).

9.4.2.2 Example: MERIT-HF Study

This study (MERIT-HF Study Group, 1999) evaluated the effect of meto-prolol CR/XL on CHF compared to placebo. Primary endpoints were: 1) all-cause mortality; 2) all-cause mortality + all-cause hospitalization. An α-level of 0.05 (two-sided) was allocated to these endpoints as 0.04 and 0.01, respectively. The trial was terminated for a statistically significant reduction in all-cause mortality based on a pre-planned interim analysis; the HR was 0.66, with nominal $p<0.0001$, and the HR for the mortality-hospitalization composite was 0.81 ($p = 0.00012$). Results were consistent across 12 pre-defined subgroups, which did not include region or country.

During the NDA review (FDA Medical Reviews for Toprol-XL metoprolol succinate, 2000; FDA Statistical Review and Evaluation for Toprol-XL metoprolol succinate, 2000), the statistical reviewer conducted a subgroup analysis by region (US vs Europe) and noted a strong suggestion of a treatment-by-region interaction ($p = 0.006$) for all-cause mortality: in Europe, HR = 0.55 ($p = 0.0001$), while in the US, HR = 1.05 ($p = 0.80$). For the composite, effects were similar (0.84 vs 0.81) across both regions.

FDA conducted extensive exploratory analyses to explore the poorer US mortality effect (FDA Statistical Review and Evaluation for Toprol-XL metoprolol succinate, 2000). There were imbalances in racial and gender composition between regions, with females and blacks more heavily represented in the US than in Europe. However, the HR in the US excluding non-white patients was even higher than 1.05. While the HR in women was substantially higher than in men (0.92 vs 0.61) for the overall trial population and the difference was even more marked in the US (1.45 vs 0.95), this difference was not consistently demonstrated in all European countries. No plausible covariates stood out to explain the US mortality result. FDA interpreted that the absence of observed mortality benefit in the US was perhaps due to chance, but was more likely caused by inter-country differences in gender distribution of randomized patients, cause of deaths in CHF, or other demographic or medical practice differences.

Wedel et al. (2001) examined predefined and post-hoc subgroups in MERIT-HF. A treatment-by-country analysis yielded an interaction p-value of 0.22. The reason for not combining non-US countries into a single region was because these countries did not represent a homogeneous group regarding background epidemiologic characteristics, socio-economic characteristics, or standard of care. In addition, such post-hoc groupings can be very prone to biased judgments and interpretations. Through examination of outcomes across a large number of predefined and post-hoc subgroups, the authors concluded that the apparent anomaly in the US mortality results was not highly inconsistent with the overall treatment effect and within the level of variation one could expect, and likely largely a chance result. Quan et al. (2017) suggested a method to quantify the chance of observing at least one negative regional treatment effect based on the study result. Assuming all regions have identical true HR of 0.66 (the observed overall HR), the chance to observe a least one negative effect among 12 regions was 89%, so that a negative region effect could easily be observed by chance.

Ultimately, FDA reviewers emphasized that the US patient population had not been intended to be used to evaluate the overall efficacy, which had been established by the pre-specified primary analysis in the overall population (FDA Medical Reviews for Toprol-XL metoprolol succinate, 2000). In 2009, FDA-approved metoprolol for treatment of CHF based on the MERIT-HF study, but regional differences were described in the product label (FDA Toprol package insert, 2009).

About nine years elapsed between the MERIT-HF NDA and FDA approval of metoprolol, mainly due to the suspected inconsistency issues. The current consensus of the scientific community, documented in ICH E17 (International Council for Harmonization of Technical Requirement for Pharmaceuticals for Human Use, 2017), is that the best estimate of treatment effect usually comes from an analysis of all randomized patients. Several other points should be noted as well. Region should be included in the planned subgroup analyses for MRCTs. The examination of subgroups, including those defined by region or country, should generally be on a qualitative basis and not by a quantitative estimate of treatment effect. Consistency is descriptive but should be part of a structured framework to allow transparent dialog among stakeholders.

9.4.2.3 Example: The HOPE Study

The Heart Outcomes Prevention Evaluation (HOPE) trial was a double-blind, placebo-controlled, randomized study to evaluate the effects of ramipril for preventing cardiovascular (CV) events in patients at high risk (Yusuf et al., 2000; Arnold et al., 2013). A total of 9297 high-risk patients with evidence of vascular disease or diabetes plus one other CV risk factor, and not known to have a low ejection fraction or heart failure, were randomly assigned to receive ramipril (10 mg once per day orally) or matching placebo for a mean of five years. The primary endpoint was a composite of MI, stroke, or death from CV causes.

The trial was stopped at an interim analysis based on a recommendation from its DMC due to clear evidence of benefit for ramipril (crossing of monitoring boundaries in two consecutive reviews; see Arnold et al., 2013). A primary event occurred in 14.0% of ramipril patients and 17.8% of placebo patients, a 22% risk reduction (HR=0.78, 95% CI: 0.70–0.84, $p < 0.001$). The results were also significant for each component of the composite endpoint. Some subpopulations had been pre-defined in the protocol based upon, for example, presence or absence of diabetes, CV disease, hypertension, microalbuminuria; also, gender, and age. The effect of ramipril on the primary endpoint was consistent across all the subpopulations.

This trial had been conducted in 4 regions and 18 countries (FDA, Arnold et al., 2013). Canada had by far the largest enrollment (59%), followed by the US (9%). Two other regions provided the remainder of the population: Europe (14 countries totaling 21%) and Latin America (3 countries totaling 11%). Yusuf and Wittes (2016) described considerable country variations in treatment effect. Canada, with the highest enrollment, had almost the same observed effect as the overall estimate (RR = 0.78). Countries with low enrollment showed much larger effect variations; some yielded outcomes favoring placebo over ramipril. This variation, however, may just be due to the randomness resulting from the small country sample sizes and thus should not be over-interpreted, as pointed out by the authors. Had regional effects been included in the protocol as a predefined subpopulation, a prior assessment of the likelihood of a qualitative treatment-by-region interaction (i.e., a directional treatment difference across regions) could have been provided. Also, a DSMB charter can advise a monitoring committee to look closely at the pattern of regional results before making a decision to halt a trial early when evidence of efficacy is lacking in some regions.

9.4.2.4 Example: The CLEOPATRA Study

The CLEOPATRA (CLinical Evaluation Of Pertuzumab And TRAstuzumab) trial was a randomized, double-blind, placebo-controlled, phase 3 study involving patients with human epidermal growth factor receptor 2 (HER2) positive metastatic breast cancer (Baselga et al., 2012). Patients were randomly assigned in a 1:1 ratio, to the Pertuzumab (pertuzumab plus trastuzumab plus docetaxel) group or the control (placebo plus trastuzumab plus docetaxel) group, with stratification by geographic region (Asia, Europe, North America, or South America) and prior treatment status (prior chemotherapy vs. none). The primary endpoint was progression-free survival (PFS).

A total of 808 patients were enrolled at 204 centers in 25 countries. The Pertuzumab group had a significantly improved PFS with median 18.5 months, compared to 12.4 months for control (HR = 0.62; 95% CI: 0.51–0.75; $p < 0.0001$).

The sponsor analyzed the subgroup of 53 Japanese patients, comprising only 6.6% of the trial population (Pharmaceuticals and Medical Devices Agency, 2013). It had been hoped that the Japanese patients would show a consistent trend with the overall results (i.e., HR for Japan less than 1.00). The final PFS analysis in the Japanese population yielded HR = 1.62 (95% CI: 0.70–3.78), which did not meet the pre-specified consistency criterion.

The considerations which led to the small enrollment in Japan in this study are unclear. However, from a design point of view, the chance for a region with 6.6% of the sample size to yield a negative result is about 25% when power is planned at 80% for the alternative hypothesis. PMDA acknowledged that the failure to meet the consistency criteria was possibly caused by the small sample size, as well as by imbalances in prognostic factors between treatments among these patients. Ultimately PMDA concluded that CLEOPATRA had failed to confirm consistency for the following reasons: (a) multivariate analyses suggested the presence of interactions of treatment effect with the country (Japan vs. others), and (b) the estimated HRs in the Japanese population based on multivariate analyses taking account of prognostic factors also failed to clearly show the efficacy of pertuzumab.

On the other hand, the overall results showed internal consistency across endpoints, demonstrating benefit not only for the primary endpoint of PFS but also for the secondary (and clinically more important) endpoint, overall survival (Swain et al., 2013). The pertuzumab arm had a 34% reduction in the risk of death during the course of the study (HR = 0.66; 95% CI 0.52–0.84; p = 0.0008). PMDA (Pharmaceuticals and Medical Devices Agency, 2013) also cited strong benefit for pertuzumab both inside and outside of Japan, without providing specifics and finally concluded that pertuzumab would be positioned as a treatment option for Japanese patients, based on the overall results and further comprehensive review (e.g., the similarity of the medical environment for breast cancer and pharmacokinetic profile between the Japanese and non-Japanese populations).

9.4.2.5 Example: The LEADER Trial

LEADER was a multicenter, international, randomized, double-blind, placebo-controlled trial investigating the long-term effects of Victoza® compared to placebo, both in addition to standard of care, in people with type 2 diabetes at high risk of major CV events (FDA, 2017a; Nordisk, 2017).

LEADER enrolled 9,340 participants from 32 countries. The primary endpoint was the first occurrence of a composite of major adverse CV events (MACE) comprising CV death, non-fatal MI, or non-fatal stroke. The LEADER study was required by FDA to evaluate whether the use of Victoza was associated with unacceptably high CV risk. For the primary analysis, a Cox proportional hazards model was used to test for non-inferiority against a pre-specified risk margin of 1.3 for the HR for MACE, and to test for superiority if non-inferiority was demonstrated. The trial results in fact indicated benefit for Victoza, i.e., an estimated 13% reduction in primary outcomes compared to placebo (HR = 0.87, 95% CI: 0.78–0.97; non-inferiority $p < 0.001$, superiority $p = 0.001$; see Marso et al., 2016).

The sponsor performed a number of pre-specified subgroup analyses, including region. No CV advantage was suggested for patients from North America (HR = 1.01, 95% CI: 0.84–1.22), and an interaction test yielded p = 0.20. The observation for North America was driven by the US, which contributed 88% of the region sample size (US: HR = 1.03, 95% CI: 0.84–1.25; Canada: HR = 0.80, 95% CI: 0.42–1.52).

Factors related to patient characteristics or exposure time were investigated for imbalances. Post-hoc analyses found that the difference between the US and non-US populations remained after adjustment for covariates and interaction. The rate of first MACE in placebo patients was similar for the US and non-US populations, indicating no differences in background CV risk profile. Analyses of exposure time to treatment showed that the mean proportion of time on trial product was lower in the US (73%) than in the non-US population (87%). Correspondingly, the proportion of patients on treatment decreased more over time in the US population in both treatment groups.

The signal of regional interaction, and in particular the US finding, were investigated in post-hoc analyses using traditional interaction terms, and some modeling and examination of baseline characteristics. At the end, no clear explanation was found and the "play of chance" was not ruled out.

At an FDA Advisory Committee meeting, FDA (FDA, 2017a) addressed the signal of inconsistency from the US: "Several analyses were conducted to explain these findings, but it is important to emphasize that these were exploratory and there still remains a possibility that the subgroup findings could be explained by chance alone." The sponsor's background document described: "In summary, the pre-specified subgroup analysis of time to first MACE by region provided no strong evidence to support a regional difference (interaction $p = 0.20$). Further analyses... showed that exposure time to trial product was lower for the US compared to the non-US populations. On-treatment analyses of time to first MACE yielded hazard ratio estimates in the US consistent with that of the overall population. This supports that the US population is not different from the overall population with respect to cardiovascular risk reduction with liraglutide." Based on the LEADER results, the FDA approved a new indication for Victoza® (liraglutide) to reduce the risk of major adverse CV events, heart attack, stroke, and CV death, in adults with type 2 diabetes and established CV disease.

We conclude with an example that illustrates region differences of a type that could plausibly lead to effect differences in trials and that trial planners should be alert to.

9.4.2.6 Example: The MAGIC Study

The Magnesium in Coronaries (MAGIC) trial was a randomized, double-blind study in 6213 patients with acute ST-elevation myocardial infarction (STEMI), assigned to receive either magnesium sulphate or placebo. The primary endpoint was 30-day all-cause mortality. Randomization was stratified by patient eligibility for reperfusion therapy. The overall results did not show a difference between the magnesium and placebo groups, with odds ratio (95% CI): 1.0 (0.9–1.2) (MAGIC Investigators, 2002).

Post-hoc investigation focused on three geographic regions identified based on differences in risk factors, background treatment, and local medical practice (Domanski et al., 2004):

- Region 1 = US, Canada: 5% of total enrollment;
- Region 2 = Eastern Europe (Bulgaria, Georgia, Russia): 91%;
- Region 3 = Austria, Belgium, Chile, Hungary, Israel, the Netherlands, New Zealand, Venezuela: 4%.

Odds ratios (95% CIs) for mortality for the three regions were 1.4 (0.6–3.1), 1.0 (0.8–1.1), 1.7 (0.8–3.6), respectively.

Eastern Europe showed a higher prevalence at the entry of risk factors prognostic for mortality compared to the other two regions (which were generally fairly similar to each other), including hypertension (73.6% vs 54.3%), prior MI (27.0% vs 18.7%), heart failure history (10.6% vs 6.0%) anterior location of index MI (57.0% vs 47.2%), and presence of pulmonary congestion (12.4% vs 6.9%). There was substantial regional variation in reperfusion therapy and concurrent medications; e.g., less than 1% of patients in Region 2 received primary angioplasty, versus 27% in the other regions; beta-blockers were also less frequently used in Region 2 (51% vs 70%), as was lipid-lowering therapy (1% vs 29%). The patterns of regional differences were generally similar to those seen in other international trials, such as the HERO-2 study (Domanski et al., 2004), which showed a higher prevalence of risk factors and less reperfusion therapy in Russia compared to western countries.

It is unclear whether the regional variation seen in the estimated mortality treatment effect is due to more than chance, because of the limited outcome information available from the small regions (e.g., only 27 and 35 primary events in Regions 1 and 3, respectively). However, it is quite clear that there were substantial regional differences in the state of patients' CV risk prior to enrollment and in the nature of therapies after enrollment, which could be expected to affect cardiac mortality and could potentially introduce effect differences for certain types of treatments.

MAGIC thus provides a useful illustration of underlying region differences due to intrinsic and extrinsic factors that would be critical to understanding while designing a clinical trial. Relevant questions include the following: should a single trial targeting an overall common treatment effect even be conducted across regions that are so fundamentally different, whether in patient characteristics, clinical practices, etc.? If so, what are the implications for the design, analysis, and interpretation of its results? What procedures might be considered to standardize inclusion criteria and background therapy to make the trial population more homogeneous and the results more interpretable, etc. Failure to sufficiently investigate and understand such issues in advance and carefully address them during trial planning could lead to highly ambiguous or uninterpretable results.

9.5 Discussion

MRCTs have become an important component of strategy in global drug development. To fully realize the advantages of MRCTs, consistency across regions needs to be properly addressed. Lessons learned from the review of the examples we have shown are that the consistency issue needs to be managed at every stage of an MRCT, from design, to monitoring during the trial, to analysis, and ultimately to interpretation.

At the design stage of MRCTs, the consistency assessment should be described in a structured framework to allow transparent dialog among stakeholders. The agency responsible for each region will naturally focus strongly on the similarity of effects in its region compared to others. However, region sample sizes will generally not allow this to be done simply and definitively. When many regions are defined within a study, sample sizes for some will likely be quite small. As a result, it may not be possible to obtain reliable estimates in all regions, and consistency may not be appropriately assessed (Tanaka et al., 2012; Yusuf and Wittes, 2016). As an illustration, for a conventionally designed MRCT with power, 90% where the hypothesized effect is true for all regions, the chances to observe a negative estimate for a region comprising 5%, 10%, 15%, and 20% of the total, are 23%, 15%, 10%, and 7%, respectively. If there are four regions in an MRCT, the chance to see a negative treatment effect estimate in at least one is nearly 50% if the region sample sizes are equal and higher for other sample size distributions. A clear definition of region, and rationale for the choice, needs to be described in the protocol. The pooling of geographic regions based on the commonality of intrinsic and extrinsic factors should be considered at the design stage (International Council for Harmonization of Technical Requirement for Pharmaceuticals for Human Use, 2017).

Proper stratification for major confounding extrinsic and intrinsic factors including region can enhance the homogeneity of effects across the study population. For some indications, main endpoints may be subjective (e.g., the central nervous system area). In these cases, appropriate measures are necessary to account in the protocol for differences across cultures, medical practices, and other factors that potentially differ across regions, before trial initiation. Evidence of disease is collected prospectively. After trial initiation, implementation of remedies during the course of the trial requires protocol amendments and clear communications to the sites; such post-initiation changes are often very costly, time consuming, and ineffective. During the course of the TOPCAT trial, although a proposal was presented to the SC, it was considered too late to implement the recommendation. Therefore, closely monitoring the blinded data is an effective tool to identify issues such as region imbalance for baseline covariates and evidence of disease, and inconsistency of primary outcomes across regions. A mutually acceptable way for the sponsor and sites to re-evaluate site enrollment targets, including stopping enrollment, should be established before the trial start. Timely identification of these issues is crucial for correcting them or mitigating their impact. The regional inconsistency issue in TOPCAT was reflected in blinded interim data and might have been addressed sooner; the aspirin dose region imbalance in PLATO might similarly have been identified, and actions considered, based on blinded accruing data. At the end of the trial and before unblinding, the statistical analysis plan should address regional imbalances of intrinsic and extrinsic factors identified via blinded data reviews. This may facilitate a more objective interpretation of the trial results.

Interim monitoring of unblinded data may also offer opportunities to identify and mitigate inconsistency. The DMC needs to decide what information to communicate to the SC to make proper decisions, while at the same time maintaining study integrity. This requires careful and timely communication between the DMC and other parties.

Despite appropriate proactive efforts, inconsistency may still be observed. There are several tools to assess whether such inconsistency is by chance due to small sample sizes or a large number of regions. One such toolset is known as *Hill's Criteria of Causality* (Hill, 1965). These criteria move beyond p-values, providing concepts that can contribute to evidence of a causal relationship, particularly in assessing the evidence of an unexpected regional finding. In this paper, we cited examples of these principles, including internal consistency (MERIT and CLEOPATRA), external consistency (BiDil), and biological plausibility (TOPCAT metabolite results and gefitinib EGRF findings). These concepts can help provide an objective set of criteria for assessing a regional finding.

Other cases may remain challenging to interpret and may take more time and experience before underlying causes are understood when inconsistent results cannot be explained by measured covariates. For example, it was more than eight years after the completion of INTACT trials before the identification of EGFR as a factor that could lead to inconsistency between Asian and non-Asian patients. Sometimes, convincing biological explanations for inconsistency remain elusive. In PLATO, the inconsistency between US and non-US may be related to aspirin dosage, but there are still not persuasive biological explanations for this interaction up to the present. In the BiDil development, it was suggested consistently in the results of three trials that BiDil is more effective in black patients, but again, strong biological rationale remains absent.

The inconsistency of results in MRCTs poses a dilemma for regulatory agencies when deciding whether a product should be approved in their geographic area of responsibility. For drugs intended to treat life-threatening diseases, the stakes for a correct decision are high. On one hand, if an ineffective or unsafe product enters the market, patients can suffer; on the other hand, if an effective treatment is blocked or delayed, lives could similarly be negatively affected. We saw this play out in different ways in three of our examples. MHLW approved gefitinib for treatment of NSCLC on the basis of the INTACT 1 and 2 trials; although biological explanations for the regional inconsistency were lacking, the replication in two studies may have been the trigger for approval. FDA did not consider that BiDil was approvable based on the results of V-HeFT I and II, but did approve it following A-HeFT, a landmark decision for race-specific drug approval. In PLATO, the FDA-approved ticagrelor, although with a warning in the label based on ad hoc analysis results. These three examples illustrate questions that arise when inconsistency is observed in study results: what evidence may constitute the consideration for approval of a drug, or approval with a label warning, or with a commitment to perform additional research?

The example of gefitinib for NSCLC set a precedent for approval of a drug whose effectiveness is observed on (a region with) a minority population, consistently in two studies. In case a drug is deemed to be effective only in some regions or subgroups, the treatment effect estimates are biased and need to be corrected. Methods such as the drop-min approach (Chen et al., 2017) provide bias-corrected inferences based on the data of all patients and thus are in compliance with the important principle of intention-to-treat.

References

Arnold JM, Yusuf S, Young J, et al. Prevention of heart failure in patients in the heart outcomes prevention evaluation (HOPE) study. *Circulation*. 2013;107(9):1284–1290.

Baselga J, Cortés J, Kim SB, et al. Pertuzumab plus trastuzumab plus docetaxel for metastatic breast cancer. *N Engl J Med*. 2012;366:109–119.

Bonaca MP, Bhatt DL, Cohen M, et al. Long-term use of ticagrelor in patients with prior myocardial infarction. *N Engl J Med*. 2015;372:1791–1800.

Bristow MR, Enciso JS, Gersh BJ, et al. Detection and management of geographic disparities in the TOPCAT trial: lessons learned and derivative recommendations. *JACC Basic Transl Sci*. 2016;1(3):180–189.

Carroll, K. Trial 709 The ISEL Study (IRESSA® Survival Evaluation in Lung Cancer). 2004. http://slideplayer.com/slide/9506279/.

Carroll KJ, Fleming TR. Statistical evaluation and analysis of regional interactions: the PLATO trial case study. *Stat Biopharm Res*. 2013;5(2):91–101.

Carson P, Ziesche S, Johnson G, Cohn JN. Racial differences in response to therapy for heart failure: analysis of the vasodilator-heart failure trials. *J Card Fail*. 1999;5:178–187.

Chen J, et al. Consistency of treatment effect across regions in multiregional clinical trials, Part 1: design considerations. *Drug Inf J*. 2011;45:595–602.

Chen J, Quan H, Binkowitz B, et al. Assessing consistent treatment effect in a multiregional clinical trial: a systematic review. *Pharm Stat*. 2010;9:242–253.

Chen F, Li G, Lan KKG. Inconsistency and drop-minimum data analysis. *Stat Med*. 2017;36:416–425.

Cohn JN, Tognoni G. A randomized trial of the angiotensin-receptor blocker valsartan in chronic heart failure. *N Engl J Med*. 2001;345:1667–1675.

Cohn JN, Archibald DG, Ziesche S, et al. Effect of vasodilator therapy on mortality in chronic congestive heart failure: results of a veterans administration cooperative study. *N Engl J Med*. 1986;314:1547–1552.

Cohn JN, Johnson G, Ziesche S, et al. A comparison of enalapril with hydralazine–isosorbide dinitrate in the treatment of chronic congestive heart failure. *N Engl J Med*. 1991;325:303–310.

de Denus S, O'Meara E, Desai AS, et al. Spironolactone metabolites in TOPCAT - new insights into regional variation. *N Engl J Med*. 2017;376:1690–1692.

Domanski M, Antman E, McKinlay S, et al. Geographic variability in patient characteristics, treatment and outcome in an international trial of magnesium in acute myocardial infarction. *Controlled Clin Trials*. 2004; 25: 553–562.

Exner DV, Dries DL, Domanski MJ, Cohn JN. Lesser response to angiotensin-converting-enzyme inhibitor therapy in blacks as compared with white patients with left ventricular dysfunction. *N Engl J Med*. 2001;344 (18):1351–1357.

FDA. FDA Briefing Document: Endocrinologic and Metabolic Drugs Advisory Committee (EMDAC) Meeting, Victoza (liraglutide) injection, for subcutaneous use. 2017a. Accessible from https://www.fda.gov/downloads/AdvisoryCommittees/CommitteesMeetingMaterials/Drugs/EndocrinologicandMetabolicDrugsAdvisoryCommittee/UCM563334.pdf.

FDA. Endocrinologic and Metabolic Drugs Advisory Committee (EMDAC) Meeting, Victoza (liraglutide) injection, for subcutaneous use – FDA Slides. 2017b. Accessible from https://www.fda.gov/downloads/AdvisoryCommittees/CommitteesMeetingMaterials/Drugs/EndocrinologicandMetabolicDrugsAdvisoryCommittee/UCM566062.pdf.

FDA BiDil package insert. 2005. Accessible from https://www.accessdata.fda.gov/drugsatfda_docs/label/2005/020727lbl.pdf.

FDA Brilinta package insert. 2011. Accessible from http://www.azpicentral.com/brilinta/brilinta.pdf.

FDA Medical Review(s) for Toprol-XL (metoprolol succinate). 2000. Accessible from https://www.accessdata.fda.gov/drugsatfda_docs/nda/2000/N-19–962S013_Toprol_Medr.pdf.

FDA Statistical Review and Evaluation for Toprol-XL (metoprolol succinate). 2000. Accessible from https://www.accessdata.fda.gov/drugsatfda_docs/nda/2000/N-19–962S013_Toprol_Statr.pdf.

FDA Toprol package insert. 2009. Accessible from https://www.accessdata.fda.gov/drugsatfda_docs/label/2009/019962s038lbl.pdf.

Giaccone G, Herbst RS, Manegold C, et al. Gefitinib in combination with gemcitabine and cisplatin in advanced non–small-cell lung cancer: a Phase III trial - INTACT 1. *J Clin Oncol.* 2004;22:777–784.

Hama R, Sakaguchi K. The gefitinib story. 2004. Accessible from http://npojip.org/english/The-gefitinib-story.pdf.

Herbst RS, Giaccone G, Schiller JH, et al. Gefitinib in combination with paclitaxel and carboplatin in advanced non–small-cell lung cancer: a phase III trial - INTACT 2. *J Clin Oncol.* 2004;22:785–794.

Hill AB. The environment and disease: association or causation. *Proc R Soc Med.* 1965;58:295–300.

https://www.nejm.org/doi/full/10.1056/NEJMe2034294?query=TOC.

https://www.fda.gov/media/78504/download.

https://gisanddata.maps.arcgis.com/apps/opsdashboard/index.html#/bda759474 0fd40299423467b48e9ecf6.

International Council for Harmonization of Technical Requirement for Pharmaceuticals for Human Use, (1998) ICH E9: statistical principles for clinical trials. Accessible from https://www.fda.gov/downloads/drugs/guidancecomplianceregulatoryinformation/guidances/ucm073137.pdf.

International Council for Harmonization of Technical Requirement for Pharmaceuticals for Human Use, 2017. ICH E17: general principles for planning and design of multi-regional clinical trials. Accessible from http://www.ich.org/fileadmin/Public_Web_Site/ICH_Products/Guidelines/Efficacy/E17/E17EWG_Step4_2017_1116.pdf.

Li G, Chen J, Quan H, Shentu Y. Consistency assessment with global and bridging development strategies in emerging markets. *Contemp Clin Trials.* 2013;36(2):687–696.

Maemondo M, Inoue A, Kobayashi K, et al. Gefitinib or chemotherapy for non-small-cell lung cancer with mutated EGFR. *N Engl J Med.* 2010;362(25):2380–2388.

MAGIC Investigators. Early administration of magnesium to high risk patients with acute myocardial infarction in the magnesium in coronaries (MAGIC) trial: a randomized, controlled trial. *Lancet.* 2002;360:1189–1196.

Marso SP, Daniels GH, Brown-Frandsen K, et al. Liraglutide and cardiovascular outcomes on Type 2 diabetes. *N Engl J Med.* 2016;375:311–322.

MHLW (Ministry of Health, Labour and Welfare of Japan). Basic principles on global clinical trials 2007. (Available at: http://www.pmda.go.jp/files/000153265.pdf) [Accessed date: November 14, 2015].

MERIT-HF Study Group. Effect of metoprolol CR/XL in chronic heart failure: Metoprolol CR/XL randomized intervention trial in congestive heart failure (MERIT-HF). *Lancet.* 1999;353:2001–2007.

Novo Nordisk. Novo Nordisk Briefing Document: Endocrinologic and Metabolic Drugs Advisory Committee (EMDAC) Meeting, Victoza® (liraglutide) injection, LEADER: Liraglutide Effect and Action in Diabetes: Evaluation of Cardiovascular Outcome Results. 2017. Accessible from https://www.fda.gov/downloads/AdvisoryCommittees/CommitteesMeetingMaterials/Drugs/Endo-crinologicandMetabolicDrugsAdvisoryCommittee/UCM563335.pdf.

Pharmaceuticals and Medical Devices Agency. Report on the deliberation results of Parjet. 2013. https://www.pmda.go.jp/files/000153631.pdf.

Pfeffer MA, Claggett B, Assmann SF, et al. Regional variation in patients and outcomes in the treatment of preserved cardiac function heart failure with an aldosterone antagonist (TOPCAT) trial. *Circulation* 2015;131(1):34–42.

Pitt B, Pfeffer MA, Assmann SF, et al. Spironolactone for heart failure with preserved ejection fraction. *N Engl J Med*. 2014;370:1383–1392.

Quan H, Li M, Chen J, et al. Assessment of consistency of treatment effects in multiregional clinical trials. *Drug Inf J*. 2010;44:617–632.

Quan H, Mao X, Tanaka Y, et al. Example-based illustrations of design, conduct, analysis and result interpretation of multi-regional clinical trials. *Contemp Clin Trials*. 2017;58:13–22.

Roberts D. The color coded pill. In *Fatal Invention: How Science, Politics, and Big Business Re-create Race in the Twenty-first Century* (https://books.google.comlbooks/about/Fatal_Invention.html?id=_TsaXOpTCSC). The New Press. ISBN 978-1-595-58834-0.

Swain SM, Kim SB, Cortés J, et al. Overall survival benefit with pertuzumab, trastuzumab, and docetaxel for HER2-positive metastatic breast cancer in CLEO-PATRA, a randomised Phase 3 study. *Lancet Oncol*. 2013;14(6):461–471.

Tanaka Y, Li G, Wang Y, Chen J. Qualitative consistency of treatment effects in multiregional clinical trials. *J Biopharm Stat*. 2012;22:988–1000.

Thatcher N, Chang A, Parikh P, et al. Gefitinib plus best supportive care in previously treated patients with refractory advanced non-small-cell lung cancer: results from a randomised, placebo-controlled, multicentre study (Iressa Survival Evaluation in Lung Cancer). *Lancet*. 2005;366:1527–1537.

Wallentin L, Becker RC, Budaj A, et al. Ticagrelor versus clopidogrel in patients with acute coronary syndromes. *N Engl J Med*. 2009;361:1045–1057.

WHO Solidarity Trial Consortium. Repurposed antiviral drugs for Covid-19—interim WHO Solidarity trial results. *N Engl J Med*. 2021;384:497–511.

Yusuf S, Wittes J. Interpreting geographic variations in results of randomized, controlled trials. *N Engl J Med*. 2016;375(23):2263–2271.

Yusuf S, Sleight PE, Pogue JF, Bosch J, Davies R, Dagenais G. Effects of an angiotensin-converting-enzyme inhibitor, ramipril, on cardiovascular events in high-risk patients. *N Engl J Med*. 2000;342(3):145–153.

10

Leveraging Foreign Clinical Data Extrapolation to Accelerate Global Drug Development: A Case Study in Hematological Oncology

Hongjie Zhu, Jingjing Ye, and Xiang Guo

10.1 Introduction

Globalization of clinical drug development has led to the popularity of multi-regional clinical trials (MRCTs). Possibilities also exist, as indicated in the International Conference on Harmonisation-E5 (R1) and United States (US) Code of Federal Regulations Title 21, that data from clinical trials conducted solely in foreign countries can be found acceptable given the conditions are satisfied: the trials are in compliance with the Good Clinical Practice, the investigators are competent, and the data can be validated and extrapolated to the new region. Historically, there have been examples that the US Food and Drug Administration (FDA) accepts extrapolation from European clinical trials, given the similarity in the population, medical practice, and regulation of the two regions, while on the other hand, fewer cases were observed from the other regions, such as Asia. This chapter illustrates foreign data extrapolation with the development of Zanubrutinib (BRUZINKA®). The accelerated approval of the compound with orphan drug designation in the relapsed or refractory mantle cell lymphoma (MCL) indication has facilitated US patients' access to the next generation Bruton's Tyrosine Kinase (BTK) inhibitor with demonstrated high rates of durable response and favorable safety profile.

Zanubrutinib is a novel, irreversible BTK inhibitor developed by BeiGene. It was designed to improve potency and target selectivity while achieving maximal exposure (Guo et al. 2009; Song et al. 2020). It received a US FDA breakthrough designation for the treatment of adult patients with MCL who

DOI: 10.1201/9781003109785-10

have previously received at least 1 prior therapy in January 2019. The NDA application of Zanubrutinib for the indication was accelerated approved by the agency on November 14, 2019, less than 3 months since the agency's acceptance of the application on August 21, 2019, with post-marketing requirements.

The first-in-human study of the compound, BGB-3111-AU-003 (referred to as Study AU003 in the following content), was initiated in August 2014. It is a Phase I/II, dose-selection, pharmacokinetics (PK)/pharmacodynamics, safety, and efficacy study in adult patients with relapsed/refractory (R/R) or treatment-naive B cell lymphoid malignancies, and conducted in Australia, New Zealand, Italy, South Korea, United Kingdom, and the US (ClinicalTrials.gov identifier NCT02343120). After a dose-escalation part to determine the maximum tolerated or recommended Phase 2 dose, the study expanded to multiple indications, including MCL (Tam et al. 2019b), chronic lymphocytic leukemia, or small lymphocytic lymphoma (Tam et al. 2019a), and Waldenström macroglobulinemia (Trotman et al. 2020). The basket trial design was able to provide efficiency in operation and establish solid data supporting the fast development of the compound simultaneously in several indications. Concurrently, a separate Phase I study BGB-3111-1002 was conducted in China to confirm the dose for Chinese patients. Multiple pivotal and non-pivotal Ph II and III studies were then initiated in China alone or globally.

In the remaining content of the chapter, we describe several factors of the initial zanubrutinib submission in the US, which we think play important roles in the approval of the NDA in R/R MCL.

10.2 Strong Unmet Medical Needs for R/R MCL Patients

At the time of the submission, limited treatment options were available for R/R MCL patients in the US. Two drugs received regular approval, namely bortezomib (Velcade®) and lenalidomide (Revlimid®). However, the overall response rates (ORRs) are only 31% and 26%, respectively, with the corresponding 9.3 and 16.6 months of duration of responses (Velcade [bortezomib] US prescribing information [USPI] 2018; Revlimid [lenalidomide] USPI 2019). Strong unmet medical needs still exist. Two BTK inhibitors, including the first-in-class BTK inhibitor ibrutinib (Imbruvica®) and a second BTK inhibitor acalabrutinib (Calquence®) had accelerated approvals for the treatment of R/R MCL, but the clinical benefit of the two drugs is required to be verified by confirmatory trials.

10.3 Consistent Efficacy of Zanubrutinib Demonstrated in China and Global Patients

The submission was supported by the drug efficacy consistently demonstrated in two studies considered as pivotal: the aforementioned AU003 study and a China-only Phase 2 Study BGB-3111-206 (NCT03206970, referred to as Study 206 in the following content). The 206 study was designed as a single-arm, multicenter efficacy, and safety study of zanubrutinib in adult patients with R/R MCL who had received ≥ 1 but < 5 prior treatment regimens (Song et al. 2020). Patients who had been exposed to a BTK inhibitor before were not eligible for the study. The study was solely conducted at sites in China. Patients were treated at a dose of 160 mg twice daily in 28-day cycles for up to 3 years or until disease progression, unacceptable toxicity, death, withdrawal of consent, or study termination.

The sponsor conducted the studies in compliance with the Good Clinical Practice and quality. The protocol, amendments, and the informed consent forms were all approved by the Institutional Review Boards/Ethics Committees of participating sites and patients' rights are protected. The study data and analysis of the two pivotal studies were submitted to the agency and considered acceptable (FDA CDER 2019). In the 206 study, a relatively small number (8 out of 86) of patients reported major protocol deviations. Most of the deviations are the use of prohibited medications, which, however, were all prohibited due to the potential for QTc elevation and not expected to impact efficacy evaluation after review. No major protocol deviations were reported among the R/R MCL patients in the AU003 study.

It is important to highlight that the baseline characteristics of the single-arm 206 study conducted in China show that the recruited patients in the study represent a deeply treated population at the late stage of the disease. At the study entry, 34% of the patients had three or more prior systemic therapies with a median number of prior lines of therapies of two. Seventy-four percent of them are at Ann Arbor Stage IV, and the vast majority (84%) had intermediate- or high-risk Biologic Mantle Cell Lymphoma International Prognostic Index scores (Song et al. 2020). It is therefore considered that the study population was comparable to the expected characteristics of patients with R/R MCL in the US (FDA CDER 2019). Of note, other than the race, the population is also generally consistent with the phase II studies of ibrutinib and acalabrutinib, despite some noted differences in age distribution and prior treatment history (Song et al. 2020).

For both studies, the primary efficacy endpoint is overall response rate (ORR) assessed according to the criteria in the Lugano classification (Cheson et al. 2014) by an Independent Review Committee (IRC). The response assessment of the IRC was further adjudicated by the FDA reviewers. Although there were discrepancies in the complete response assessment in the 206 study, the assessments of achieving the primary endpoint of overall response (partial and complete responses) were consistent. The discrepancies in the complete response assessment were mainly due to the requirement of evidence for bone marrow disease clearance by histology or gastrointestinal disease clearance by endoscopy beyond the positron emission tomography results (FDA CDER 2019). However, even after downgrading eight complete responders to partial responders, the resulting complete response rate in study 206 is still as good as 59% (FDA CDER 2019). Additionally, the efficacy of zanubrutinib is further supported by multiple secondary efficacy endpoints, such as the duration of response, time to response, and progression-free survival. These endpoints were commonly used in the studies of other BTK inhibitors in the indication (Wang et al. 2013, 2018).

The sample size of the expansion cohorts of Study AU003 was determined based on the dual objectives of evaluating the safety and efficacy of the study drug, although formal hypothesis testing on the primary efficacy endpoint was not planned. The planned sample size of 380 patients across multiple indications of the study supported the rigorous evaluation of the compound safety profile. The efficacy analysis set eventually includes 32 R/R MCL patients that were treated by zanubrutinib at the label recommended doses of 160 mg twice daily or 320 mg daily. On the other hand, the 206 study, as was initially designed as a pivotal study to support the indication registration, pre-specified a formal hypothesis testing on the primary endpoint to rule out a historical ORR of 40% at one-sided 0.025 using a binomial exact test. The study was planned to enroll 80 patients in order to provide sufficient safety evaluation, which then provides over 99% power to rule out the historical control if the true rate is 70%. The planned dose of all patients to be treated in the study is 160 mg twice daily. The primary efficacy analysis set thus includes all patients who received any dose of the study drug. The study eventually included 86 patients in the analysis set.

The two studies conducted in China and globally reported consistent efficacy results in ORR and duration of response. The ORR was 84% (95% CI: 74%, 91%) for the 206 study and 84% (95% CI: 67%, 95%) for the 003 study, and the median duration of response was 19.5 months (16.6, NE) for 206 and 18.5 months (12.6, NE) for AU003 (FDA CDER 2019; Song et al. 2020). The pre-specified hypothesis testing with the null hypothesis of 40% ORR was rejected with a highly significant p-value <0.0001 in the 206 study (Song et al. 2020). Further assessing the consistency in the ORRs obtained from the two regions with a Bayesian method, assuming independent vague priors of *beta*(0.5,0.5) for the ORRs and binomial distributions for the numbers of responders, the equal-tailed posterior 95% credible interval of the difference of the ORRs ($ORR_{AU003}-ORR_{206}$) is (−16%, 14%). The result showed strong support with a high probability that the efficacy benefit of patients of the two regions from the compound was similar, although it is acknowledged that the cross-study comparison is limited by various observed and unobserved confounding effects. Subgroup evaluation on a number of patient baseline characteristics in the 206 study further shows consistent outcome in the primary efficacy endpoint (Song et al. 2020).

10.4 Comparable PK Profile Between Asian and Non-Asian Patients

The PK profile of zanubrutinib was comparable between Asians and non-Asians (Ou et al. 2019). A two-compartment population pharmacokinetic model was built on a pooled dataset including patients with B-cell malignancies and healthy volunteers from 9 clinical studies. The impact of covariates on zanubrutinib PK was evaluated, including race, age, body weight, sex, tumor type, health status, etc. No clinically significant difference in the PK of zanubrutinib was observed on race (Asian, Caucasian, and Others), which supported the bridging between the Asian and non-Asian populations.

10.5 Safety Profile of Zanubrutinib Supported by a Large Safety Pool

The evaluation of the safety profile of the compound to support the submission was based on a database of 641 patients treated with the drug monotherapy across multiple indications at the recommended dose regimens in the label. Other than AU003 and 206 studies, another 3 China studies were also included in the safety pool. Most (61%) of the patients were exposed to zanubrutinib for greater than one year. A primary focus of the FDA's safety review was also the patient population with R/R MCL who received the recommended two-dose regimens ($n = 118$). The common adverse reactions can be found in the product USPI and were generally as expected for the class of BTK inhibitors, and lower frequencies of Grade 3 or higher events, such as diarrhea, neutropenia, thrombocytopenia, atrial fibrillation/flutter, and hemorrhage were reported for zanubrutinib compared to those for ibrutinib (Imbruvica [ibrutinib] USPI 2018; Brukinsa [zanubrutinib] USPI 2019). The sponsor specifically analyzed and compared AEs in the Asian vs. non-Asian patients. Asian patients account for 50% and 75% of the overall safety pool and the R/R MCL patients pool, respectively. By comparing the rate of all grades, Grade 3+, and serious AEs, as well as

AEs leading to treatment discontinuation or death, it can be concluded that there is no notable difference between the two populations.

10.6 Discussion

In this chapter, we discussed the case of Zanubrutinib that obtained its initial US approval based on a pivotal China study. The strong unmet medical needs in the pursued indication, quality of the study conduct, data collection and analysis, favorable benefit-risk ratio based on very promising response rates and expected safety results demonstrated in a sample of patients with comparable characteristics to the US patients, adequate safety data for the evaluation, as well as the supportive PK profile comparison between the populations are all considered contributing to the positive review of the submission from the regulatory agency. The pivotal studies, however, shared the same limitations as other single-arm trials, for which the sponsor has committed a randomized Phase III study with the progression-free survival as the primary endpoint. The study is still ongoing at the time this chapter is written.

References

Brukinsa (zanubrutinib) [US prescribing information]. 2019. Camana Bay Grand Cayman: BeiGene, Ltd.

Cheson, B.D., Fisher, R.I., Barrington, S.F., et al. 2014. Recommendations for initial evaluation, staging, and response assessment of Hodgkin and non-Hodgkin lymphoma: the Lugano classification. *J Clin Oncol* 32: 3059–3068.

Guo, Y., Liu, Y., Hu, N., et al. 2009. Discovery of Zanubrutinib (BGB-3111), a novel, potent, and selective covalent inhibitor of Bruton's tyrosine kinase. *J Med Chem* 62:7923–7940.

Imbruvica (ibrutinib) [US prescribing information]. 2019. Sunnyvale, CA: Pharmacyclics LLC; Horsham, PA: Janssen Biotech, Inc.

Ou, Y., Wang, K., Liu, L., et al. 2019. Exposure-response relationship of the Bruton tyrosine kinase inhibitor, zanubrutinib (BGB-3111) in patients with hematologic malignancies. *Blood* 134 (Supplement_1): 5063. doi:10.1182/blood-2019-129580

Revlimid (lenalidomide) [US prescribing information]. 2019. Summit, NJ: Celgene Corporation.

Song, Y., Zhou, K., Zou, D., et al. 2020. Treatment of patients with relapsed or refractory mantle-cell lymphoma with zanubrutinib, a selective inhibitor of Bruton's tyrosine kinase. *Clin Cancer Res* 26:4216–4224.

Tam, C.S., Trotman, J., Opat, S., et al. 2019a. Phase 1 study of the selective BTK inhibitor zanubrutinib in B-cell malignancies and safety and efficacy evaluation in CLL. *Blood* 134:851–859.

Tam, C.S., Wang, M., Simpson, D., et al. 2019b. Updated safety and efficacy data in the phase 1 trial of patients with mantle cell lymphoma (MCL) treated with Bruton's tyrosine kinase (BTK) inhibitor zanubrutinib (BGB-3111). *Hematol Oncol* 37: 245–247.

Trotman, J., Opat, S., Gottlieb, D.J., et al. 2020. Zanubrutinib for the treatment of patients with Waldenström macroglobulinemia: three years of follow-up. *Blood* 136:2027–2037.

U.S. Food and Drug Administration Center for Drug Evaluation and Research. 2019. Zanubrutinib NDA 213217 multi-disciplinary review and evaluation. https://www.accessdata.fda.gov/drugsatfda_docs/nda/2019/213217Orig1 s000MultidisciplineR.pdf

Velcade (bortezomib) [US prescribing information]. 2018. Cambridge, MA: Millennium Pharmaceuticals, Inc.

Wang, M.L., Rule, S., Martin, P., et al. 2013. Targeting BTK with ibrutinib in relapsed or refractory mantle-cell lymphoma. *N Engl J Med* 369:507–516.

Wang, M.L., Rule, S., Zinzani, P.L., et al. 2018. Acalabrutinib in relapsed or refractory mantle cell lymphoma (ACE-LY-004): a single-arm, multicentre, phase 2 trial. *Lancet* 391:659–667.

11

Analysis Models for Multi-regional Clinical Trials

Gang Li, Hui Quan, and Gordon KK Lan

11.1 Introduction

In recent years, multiregional clinical trial (MRCT) is becoming a preferred strategy to develop new medicines. It is generally agreed upon that the between-region variability needs to be accounted for in the statistical design and analysis. Besides the conventionally used fixed-effect model (FEM), two random effect models, continuous random effect model (CREM), and discrete random effect model (DREM) are also proposed for this purpose. CREM is a model commonly used for meta-analysis and is proposed by Hung (2007) and Hung, Wang and O'Neill (2010) for designing MRCTs; its operating details are provided by Quan et al. (2010), Quan et al. (2013, 2017). Lan and Pinheiro (2012) introduce a discrete random effect model (DREM). As the features of the FEM are well known, in this chapter, we focus on the comparisons and evaluations of these two random effect approaches. CREM and DREM adopt totally different random mechanisms. CREM assumes the regional treatment effects are normally distributed, while DREM assumes the regional sample sizes follow a multinomial distribution. In section 11.2, we describe the CREM approach. In section 11.3, we give an intuitive interpretation of DREM. In section 11.4, we assess the performances of the two approaches via simulation. Quan et al. (2017) discuss the impacts of the factors including between-region variability, number of regions, and extremity of sample size allocation between regions on the design and analysis of MRCTs. Simulated data are generated from CREM and from DREM, respectively in the framework of these factors. Section 11.5 uses an MRCT example to illustrate the applications of the three models. In section 11.6, we discuss the considerations on the choices of analysis methods.

DOI: 10.1201/9781003109785-11

11.2 The Continuous Random Effect Model

We start by defining some notation. Suppose a multiregional trial is conducted in K regions to compare a new treatment (T) to control (C) and on a continuous and normally distributed endpoint. Region i has the sample sizes $n_i^T = n_i^C = n_i$ and mean responses $\bar{X}_i^T$ and $\bar{X}_i^C$ for the treatment and control, respectively. Let $\hat{\Delta}_i = \bar{X}_i^T - \bar{X}_i^C$ be the response difference between T and C, and denote $w_i = \frac{n_i}{N}$ and $N = \sum_{i=1}^K n_i$. From a theoretical point of view, we need only consider $\hat{\Delta}_i$, $i = 1, ..., K$. The overall treatment effect is estimated as

$$\hat{\Delta} = \frac{\sum_{i=1}^K n_i \hat{\Delta}_i}{N} = \sum_{i=1}^K w_i \hat{\Delta}_i. \tag{11.1}$$

In a classical FEM, the true treatment effect Δ is treated as a fixed parameter across regions. Sample size n_i's are also treated as fixed numbers and $\hat{\Delta}_i \sim N(\Delta, 2\sigma^2/n_i)$. Nonetheless, in the CREM (see Quan et al. 2013), the regional treatment effects Δ_i's are considered as random variables and follow

$$\Delta_i \sim N(\Delta, \tau_C^2). \tag{11.2}$$

In CREM, $\hat{\Delta}_i \mid \Delta_i \sim N(\Delta_i, 2\sigma^2/n_i)$ where σ^2 is the variance of study endpoint. Thus, under a DFEM (Discrete Fixed Effect Model) where Δ_i is treated as a fixed parameter rather than a random variable

$$\hat{\Delta} \sim N\left(\Delta', \frac{2\sigma^2}{N}\right),$$

where $\Delta' = \sum_{i=1}^K W_i \Delta_i$

Clearly, τ_C^2 is a measure of the between-region variability. The marginal distribution of $\hat{\Delta}_i$ under the CREM is $\hat{\Delta}_i \sim N(\Delta, \tau_C^2 + 2\sigma^2/n_i)$ and

$$\Delta \sim N(\Delta, \sigma_C^2), \text{ where } \sigma_C^2 = \frac{2\sigma^2}{N} + \tau_C^2 \sum_{i=1}^K w_i^2. \tag{11.3}$$

A more efficient estimator for quantifying the overall treatment effect under the CREM, which will be referred to as eCREM is

$$\tilde{\Delta} = \frac{\sum_{i=1}^K a_i \hat{\Delta}_i}{\sum_{i=1}^K a_i} \sim N(\Delta, \tilde{\sigma}_C^2), \tag{11.4}$$

where $\tilde{\sigma}_C^2 = \frac{1}{\sum_{i=1}^K a_i}$ and $a_i = 1/\left(\tau_C^2 + \frac{2\sigma^2}{n_i}\right)$ is the inverse of the variance of $\hat{\Delta}_i$ under the CREM. An estimator of τ_C^2 can be as

$$\hat{\tau}_C^2 = \max\left(0, \frac{\frac{N}{2\hat{\sigma}^2}\sum_{i=1}^K w_i(\hat{\Delta}_i - \hat{\Delta})^2 - (K-1)}{\frac{N}{2\hat{\sigma}^2}(1 - \sum_{i=1}^K w_i^2)}\right). \tag{11.5}$$

where $\hat{\sigma}^2$ is an estimate of σ^2, the variance of the study endpoint.

11.3 An Intuitive Interpretation of DREM

DREM is proposed by Lan and Pinheiro (2012), where patients are assumed to be randomly drawn from the K regions. Therefore, the regional sample sizes are treated as random variables jointly follow a multinomial distribution. Here we introduce DREM in a more intuitive way. In a MRCT, the proportion of regional sample size may be pre-assigned mainly based on regulatory and operational considerations. The enrollment of the trial will stop when the total sample size reaches the target number and the actual proportion may vary with the enrollment speed of each region. Basically, the regional sample sizes can still be considered as a random vector.

Assume the sample size vector of a K-region trial $N = (N_1, \ldots, N_K)$ is a multinomial random vector such that $N_1 + \ldots + N_K = N$, with parameters $(W_1, \ldots, W_K)$ where $W_1 > 0, \ldots, W_K > 0$ and $W_1 + \ldots + W_K = 1$. Then

$$P\{N = (n_1, \ldots, n_K)\} = \frac{N!}{n_1! \ldots n_K!} W_1^{n_1} \ldots W_K^{n_K}.$$

$E(N_i) = NW_i$, $Var(N_i) = NW_i(1 - W_i)$, and $Cov(N_i, N_j) = -NW_iW_j$, for $i \neq j$.

Ideally, $(W_1, \ldots, W_K)$ represents the planned sample size proportions of regions. Given $N = n = (n_1, \ldots, n_K)$, the estimators of treatment effects $\hat{\Delta}_i$ and $\hat{\Delta}_j$ from regions i and j, $i \neq j$, are independently normally distributed, $\hat{\Delta}_i | n_i \sim N(\Delta_i, 2\sigma^2/n_i)$. Here, Δ_i is a fixed parameter as in the discrete FEM.

The overall treatment effect $\Delta' = \sum_{i=1}^K W_i \Delta_i$ can be estimated as

$$\hat{\Delta} = \sum_{i=1}^K w_i \hat{\Delta}_i \sim N(\Delta', \sigma_D^2), \tag{11.6}$$

where $w_i = n_i/N$, $\sigma_D^2 = \frac{2\sigma^2 + \tau_D^2}{N}$ and $\tau_D^2 = \sum_{i=1}^K W_i(\Delta_i - \Delta')^2$. Similar to τ_C^2, τ_D^2 is also a measure of between-region variability and is estimated by

$$\hat{\tau}_D^2 = \max\left(0, \sum_{i=1}^{K} \frac{n_i}{N}(\hat{\Delta}_i - \hat{\Delta})^2 - (K-1)\frac{2\hat{\sigma}^2}{N}\right), \tag{11.7}$$

as it is shown in Appendix 2: $E\left(\sum_{i=1}^{K} \frac{n_i}{N}(\hat{\Delta}_i - \hat{\Delta})^2\right) = \tau_D^2 + (K-1)\frac{2\sigma^2}{N}$, the second term can be ignored when N is large.

11.4 Operation Characteristics of CREM and DREM

From (11.3), for a large N, $\sigma_C^2 \approx \tau_C^2 \sum_{i=1}^{K} w_i^2 \geq \tau_C^2/K$. CREM and DREM assume different random mechanisms. However, they are closely related. From (11.5) and (11.7),

$$\hat{\tau}_C^2 = \frac{\hat{\tau}_D^2}{1 - \sum_{i=1}^{K} w_i^2} \text{ or } \hat{\tau}_D^2 = \hat{\tau}_C^2\left(1 - \sum_{i=1}^{K} w_i^2\right). \tag{11.8}$$

From (11.4) and (11.5), the variance of CREM estimator $\tilde{\sigma}_C^2$ is

$$\tilde{\sigma}_C^2 = \frac{1}{\sum_{i=1}^{K} a_i} = \frac{1}{\sum_{i=1}^{K} 1/\left(\tau_C^2 + \frac{2\sigma^2}{n_i}\right)} \geq \frac{\tau_C^2 + \frac{2K\sigma^2}{N}}{K} = \frac{\tau_C^2}{K} + \frac{2\sigma^2}{N}. \text{ It is shown in Appendix 3}$$

$$\tilde{\sigma}_C^2 \geq \frac{\hat{\tau}_D^2}{K-1}. \tag{11.9}$$

The equality in (11.9) holds only when $w_1 = \ldots = w_K$.

11.4.1 Sample Size Requirement for Different Models

We can always compare the sample size requirement for different models. For eCREM, the corresponding sample size $\tilde{N}_C$ based on (11.3) for $1 - \beta$ power at a one-sided level α is the solution of (Quan et al. 2013)

$$\sum_{i=1}^{K} 1/\left(\tau_C^2 + \frac{2\sigma^2}{\tilde{N}_C w_i}\right) = (z_\alpha + z_\beta)^2/\Delta^2,$$

where z_α is the α quantile of the standard normal distribution.

When $\tau_C^2 = 0$ and $\Delta' = \Delta$, $\tilde{N}_C$ is also the required sample size for a DFEM or the classical FEM. For a DREM, the required sample size for detecting $\Delta' = \Delta$ based on (11.6) is

$$N_D = (2\sigma^2 + \tau_D^2)(z_\alpha + z_\beta)^2 / \Delta^2.$$

We will assume asymptotically $\tau_D^2 = \tau_C^2(1 - \sum_{i=1}^{K} W_i^2)$ from (11.8), which will be used in the formula for N_D calculation where W_i is set to be $w_i = n_i/N$ as W_i is unknown. Note that

$\sum_{i=1}^{K} w_i E(\hat{\Delta}_i - \hat{\Delta})^2 = \frac{2\sigma^2(K-1)}{N} + \tau_C^2(1 - \sum_{i=1}^{K} w_i^2)$. The first term will be close to zero when the sample size is large.

As discussed in Quan et al. (2017), the definition of regions has a great impact on the overall sample size required for a CREM design, while there is no impact for the DFEM and very little impact for DREM. This phenomenon will be seen in the following example as well.

Assume $\sigma = 1$, $\Delta = 0.25$, $\alpha = 0.025$, $1-\beta = 0.9$, we assess how the sample size varies with $\tau_C/\sigma = 0.05$ and 0.1, $K = 3, 4, 6, 10, 15$; and three cases of w_i: one is for equal $w_i = 1/K$, and the other 2 are for unequal w_i's. The sample size for the DFEM is 337 and for the DREM is also 337. The results of $\tilde{N}_C$ are presented in Figure 11.1. Note that τ_C has a great impact on $\tilde{N}_C$, e.g., in Case 3 and $K = 3$, $\tilde{N}_C$ increases from 434 to 1137. $\tilde{N}_C$ is a decreasing function of the number of regions K and is larger than N_D even when τ_C is as small as 0.05.

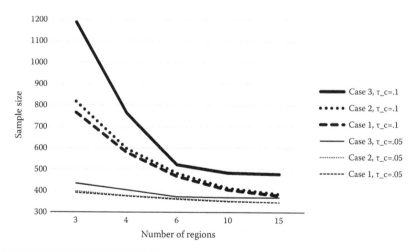

*Case 1: equal W_i; the 2 unequal W_i cases:		
	W_i case 2	W_i case 3
$K=3$	$w_1:w_2:w_3 = 3:2:1$	$w_1:w_2:w_3 = 6:2:1$
$K=4$	$w_1:w_2:w_3:w_4 = 2:2:1:1$	$w_1:w_2:w_3:w_4 = 6:2:1:1$
$K=6$	$w_1:\ldots:w_6 = 2:2:2:1:1:1$	$w_1:w_2:w_3:\ldots:w_6 = 4:2:1:1:1:1$
$K=10$	$w_1:\ldots:w_5:w_6:\ldots:w_{10} = 2:\ldots:2:1:\ldots 1$	$w_1:w_2:w_3:\ldots:w_{10} = 8:4:1:\ldots 1$
$K=15$	$w_1:\ldots:w_7:w_8:\ldots:w_{15} = 2:\ldots:2:1:\ldots 1$	$w_1:w_2:w_3:w_4:\ldots:w_{15} = 16:8:4:1:\ldots 1$

FIGURE 11.1

Sample size $\tilde{N}_C$ under different numbers of regions ($\sigma = 1$, $\Delta = 0.25$, $\alpha = 0.025$, $1-\beta = 0.9$, $\tau_C/\sigma = 0.05$ and 0.1).

Case 3 gives much more weight to regions 1 and 2 than 3, this is similar to reduce the number of regions. As a result, when K increases from 10 to 15, $\tilde{N}_C$ does not decrease as much as for the other 2 cases.

11.4.2 The Performances of the Two Random Effect Models Using Data Generated from CREM Model

Simulations with 1,000,000 repetitions are performed to compare the two random effect models. In the simulation, data are first generated using the CREM model based on the settings and respective sample size from Section 3.1. In these simulations, the estimate of σ^2, the variance of the endpoint is assigned to 1 and assumed to be known, because its estimate should be stable as the sample sizes are fairly large so we just need to generate the mean values of each region rather than individual patients' responses. We evaluate the estimates of τ_C and the resulted Type I error rate and power. For CREM, the evaluation is on the efficient CREM test statistic in (11.4), which is labeled as eCREM. For $\alpha = 0.025$, we consider a test is valid if its actual type I error rate is less than 0.03 or within a 20% inflation from 0.025.

Figure 11.2. A displays estimated τ_C vs K curves. τ_C is overestimated when τ_C is small (e.g., $\tau_C = 0.05$) and underestimated when τ_C is large (e.g., $\tau_C = 0.1$) for all 3 Cases of W_is. The reason for the overestimation when τ_C is small probably is due to the truncation based on (11.5). In general, the estimated τ_C increases with K. Using $true\tau_C$, the simulated type I error rate and power for eCREM are close to the nominal level 0.025 and 90%, respectively. However, based on its estimate $\hat{\tau}_C$, the simulated type I error rate and power of eCREM may be quite different from their respective nominal levels when $\tau_C = 0.1$ as displayed in Figure 11.3. As Figure 11.3.A suggests the type I error rate decreases as K increases for eCREM and is below 0.03 (i.e., within a 20% inflation from the nominal level 0.025) when $\tau_C = 0.05$. However, when $\tau_C = 0.1$, it exceeds 0.03 for $K \leq 6$. Figure 11.3.B indicates that the power of eCREM increases with K and can be several percent below the target level of 90%. Figure 11.4 displays type I error rate and power vs K curves of DREM. The type I error rate exceeds 0.03 in general except when $\tau_C = 0.05$ and $K \geq 6$. The power of DREM is above 90% as Figure 11.4.B indicates with an inflated type I error rate.

The variance of eCREM $\tilde{\sigma}_C^2$ does not exceed σ_C^2 (see (11.3)). Figure 11.5 presents the estimated of ratio $\sigma_C^2 / \tilde{\sigma}_C^2$, a higher ratio indicates a more loss of efficiency relative to eCREM.

In summary, if data follows the CREM and $\tau_C = 0.05$, $\hat{\tau}_C$ tends to be an overestimate; as a consequence, eCREM over-controls type I error rate and loses power. In contrast, when $\tau_C = 0.1$ and the number of regions is not large enough, $\hat{\tau}_C$ tends to be an under-estimate; consequently, eCREM inflates type I error rate and is not valid. DREM is only valid when $\tau_C = 0.05$ and $K \geq 6$. In addition, the type I error rate decreases as K increases for both CREM and DREM.

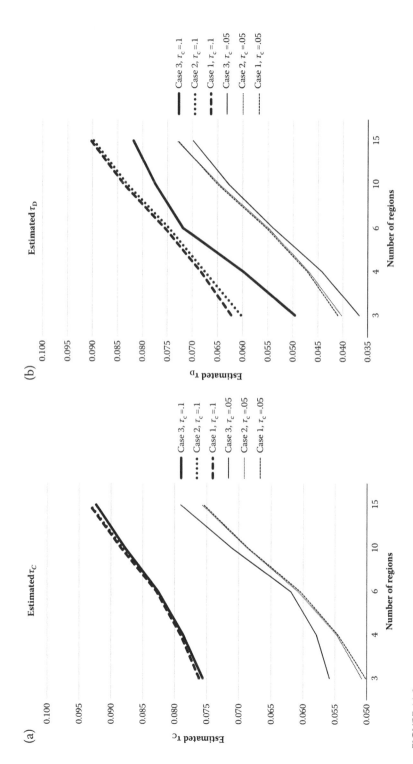

FIGURE 11.2

Estimates of τ_C and τ_D, when data are from *CREM* ($\sigma = 1$, $\alpha = 0.025$, $1-\beta = 0.9$, $\tau_C = 0.05$ and 0.1)*.

*The corresponding sample sizes for each Case and K are from Figure 11.1.

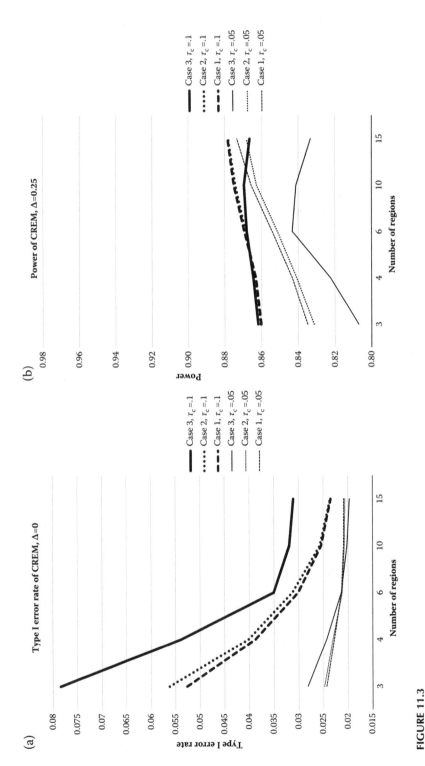

FIGURE 11.3
Type I error rates and power of CREM, when data are from CREM ($\sigma = 1$, $\alpha = 0.025$, $1-\beta = 0.9$, $\tau_C = 0.05$, and 0.1)*.

*The corresponding sample sizes for each Case and K are from Figure 11.1.

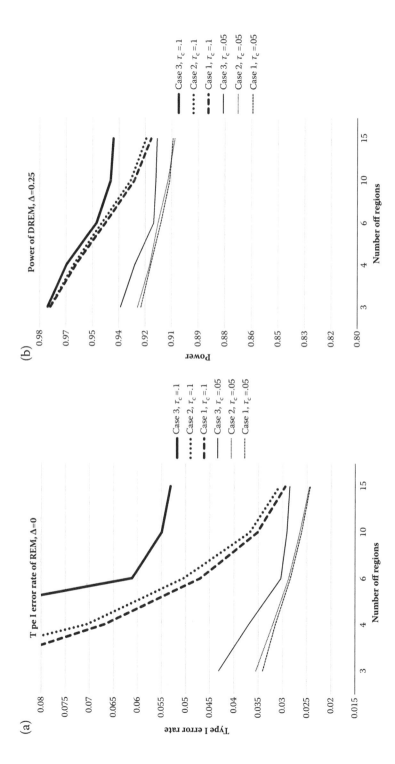

FIGURE 11.4

Type I error rate and power of DREM, when data are from CREM ($\sigma = 1$, $\alpha = 0.025$, $1-\beta = 0.9$, $\tau_C = 0.05$, and 0.1)*.

*The corresponding sample sizes for each **Case** and **K** are from **Figure 11.1**.

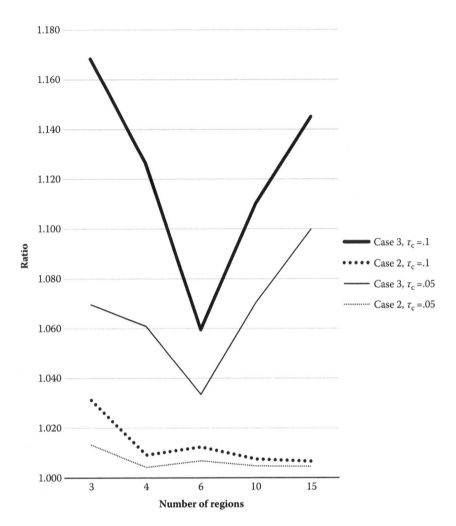

FIGURE 11.5
A comparison of $\hat{\sigma}_C$ and $\tilde{\sigma}_C$, when data are from *CREM* ($\sigma = 1$, $\tau_C = 0.05$, and 0.1)*.

*The corresponding sample sizes for each Case and K are from Figure 11.1.

11.4.3 The Performances of the Two Random Effect Models Using Data Generated from DREM Model

In the simulation, $\sigma = 1$, $\alpha = 0.025$, $1-\beta = 0.9$, $\Delta' = 0.25$ for power and $\Delta' = 0$ for Type I error rate evaluations. The total sample size $N=337$ and the regional sample size is multinomial with $N = 337$ with three case of W_i in section 11.4.1 considered. For region i, we construct the regional treatment effect $\Delta_i = \Delta' + d_i$, where $d_1, \ldots, d_K$ satisfy

$$\sum_{i=1}^{K} d_i \cdot W_i = 0 \text{ and } \sum_{i=1}^{K} d_i^2 \cdot W_i = \tau_D^2.$$

Therefore, the variability among regions is τ_D^2. The following 3 patterns of $d_1, \ldots, d_K$ are evaluated:

Pattern 1, $d_i = \tau_D \frac{i - D_{W1}}{S_{W1}}$, where $D_{W1} = \sum_{i=1}^{K} i \cdot W_i$ and

$$S_{W1} = \sqrt{\sum_{i=1}^{K} i^2 \cdot W_i - D_{W1}^2};$$

Pattern 2, $d_i = \tau_D \frac{i^{1.5} - D_{W2}}{S_{W2}}$, where $D_{W2} = \sum_{i=1}^{K} i^{1.5} \cdot W_i$ and

$$S_{W2} = \sqrt{\sum_{i=1}^{K} i^3 \cdot W_i - D_{W2}^2};$$

Pattern 3, $d_i = \tau_D \frac{(K - i + 1)^{1.5} - D_{W3}}{S_{W3}}$, where $D_{W3} = \sum_{i=1}^{K} (K - i + 1)^{1.5} \cdot W_i$ and

$$S_{W3} = \sqrt{\sum_{i=1}^{K} (K - i + 1)^3 \cdot W_i - D_{W3}^2}.$$

Pattern 1 represents a uniform difference pattern, while patterns 2 and 3 are skewed ones. The results for patterns 2 and 3 are similar to these of pattern 1. Here we discuss only pattern 1 for $\tau_D = 0.05$ and 0.2. Simulations again are conducted with 1,000,000 repetitions.

Figure 11.6 displays the curves of the estimates of τ_D and τ_C vs K (although the interpretation of τ_C is unclear) for cases 1–3 and $\tau_D = 0.05$ and 0.2. Figure 11.6.A suggests that τ_D is under-estimated when $\tau_D = 0.2$ and the curves of cases 1–3 almost overlap; in contrast, when $\tau_D = 0.05$, τ_D is over-estimated for all $K \geq 4$ and cases 1–3, again the 3 curves almost overlap. The estimate of τ_C decreases and seems to converge to a value as K increases. However, the impact of the estimates of τ_D and τ_C on type I error rate and power of DREM and CREM is quite different. As Figure 11.7 displays, both type I error rate and power are close to their respective nominal levels. This is because the τ_D adds only a very small proportion to $\sigma_D^2 = \frac{2\sigma^2 + \tau_D^2}{N}$ in (11.6), the variance of DREM test statistic, in the evaluations, even for $\tau_D = 0.2$, $\tau_D^2/(N\sigma_D^2) = 0.04/2.04$, about 2% of $N\sigma_D^2$. Figure 11.8 evaluates the type I error rate and power of CREM. Figure 11.8.A indicates that when $\tau_D = 0.05$, CREM has an error rate below the nominal level of 0.025 and increases with K reaching to 0.025 when $K = 15$ in all 3 Cases; its corresponding power also increases with K, from ~86% to 90% (see Figure 11.8.B). However, when $\tau_D = 0.2$, CREM has an error rate serious below the nominal level of 0.025 for cases 1 and 2; the consequence of seriously below the nominal type I error rate is a drastic loss of power, e.g., when $K = 3$ in Case 1, the power is 47% (see Figure 11.7.B). For Case 3 and $\tau_D = 0.2$, CREM has the Type I error rate below 0.025 if $K \leq 6$; but exceeds 0.04 if $K \geq 10$. It is worth noting that the type I error rate increases with K. This is in the opposite situation in

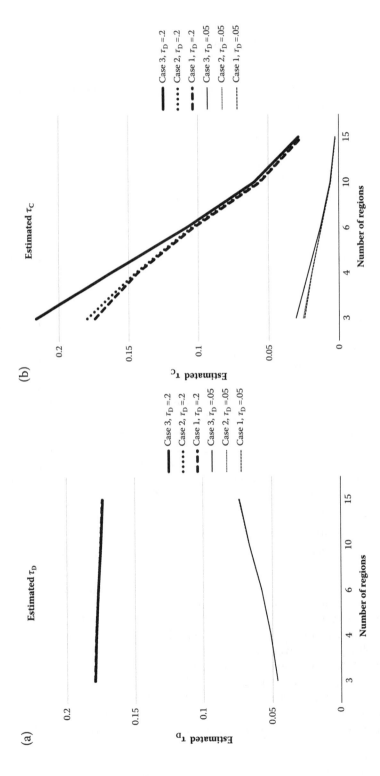

FIGURE 11.6
Estimates of τ_D and τ_C, when data are from *DREM* ($\sigma = 1$, $\alpha = 0.025$, $1-\beta = 0.9$, $\tau_D = 0.05$, and 0.2, and $N = 337$).

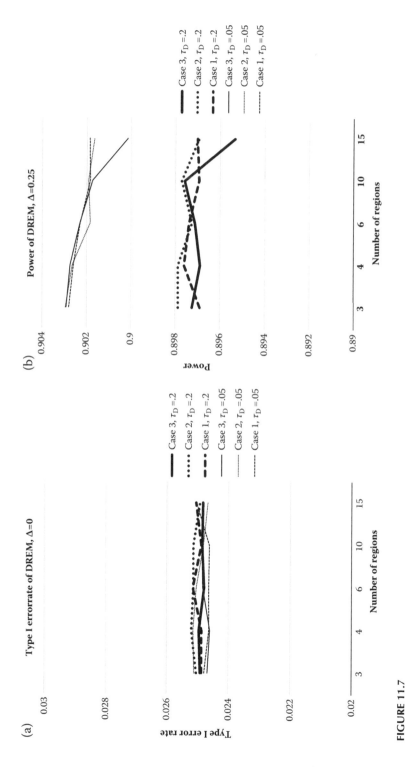

FIGURE 11.7

Type I error rate and power of DREM, when data are from DREM ($\sigma = 1$, $\alpha = 0.025$, $1-\beta = 0.9$, $\tau_D = 0.05$, and 0.2, and $N = 337$).

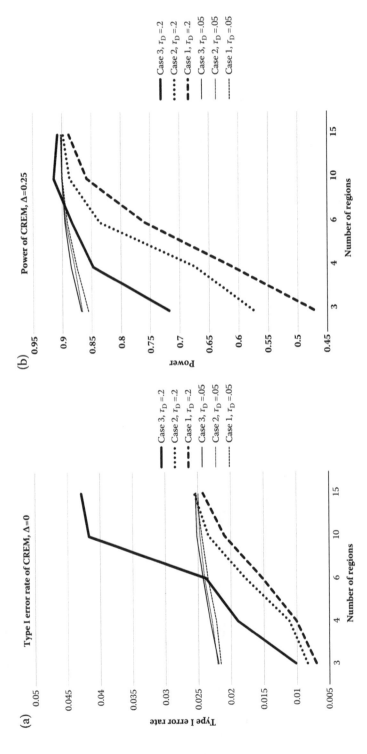

FIGURE 11.8
Type I error rate and power of CREM, when data are from DREM ($\sigma = 1$, $\alpha = 0.025$, $1-\beta = 0.9$, $\tau_D = 0.05$ and 0.2, and $N = 337$).

Figure 11.3, where the type I error rate decreases with K for data from CREM. As Case 3 presents type I error rate problems, Figure 11.9 plots for different K the curve of the type I error rate (and power) vs τ_D in Case 3. When $K = 3$, 4, and 6, the type I error rate is under control for τ_D between 0.05 to 0.2, but there is a substantial loss in power for $K = 3$. For $K = 10$ and 15, however, the Type I error rate exceeds 0.03, 20% more than the nominal level 0.025 for $\tau_D \geq 0.15$.

In summary, if data follows DREM, the DREM approach controls the Type I error rate and has power close to its target for τ_D ranges from 0.05 to 0.2. This is because the total variance of the DREM test statistic is $2\sigma^2 + \tau_D^2$, when $\sigma = 1$ and $\tau_D = 0.2$, $2\sigma^2 + \tau_D^2 = 2.04$, τ_D contributes 2% to the total variance. As for eCREM, when $\tau_D = 0.05$, it has a type I error rate a little below but close 0.025 and power also close to 90%. However, when $\tau_D = 0.2$, the test is still valid but loses power in Cases 1 and 2; in Case 3, its type I error rate < 0.025 for $K \leq 6$ and > 0.03 (invalid) for $K \geq 10$.

11.5 Example

The Metoprolol Controlled-Release Randomized Intervention Trial in Heart Failure (MERIT-HF) (MERIT-HF Study Group 1999) was an MRCT conducted to evaluate the treatment effect of once-daily metoprolol controlled or extended release in patients with Congestive Heart Failure (CHF). One of the primary endpoints was total mortality. A total of 3991 patients were enrolled from 14 countries. The trial used an adaptive design with four prespecified interim analyses. Based on the recommendation of the DMC, the trial was stopped early at the second pre-planned interim analysis with an observed overall hazard ratio on total mortality via the fixed effects model of 0.66 (95% confidence interval (0.53, 0.81), and nominal $p = 0.00015$).

Here we use the MERIT-HF trial as an example for illustration of CREM and DREM. As the individual patient data of this trial are not accessible, Tables 4 and 5 of Quan et al. (2013), which provide summary results on mortality for MERIT-HF in each country/region, respectively, are used in our analysis, e.g., the weight of a region is the number of events vs 362, the total number of events of the study. Therefore, the results obtained here are numerically slightly different from those based on individual patient data. Using this approach, we obtain the standard deviation of $\log(\widehat{HR})$ as 0.11. Thus, $\hat{\sigma} = 0.11 * \sqrt{362} = 2.093$.

For this MRCT, two countries had zero events in the metoprolol arm. Wedel et al. (2001) separately combined them with another two countries to form a total of 12 regions. In our illustration, the regions are handled in three different ways: 1) $K = 12$, the 12 regions defined by Wedel et al. (2001), 2) $K = 4$, 4 geographic regions including the United States, Eastern Europe

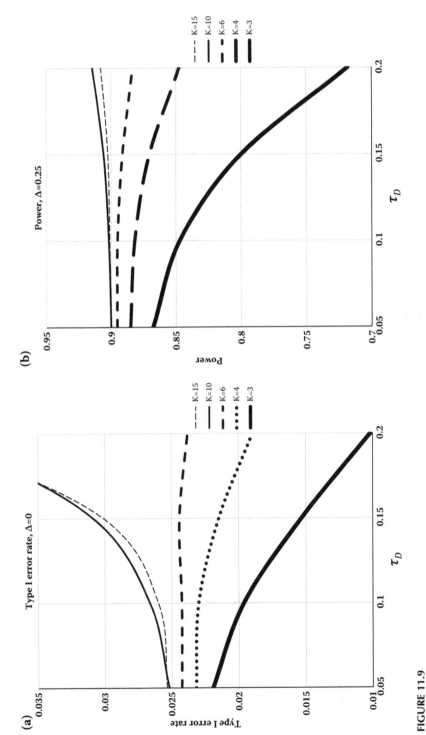

FIGURE 11.9
Type I error rate and power of CREM in Case 3 and Pattern 1, when data are from *DREM* ($\sigma = 1$, $\alpha = 0.025$, $1-\beta = 0.9$, and $N = 337$).

TABLE 11.1

Results on mortality from CREM and DREM for MERIT-HF[*]

				$\hat{\sigma}$ of $log(\widehat{HR})$	$\widehat{HR}$	95% CI
Originally reported[†]					0.66	(0.53, 0.81)
Estimated from FEM[‡]				0.1100	0.647	(0.521,0.803)
eCREM	K	$\hat{\tau}_C$	$\hat{\tau}_C/\hat{\sigma}$	$\hat{\sigma}_C$		
	12	0.271	0.129	0.1449	0.624	(0.470, 0.829)
	4	0.306	0.146	0.1902	0.654	(0.450, 0.950)
	2	0.452	0.216	0.2928	0.737	(415, 1.309)
DREM		$\hat{\tau}_D$	$\hat{\tau}_D/\hat{\sigma}$	$\hat{\sigma}_D$		
	12	0.251	0.120	0.1108	0.647	(0.521, 0.804)
	4	0.262	0.125	0.1109	0.647	(0.521, 0.804)
	2	0.286	0.137	0.1110	0.647	(0.520, 0.804)

[*] This table is for illustration purpose because results are based on a summary on each country and numerically different from those based on individual patient data.
[†] From MERIT-HF Study Group (1999).
[‡] Estimated based on Tables 4 and 5 of Quan et al. (2013), estimated $\hat{\sigma}$ = 2.093.

(Czech Republic, Hungary, and Poland), Nordic countries (Denmark, Finland, Iceland, Norway, and Sweden), Western Europe (Belgium, Germany, The Netherland, Switzerland, and United Kingdom Western); and 3) $K = 2$, the United States vs non-United States.

Table 11.1 reports the analysis results for both CREM and DREM as well as the estimate from the discrete FEM combining the treatment effect from each region, which had the same point estimate of hazard ratio (HR) as DREM. For CREM, as K decreases, the hazard ratio estimate $\widehat{HR}$ increases, so the between-region variability $\hat{\tau}_C^2 . \hat{\sigma}_C$ is doubled. The treatment effect of the hazard ratio estimate $\widehat{HR}$ was 0.624 with 95% confidence (95%CI) (0.470, 0.829) for $K = 12$ changed to 0.737 with 95%CI (0.415, 1.309) including 1 when $K = 2$, i.e., the treatment effect changed from significant to non-significant.

For DREM, as K decreases, the between-region variability $\hat{\tau}_D^2$ increased slightly and the hazard ratio estimate $\widehat{HR}$ stayed the same. The impact to $\hat{\sigma}_D$ was little. The upper bound of the 95% CIs <1, consistently showing the superiority of metoprolol to placebo.

11.6 Discussion

It is generally agreed upon that between-region variability needs to be accounted for in the statistical analysis. CREM treats regional treatment effects to be random variables while the DFEM and DREM treat the regional treatment effects to be fixed parameters. On the other hand, both the DFEM and CREM consider the regional sample sizes as fixed numbers, while the DREM considers the regional sample sizes as random variables jointly follow a multinomial distribution when patients are randomly drawn from the regions. Because results derived from different models are based on different assumptions and have different interpretations (Quan et al. 2017), it is not straightforward to compare the "performances" of different models. Therefore, our simulation evaluates the performance in Type I error rate and power against their respective assumptions. We consider a test is not valid if it inflates the type I error rate more than 20% from the nominal level.

When data truly follows CREM, the validity of CREM and DREM depends on $\hat{\tau}_C/\hat{\sigma}$. If $\hat{\tau}_C/\hat{\sigma} \leq 0.05$, $\hat{\tau}_C$ tends to be over-estimated. As a consequence, CREM over-controls the type I error rate and loses the power; DREM is valid only when $K \geq 6$ and may recover the CREM power loss. However, when $\hat{\tau}_C/\hat{\sigma} \geq 0.1$, both CREM and DREM inflate type I error rate by more than 20% from the nominal level and are not valid.

On the other hand, when data are from DREM, the DREM approach controls the Type I error rate and has power close to its target for τ_D ranges from 0.05 to 0.2. The validity of CREM, however, depends on τ_D/σ. When $\hat{\tau}_D/\hat{\sigma} \leq 0.05$, CREM has a type I error rate a little below but close 0.025 and power also close to 90%; but, when $\tau_D/\sigma \geq 0.2$, the type I error rate is over-controlled and loses power for $K \leq 6$ and inflated for $K \geq 10$, especially when some regions have sample sizes substantially higher than the others.

CREM and DREM are two different approaches to account for between-region variability, assuming different random mechanisms. From the above two paragraphs, we see that when data follows CREM, CREM is more appropriate in general, and the same is true with DREM and its data. However, we cannot verify in practice from which model the data comes. We need to examine the between region variability $\hat{\tau}_C/\hat{\sigma}$ or $\hat{\tau}_D/\hat{\sigma}$ and the number of regions K.

When between-region variability is small, i.e., the treatment effects among regions are similar, regardless of the mechanism, both approaches perform similarly to FEM, where the treatment effects of all regions are the same. However, as between-region variability ($\hat{\tau}_C/\hat{\sigma}$ or $\hat{\tau}_D/\hat{\sigma}$) increases, the performance of the two approaches diverge. If the data are from CREM and $\hat{\tau}_C/\hat{\sigma}$ is large, the type I error rate derived from the CREM may be inflated when the number of regions is not large enough due to the underestimation of the between regional variability. In this case, the type I error rate based on DREM is also inflated (see Figure 11.4). If the data is from DREM, CREM may not be appropriate, for not controlling the Type I error rate or losing power; but DREM is valid. Even though DREM is valid, when between region variability is too large, some of the regions are anticipated to have potential negative treatment effects. In this case, MRCT is not recommended. For example, at the design stage, assume the overall treatment effect $\Delta' = \sum_{i=1}^{K} W_i \Delta_i$ for the DREM and obtain the sample size N_D. Comparing a discrete FEM, with an overall treatment effect Δ' among all regions, the calculated sample size is N_F. Obviously $N_D > N_F$. When $\tau_D/\sigma < 0.25$, $\frac{N_D - N_F}{N_F} < 6.25\%$, i.e., a sample size increase by incorporating τ_D is less than 6.25%, within the variation of actual (enrolled) and planned sample size in practice. On the other hand, when $\frac{\tau_D}{\sigma} \geq 0.25$, there is at least a pair of regions i and j with between treatment effect difference $|\frac{\Delta_i - \Delta_j}{\sigma}| > 0.5 = 2 \frac{\Delta'}{\sigma}$, the treatment effect used in our simulation power. This is bound to show inconsistencies between regions.

The number of regions K affects the type I error rate and power as well. If K is small, the type I error rate may be inflated for both CREM and DREM when the data is from CREM. On the other hand, CREM may over-control the type I error rate when the data is from DREM. If K is large, CREM may inflate the type I error rate when the data is from CREM, especially when some regions have sample sizes substantially higher than the others.

It is also noted that when the sample size is large, DREM is similar to a discrete fixed effects model introduced by Quan et al. (2017).

Finally, the perceived major advantage of MRCTs is that they could speed up patient enrollment, thus resulting in quicker drug development and faster global approval of the drug. At the same time, the MRCT strategy is expected to maintain the sample size at a similar level, i.e., without significantly driving up the cost and slowing down the speed of the development. When the anticipated between-region variability is large enough such that it requires a drastic increase in sample size, alternative options may be considered, e.g., splitting the MRCT to include "similar" regions in the same trial. To be consistent with current practice and for easy interpretation of the trial results, a discrete fixed effects model could be proposed for an MRCT.

References

Hung HMJ. Design considerations for bridging clinical trials and global clinical trials. Presented at DIA Annual Meeting, Atlanta, GA, June 20, 2007.

Hung HMJ, Wang SJ, O'Neill RT, Consideration of regional difference in design and analysis of multi-regional trials, *Pharm. Stat.* 9 (2010) 173–178.

Lan KKG, Pinheiro J, Combined estimation of treatment effects under a discrete random effects model, *Stat. Biosci.* 4 (2012) 235–244. DOI: 10.1007/s12561-012-9054-9.

MERIT-HF Study Group, Effect of metoprolol CR/XL in chronic heart failure: Metoprolol CR/XL randomised intervention trial in congestive heart failure (MERIT-HF), *Lancet* 353 (1999) 2001–2007.

Quan H, Li M, Chen J, Gallo P, Binkowitz B, Ibia E, Tanaka Y, Ouyang P, Luo X, Li G, Assessment of consistency of treatment effects in multiregional clinical trials, *Drug Inf. J.* 44 (2010) 617–632.

Quan H, Li M, Shih JW, Ouyang SP, Chen J, Zhang J, Zhao PL, Empirical shrinkage estimator for consistency assessment of treatment effects in multiregional clinical trials, *Stat. Med.* 32 (2013) 1691–1706.

Quan, H, Mao, X, Tanaka, Y, Binkowitz, B, Li, G, Chen, J, Zhang, J, Zhao, P, Ouyang, PS, Chang, M, Example-based illustrations of design, conduct, analysis and result interpretation of multi-regional clinical trials, *Contemp. Clin. Trials* 58 (2017) 13–20.

Wedel H, DeMets D, Deedwania, P, Fagerberg B, Goldstein S, Gottlieb S, Hjalmarson A, Kjekshus J, Waagstein F, Wikstrand J, Challenges of subgroup analyses in multinational clinical trials: experiences from the MERIT-HF, *Am. Heart J.* 142 (2001) 502–511.

Appendix 1 Proof for.

Given $N = n = (n_1, \ldots, n_K) = n_1$, $\hat{\Delta}_k \sim N\left(\hat{\Delta}_k, \frac{2\sigma^2}{n_k}\right)$, and

$$\hat{\Delta} \mid N = n \sim N\left(\sum_{k=1}^{K} \frac{n_k}{N} \Delta_k, \frac{2}{N}\sigma^2\right).$$

That is, conditional on $N = n$, $\hat{\Delta}$ has mean

$$E(\hat{\Delta} \mid N) = \sum_{k=1}^{K} \frac{N_k}{N} \Delta_k \text{ and } Var(\hat{\Delta} \mid N) = \sum_{k=1}^{K} \left(\frac{N_k}{N}\right)^2 \frac{2\sigma^2}{N_k} = \frac{2}{N}\sigma^2.$$

$$Var(E(\hat{\Delta} \mid N)) = E(E(\hat{\Delta} \mid N) - \sum_{k=1}^{K} W_k \Delta_k)^2 = E\left(\sum_{k=1}^{K} \left(\frac{N_k}{N} - W_k\right)\Delta_k\right)^2$$

$$= \sum_{k=1}^{K} E\left(\frac{N_k}{N} - W_k\right)^2 \Delta_k^2 + 2\sum_{1 \le j < k \le K} E\left(\frac{N_j}{N} - W_j\right)\left(\frac{N_k}{N} - W_k\right)\Delta_j \Delta_k$$

$$= \frac{1}{N} \sum_{k=1}^{K} W_k(1 - W_k)\Delta_k^2 - \frac{2}{N} \sum_{1 \le j < k \le K} W_j W_k \Delta_j \Delta_k$$

$$= \frac{1}{N} \sum_{k=1}^{K} W_k \Delta_k^2 - \frac{\Delta^2}{N} = \frac{\tau_D^2}{N}$$

$$E(Var(\hat{\Delta} \mid N)) = \frac{2}{N}\sigma^2.$$

Therefore, $Var(\hat{\Delta}) = E(Var(\hat{\Delta} \mid N)) + Var(E(\hat{\Delta} \mid N)) = \frac{2\sigma^2 + \tau_D^2}{N}$.

Appendix 2 Proof for $E\hat{\tau}_D^2 = \tau_D^2 + (K-1)\frac{\sigma^2}{N}$ for large N

Let X_{ij} be the response of jth pair in i th region. $X_{ij} = \Delta_i + \varepsilon_{ij}$, where ε_{ij} are normally distributed independent random variables, $\varepsilon_{ij} \sim N(0, \sigma^2)$.

$\Delta = \sum_{i=1}^K W_i \Delta_i$. $\tau_D^2 = \sum_{i=1}^K W_i (\Delta_i - \Delta)^2$.

Let $\hat{\Delta}_i = \Delta_i + E_i$, where $E_i \sim N\left(0, \frac{2\sigma^2}{N_i}\right)$

Let $\hat{\Delta} = \sum_{i=1}^K \frac{N_i}{N}\hat{\Delta}_i$, $\tilde{\Delta} = \sum_{i=1}^K \frac{N_i}{N}\Delta_i$.

$$\hat{\tau}_D^2 = \sum_{i=1}^K \frac{N_i}{N}(\hat{\Delta}_i - \hat{\Delta})^2 = \sum_{i=1}^K \frac{N_i}{N}\left[(\Delta_i - \tilde{\Delta}) + \left(E_i - \sum_{j=1}^K \frac{N_i}{N}E_j\right)\right]^2$$

$$= \sum_{i=1}^K \frac{N_i}{N}[\Delta_i - \tilde{\Delta}]^2 + \sum_{i=1}^K \frac{N_i}{N}\left[E_i - \sum_{j=1}^K \frac{N_i}{N}E_j\right]^2$$

$$+ \sum_{i=1}^K \frac{N_i}{N}(\Delta_i - \tilde{\Delta})\left(E_i - \sum_{j=1}^K \frac{N_i}{N}E_j\right).$$

Conditional on $N = (n_1, ..., n_K)$, and denote $w_i = \frac{n_i}{N}$

$$E\left\{\sum_{i=1}^K \frac{N_i}{N}\left[E_i - \sum_{j=1}^K \frac{N_j}{N}E_j\right]^2 \mid N = (n_1, ..., n_K)\right\} = \sum_{i=1}^K w_i E\left[E_i - \sum_{j=1}^K w_j E_j\right]^2$$

$$= \sum_{i=1}^K w_i[(1 - w_i)^2 E(E_i)^2 + \sum_{j=1, j \neq i}^K E(w_j E_j)^2]$$

$$= \sum_{i=1}^K w_i\left[(1 - w_i)^2 \frac{2\sigma^2}{Nw_i} + \sum_{j=1, j \neq i}^K \frac{2w_j\sigma^2}{N}\right]$$

$$= \sum_{i=1}^K w_i\left[(1 - w_i)^2 \frac{1}{w_i} + (1 - w_i)\right]\frac{2\sigma^2}{N}$$

$$= \sum_{i=1}^K w_i\left[\frac{1}{w_i} - 1\right]\frac{\sigma^2}{N} = (K - 1)\frac{2\sigma^2}{N}.$$

Therefore, $E\sum_{i=1}^K \frac{N_i}{N}\left[E_i - \sum_{j=1}^K \frac{N_j}{N}E_j\right]^2 = (K - 1)\frac{2\sigma^2}{N}$.

$$\sum_{i=1}^K \frac{N_i}{N}[\Delta_i - \tilde{\Delta}]^2 = \sum_{i=1}^K \frac{N_i}{N}\left[\Delta_i - \sum_{j=1}^K \frac{N_j}{N}\Delta_j\right]^2$$

$$= \sum_{i=1}^{K} \frac{N_i}{N} \left[\left(1 - \frac{N_i}{N} \right) \Delta_i - \sum_{j=1, j \neq i}^{K} \frac{N_j}{N} \Delta_j \right]^2$$

$$= \sum_{i=1}^{K} \frac{N_i}{N} \left[\begin{array}{l} \left(\left(1 - \frac{N_i}{N} \right) \Delta_i \right)^2 + \sum_{j=1, j \neq i}^{K} \left(\frac{N_j}{N} \Delta_j \right)^2 + 2 \sum_{j=1, j \neq i}^{K} \left(1 - \frac{N_i}{N} \right) \Delta_i \frac{N_j}{N} \Delta_j + \\ 2 \sum_{j=1, j \neq i, k \neq i, j \neq k}^{K} \frac{N_j}{N} \Delta_j \frac{N_k}{N} \Delta_k \end{array} \right]$$

$$= \sum_{i=1}^{K} \left[\left(\frac{N_i}{N} - 2 \left(\frac{N_i}{N} \right)^2 + \left(\frac{N_i}{N} \right)^3 \right) \Delta_i^2 + \sum_{j=1, j \neq i}^{K} \frac{N_i}{N} \left(\frac{N_j}{N} \Delta_j \right)^2 \right.$$

$$\left. + 2 \sum_{j=1, j \neq i}^{K} \left(\frac{N_i}{N} \frac{N_j}{N} - \left(\frac{N_i}{N} \right)^2 \frac{N_j}{N} \right) \Delta_i \Delta_j + 2 \sum_{j=1, j \neq i, k \neq i, j \neq k}^{K} \frac{N_i}{N} \frac{N_j}{N} \Delta_j \frac{N_k}{N} \Delta_k \right]$$

Thus

$$E \sum_{i=1}^{K} \frac{N_i}{N} [\Delta_i - \tilde{\Delta}]^2 = \sum_{i=1}^{K} \left[\left(W_i - 2 \frac{N-1}{N} W_i^2 + \frac{(N-1)(N-2)}{N^2} W_i^3 \right) \Delta_i^2 \right.$$

$$+ \sum_{j=1, j \neq i}^{K} \frac{(N-1)(N-2)}{N^2} W_i W_j^2 \Delta_j^2$$

$$+ 2 \sum_{j=1, j \neq i}^{K} \left(\frac{N-1}{N} W_i W_j - \frac{(N-1)(N-2)}{N^2} W_i^2 W_j \right) \Delta_i \Delta_j$$

$$+ 2 \sum_{j=1, j \neq i, k \neq i, j \neq k}^{K} \frac{(N-1)(N-2)}{N^2} W_i W_j W_k \Delta_j \Delta_k \right].$$

When N is large, $\frac{(N-1)(N-2)}{N^2} \cong 1$

$$E \sum_{i=1}^{K} \frac{N_i}{N} [\Delta_i - \tilde{\Delta}]^2 = \sum_{i=1}^{K} \left[(W_i - 2W_i^2 + W_i^3) \Delta_i^2 + \sum_{j=1, j \neq i}^{K} W_i W_j^2 \Delta_j^2 \right.$$

$$\left. + 2 \sum_{j=1, j \neq i}^{K} \left(W_i W_j - W_i^2 W_j \right) \Delta_i \Delta_j + 2 \sum_{j=1, j \neq i, k \neq i, j \neq k}^{K} W_i W_j W_k \Delta_j \Delta_k \right].$$

$$= \sum_{i=1}^{K} W_i \left[(1 - W_i)^2 \Delta_i^2 + \sum_{j=1, j \neq i}^{K} W_j^2 \Delta_j^2 + 2 \sum_{j=1, j \neq i}^{K} W_j (1 - W_i) \Delta_i \Delta_j \right.$$

$$\left. + 2 \sum_{j=1, j \neq i, k \neq i, j \neq k}^{K} W_j W_k \Delta_j \Delta_k \right]$$

$$= \sum_{i=1}^{K} W_i (\Delta_i - \Delta)^2 = \tau_D^2.$$

Therefore, when N is large $E\hat{\tau}_D^2 = \tau_D^2 + (K-1)\frac{2\sigma^2}{N}$.

Appendix 3 Proof of $\tilde{\sigma}_C^2 \geq \frac{\hat{\tau}_D^2}{K-1}$.

First, We note that

$$\tilde{\sigma}_C^2 = \frac{1}{\sum_{i=1}^{K} a_i} = \frac{1}{\sum_{i=1}^{K} 1/\left(\tau_C^2 + \frac{2\sigma^2}{n_i}\right)} \geq \frac{\tau_C^2 + \frac{2K\sigma^2}{N}}{K} = \frac{\tau_C^2}{K} + \frac{2\sigma^2}{N},$$

and equality holds when $n_i = N/K$. Note also $\hat{\tau}_D^2 = \sum_{i=1}^{i=1} w_i (\hat{\Delta}_i - \hat{\Delta})^2$. So

$$\tilde{\sigma}_C^2 \geq \frac{\frac{N}{2\hat{\sigma}^2}\hat{\tau}_D^2 - (K-1)}{K\frac{N}{2\hat{\sigma}^2}(1 - \sum_{i=1}^{K} w_i^2)} + \frac{2\sigma^2}{N}$$

As $\frac{1}{1 - \sum_{i=1}^{K} w_i^2} \geq \frac{K}{K-1}$, $\tilde{\sigma}_C^2 \geq \frac{\frac{N}{2\hat{\sigma}^2}\hat{\tau}_D^2 - (K-1)}{\frac{N}{2\hat{\sigma}^2}(K-1)} + \frac{2\sigma^2}{N} = \frac{\hat{\tau}_D^2}{K-1}$.

12

Utilization of Robust Estimates of Treatment Effects via Semiparametric Models in MRCT

Ming T. Tan, Shilin Yu, and Ao Yuan

12.1 Introduction

Multiregional clinical trial (MRCT) represents the growing trend of global simultaneous drug development [Section 1 of (1)]. First, it is a clinical trial and should be consistent with principles for good clinical trial design and sound statistical methods, e.g., minimizing bias and maximizing precision. However, MRCT is more complex in all aspects of clinical trials from design, conduct, and analysis. The past decade has seen extensive efforts from government, sponsors, and academia made to address issues related to MRCT, which ultimately led to the publication of ICH E17 in 2017. Sponsors are increasingly using MRCT strategically throughout the drug-development process to meet the need for global simultaneous development and to facilitate global regulatory submission and registration, although regional differences in medical and regulatory practice indeed add the complexity in trial conduct and monitoring. The E17 document summarizes unique MRCT principles. For example, MRCT is planned assuming that the treatment applies to the whole target population using a single primary analysis approach with the strategic allocation of sample sizes to each region based on region-specific (e.g., regulatory) requirements, and it is important to identify intrinsic and extrinsic factors (covariates) early and pre-specify pooling of regions and subpopulations. The E17 document also represents a shift to a global assessment of the treatment and then across the regions (pooled region) while investigating the potential impact of intrinsic and extrinsic factors on the treatment effect.

Indeed, with these considerations, MRCT is powered to show an overall treatment effect at a given significance level; however, at the same time assuring each region under consideration has an adequate chance to show a portion of the effect size agreed upon by the regulatory authority in that region (e.g., at least 50% of the overall effect). The sample size can be determined based on methods using the formula in Chen and Quan (2016). In addition, factors that may influence trial outcomes will need to be identified in protocol. For the analysis of MRCT, treatment effects estimates may need to be obtained based on a model adjusting for pre-specified covariates. It is recognized that interpretation of trial results from different models may vary and the required sample sizes are also different. Obviously, we would like to use a robust model for such estimates, including variance estimates used for sample size determination, so they are stable under various model assumptions and the recognized increased potential for heterogeneity in MRCT.

While the need to account for heterogeneity is made clear with the E17 document, several products disapproved by the Food and Drug Administration (FDA) might provide a motivation for considering more flexible and robust semiparametric statistical models for primary analysis while accounting for non-normality and covariates that may influence the trial outcome beyond randomization. For example, the FDA advisory committee for reproductive health voted by a large margin against the approval of Sefelsa (gabapentin-ER) by Assertio Therapeutics (formerly Depomed) for the treatment of menopause hot flash although Sefelsa meant to meet the unmet need for non-hormonal based therapy for this indication. There were a series of three randomized phase III trials in postmenopausal women 18–70 years of age and who reported at least 7 moderate to severe hot flashes per day and are unable or unwilling to use hormones. The primary outcomes are changes from baseline in frequency and severity of hot flashes at 4 and 12 weeks of treatment. The analysis of the trials had utilized nonparametric methods since normality is not satisfied in the first two trials, and then parametric model adjusting for covariates in the third trial. Different models had led to inconsistent conclusions on the treatment effect. A robust modeling approach would be useful to capture the somewhat unusual distribution of the outcome. Even if it is only used internally or as an exploratory analysis in the early trial(s), it might have given insight into the design and analysis strategy for the subsequent trial(s).

The commonly used methods for MRCT analysis include a fixed or less frequently random-effects model on a (or asymptotically) normally distributed outcome at the group-level (more specifically, region-level), that is, for region i, let its true treatment effect be δ_i, its estimate be $\hat{\delta}_i$, then $\hat{\delta}_i \mid \delta_i \sim N(\delta_i, 2\sigma^2/n_i)$, where n_i is the fixed sample size at region i and the total sample size n is the sum of n_i across all regions. Then the overall treatment effect estimate $\hat{\delta} = \sum_i \hat{\delta}_i n_i / n$. A random-effects model on the $\hat{\delta}_i$ can be formulated similarly (Hung et al. 2010), however the exchangeability assumption of all the δ_i in the random-effects model is questionable. The discrete random effects model (Lan and Pinheiro 2012) assumes that patients are randomly selected from the regions. However, in reality, n_i is more fixed rather than random. This explains partly the fixed-effects model has been used more widely. Quan et al. (2013, 2014) compared fixed and random effects models in greater detail. There is now a large literature on estimating regional treatment effect(s). Yuan, Wang and Tan (2018) proposed a robust semiparametric model for trials with continuous responses as the primary endpoint to directly estimate the regional treatment effect from the model. However, most of the analyses have been at the group level as opposed to patient level (Guo et al. 2016).

In this chapter, we will introduce and review methodological advances of the approach based on robust semiparametric models on the patient-level data. The approach is to analyze MRCT as designed and use a robust fixed-effect model to estimate directly the regional treatment effects while accounting for any intrinsic or extrinsic factors. We will focus on binary outcome or endpoint, one of the most commonly encountered endpoints in clinical trials. The rest of this chapter is organized as follows. Section 12.2 reviews robust estimates of global and regional treatment effects in MRCT through semiparametric modeling and test if the treatment difference is the same across regions and introduces improved algorithm and R functions for model estimation. In Section 12.3, we illustrate the method and use the R functions to analyze semi-real data from a phase III clinical trial. We conclude with a discussion on the applications of robust modeling approach in the design and analysis of MRCT.

12.2 Robust Semiparametric Models

To introduce the robust semiparametric logistic models, we first focus on the fixed-effects case, that is, the regional effects is a fixed vector of parameters, and then discuss the random effects model later. We introduce and review recently developed semiparametric models for MRCT analysis with the binary primary endpoint. The first extends the parametric logistic model with a nonparametric non-linear term, the second extends it with a nonparametric link function originally developed for an ordinal response. It is worthwhile to note that the notations from the original papers are retained so notations for the design matrix and model parameters are model specific.

12.2.1 Model 1: Semiparametric Logistic Model with Nonparametric Non-Linear Term

The observed data is $D_n = \{(y_i, x_i, z_i): i = 1, \ldots, n\}$ iid (y, x, z), where y_i is the binary responses on the endpoint of an MRCT, x_i is the associated covariates, and $z_i = (z_{i,1}, \ldots, z_{i,2k})'$ is the treatment-region indicator, the first k components indicates the region for treatment 1 (old), the last k components indicates the region for treatment 2 (new), and k is the number of regions. For example if the i-th individual received treatment 1 and is from region j $(1 \le j \le k)$, then $z_{i,j} = 1$ and all other $z_{i,l} = 0$ for $l \ne j$; if i-th individual received treatment 2 and is from region j $(1 \le j \le k)$, then $z_{i,k+j} = 1$ and all other $z_{i,l} = 0$ for $l \ne k + j$. We introduce Model 1, the semiparametric version that includes potential non-linear effects:

$$P(y = 1 \mid x, z, \theta, h) = \frac{\exp(\beta'x + \delta'z + \lambda h(x, z))}{1 + \exp(\beta'x + \delta'z + \lambda h(x, z))} \qquad (12.1)$$

where $\theta = (\beta', \delta', \lambda)'$ and $h(\cdot)$ represents an unspecified (unknown) function not proportional to $\exp(\beta'x)$, in other words, containing no linear forms of the observed (x, z). It modifies the commonly used parametric logistic model. The function $h(\cdot)$ is intended to capture any non-linear effects and is assumed that it does not contain linear treatment effects. In particular, in a nonparametric model specification, $\beta'x$ is absorbed into $h(x, z)$. It is a general class of models that contains the index model. Often the model with parametric component $\exp(\delta'z + \beta'x)$ alone can only be correct to some extent. When $\beta = 0$ and $\delta = 0$, it gives nonparametric logistic model; when $\lambda = 0$ or $h(\cdot) \equiv c$ and x has the compact domain, $h(c)$ can be absorbed into δ, and it gives the parametric logistic model; otherwise it is generally in between the two. These features will be data-driven, i.e., the roles of β, λ, and $h(\cdot)$ in (12.1) are estimated with data. It has been shown that the semiparametric model (12.1) is identifiable, if $P(y = 1 \mid x, z, \theta_1, h_1) \equiv P(y = 1 \mid x, z, \theta_2, h_2)$, namely, $(\theta_1, h_1) = (\theta_2, h_2)$, and $\int \exp(h(t))dt = C$ for any given $0 < C < \infty$.

The log-likelihood given the observed data is

$$\begin{aligned}
\ell_n(\theta, h \mid D_n) &= \sum_{i=1}^{n} \Big(y_i \log \frac{\exp(\beta'x_i + \delta'z_i + \lambda h(x_i, z_i))}{1 + \exp(\beta'x_i + \delta'z_i + \lambda h(x_i, z_i))} \\
&\quad + (1 - y_i) \log \frac{1}{1 + \exp(\beta'x_i + \delta'z_i + \lambda h(x_i, z_i))} \Big) \qquad (12.2) \\
&= \sum_{i=1}^{n} \{ y_i (\beta'x_i + \delta'z_i + \lambda h(x_i, z_i)) \\
&\quad - \log(1 + \exp(\beta'x_i + \delta'z_i + \lambda h(x_i, z_i))) \}
\end{aligned}$$

When $\lambda = 0$ or $h(\cdot) = Const.$, it can be absorbed into the intercept term, and it reduces to classic parametric logistic model. Thus (12.2) is an extension of the existing logistic regression model.

12.2.2 Model 1 Estimation

Since the nonparametric term $h(\cdot)$ is unknown, it is an infinite-dimensional nuisance parameter (actually function). We adopted the common approach to eliminate the infinite-dimensional nuisance parameter h by finding the profile log-likelihood estimate $\tilde{\ell}_n(\theta \,|\, D_n) = \sup_h \ell_n(\theta, h \,|\, D_n)$. Also, note to compute the profile likelihood, it is known that the maximization of the nonparametric component h boils down to maximizing its values at the observation points. Therefore, we set

$$h(x_i, z_i) = h_i, \quad \sum_{i=1}^{n} y_i \exp(h_i) = 1.$$

Note that the data version of the constraint $\sum_z \int \exp(h(x, z))dx = 1$ can be approximated by $n^{-1} \sum_{i=1}^{n} \exp(h_i) = 1$. Because the y_i's are 0–1 valued, we used the constraint $\sum_{i=1}^{n} y_i \exp(h_i) = 1$ as an alternative to the former for computational convenience shown below. Denote $\mathbf{h} = (h_1, \ldots, h_n)$. Then the corresponding log-likelihood is

$$\ell_n(\theta, \mathbf{h} \,|\, D_n) = \sum_{i=1}^{n} \{y_i(\boldsymbol{\beta}'x_i + \boldsymbol{\delta}'z_i + \lambda h_i) - \log(1 + \exp(\boldsymbol{\beta}'x_i + \boldsymbol{\delta}'z_i + \lambda h_i))\}.$$

$$(12.3)$$

To eliminate the nuisance parameters h_i's, for fixed θ, we maximize the above log-likelihood over $\mathbf{h}$, to get the estimates $\hat{\mathbf{h}} = \hat{\mathbf{h}}(\theta) = (\hat{h}_1, \ldots, \hat{h}_n)$ given by (Appendix)

$$\exp(\hat{h}_i) = \geq \left(\sum_{j=1}^{n} \exp(h_j)^{-1} \exp(h_i), \quad \exp(h_i) = \frac{1}{\sqrt{1 + 4a_i} + 1}, \quad (i = 1, \ldots, n).$$

with $a_i = \exp(\boldsymbol{\beta}'x_i + \boldsymbol{\delta}'z_i)$. Here without confusion, we first defined the exp (h_i)'s, and then define $\hat{h}_i$'s through $\exp(\hat{h}_i)$'s as the scaled version of the $\exp(h_i)$'s.

Plugging the $\exp(\hat{h}_i) = \exp(\hat{h}_i(\boldsymbol{\beta}, \boldsymbol{\delta}))$'s into (12.3), we have the profile log-likelihood

$$\tilde{\ell}_n(\theta \,|\, D_n) = \sum_{i=1}^{n} \{y_i(\boldsymbol{\beta}'x_i + \boldsymbol{\delta}'z_i + \lambda \hat{h}_i) - \log(1 + \exp(\boldsymbol{\beta}'x_i + \boldsymbol{\delta}'z_i + \lambda \hat{h}_i))\}.$$

$$(12.4)$$

To estimate the true parameter $\theta_0 = (\boldsymbol{\beta}_0', \boldsymbol{\delta}_0', \lambda_0)'$, we generate the observed data under model (12.1) by the profile maximum likelihood estimator (profile MLE) $\hat{\theta} = (\hat{\boldsymbol{\beta}}', \hat{\boldsymbol{\delta}}', \hat{\lambda})'$,

$$\hat{\theta} = \arg\sup_{\theta} \tilde{\ell}_n(\theta \mid D_n).$$

Yuan et al. (2021) have shown that under common regularity conditions the profile MLE $\hat{\theta}$, as $n \to \infty$, $\hat{\theta} \overset{a.s.}{\to} \theta_0$ and it is also efficient for θ_0, and

$$\sqrt{n}\,(\hat{\theta} - \theta_0) \overset{D}{\to} N(0, \Omega^{-1}), \quad \Omega = E_{\theta_0}[i^*i^{*'}],$$

where $i^* = i^*(y, x, z \mid \theta_0)$ is the efficient score for $\theta_0 = (\beta'_0, \delta'_0, \lambda_0)'$ given in Yuan et al. (2021). The asymptotic covariance matrix Ω can also be computed by the numerical method.

12.2.3 Hypothesis Testing

To test the null hypothesis that the treatment difference is the same for all the regions, namely, H_0: $\delta_{2j} - \delta_{1j} = Const.(j = 1, \dots, k)$ vs the alternative H_1: the differences are not all equal. One test is based on the profile likelihood ratio statistic as it does not involve the computation of first-order and second-order partial derivatives of the profile likelihood. It was shown that this test statistic parallels the result of Wilks (1938) for the parametric model, and can be used to test H_0 vs H_1. For this, we define the profile likelihood ratio statistic below. Recall $\hat{\theta}$ is the profile MLE of θ under the log profile likelihood $\tilde{\ell}_n(\theta \mid D_n)$ given in (12.4), and $dim(\delta) = 2k$. H_0 is equivalent to $\delta_{1j} - \delta_{2j} = C$ for $j = 1, \dots, k$. Let $\Theta_0 = \{\beta, \delta_{11}, \dots, \delta_{1k}, \delta_{11} + C, \dots, \delta_{1k} + C\}$, and $\tilde{\theta}$ be the profile MLE of θ_0 under H_0,

$$\tilde{\theta} = \arg\sup_{\theta \in \Theta_0} \tilde{\ell}_n((\beta, \delta) \mid D_n).$$

The computation of $\tilde{\beta}$ follows that of $\hat{\theta}$. Define the profile likelihood ratio

$$\Lambda_n = 2(\tilde{\ell}_n(\hat{\theta} \mid D_n) - \tilde{\ell}_n((\tilde{\theta} \mid D_n)).$$

Yuan et al. (2021) have also shown that under the same regularity conditions and under H_0,

$$\Lambda_n \overset{D}{\to} \chi^2_{k-1},$$

where χ^2_{k-1} is the chi-squared random variable with $(k - 1)$ degrees of freedom.

However, the log-likelihood ratio statistic is known to potentially inflate the type I error. Alternatively, the score test or Wald test can be used. Let $\dot{\tilde{\ell}}_n(\theta\,|\,\hat{f}_n) = \partial\tilde{\ell}_n(\theta\,|\,\hat{f}_n)/\partial\theta$. The score test statistic is obtained by $S_n = \dot{\tilde{\ell}}_n(\hat{\theta}_0\,|\,\hat{f}_n)\Omega(\hat{\theta}_0)\dot{\tilde{\ell}}'_n(\hat{\theta}_0\,|\,\hat{f}_n)$, under H_0, asymptotically $S_n \sim \chi^2_1$.

To derive the Wald test, let $\theta = (\theta_1, \theta_2)$ with $dim\,(\theta) = d$ and $dim\,(\theta_1) = d_1$, and $\hat{\theta} = (\hat{\theta}_1, \hat{\theta}_2)$. Consider the null hypothesis H_0: $\theta_1 = \theta_{1,0}$. The Wald test statistic is given by

$$W_n = (\hat{\theta}_1 - \theta_{1,0})'Cov^{-1}(\hat{\theta}_1)(\hat{\theta}_1 - \theta_{1,0}).$$

If $Cov\,(\hat{\theta}_1)$ is known, $W_n \sim \chi^2_{d_1}$; If $Cov\,(\hat{\theta}_1)$ is estimated, $W_n/d_1 \sim F_{d_1,n-d}$.

In our parameterization, let $\hat{\mathbf{d}} = (\hat{d}_1, ...,\hat{d}_k)' = (\hat{\delta}_{21} - \hat{\delta}_{11}, ...,\hat{\delta}_{2k} - \hat{\delta}_{1k})'$. Let

$$C = \begin{pmatrix} 1 & -1 & 0 & 0 & ... & 0 \\ 0 & 1 & -1 & 0 & ... & 0 \\ 0 & 0 & ... & 0 & ... & 0 \\ 0 & 0 & ... & 0 & 1 & -1 \end{pmatrix}_{(k-1)\times k},$$

then H_0 can be written as the contrast $C\mathbf{d} = 0$. So the Wald statistic is

$$W_n = (C\hat{\mathbf{d}})'Cov^{-1}(C\hat{\mathbf{d}})C\hat{\mathbf{d}},$$

and we will use the estimated covariance, so under H_0, $W_n \sim F_{k-1,n-d}$, with $d = dim\,(\theta)$.

12.2.4 Random Effects Model

It has been recognized (e.g., Senn 1998; Fedorov and Jones 2005; Quan et al. 2013) that inference based on a fixed-effects model is trial specific and may not be generalizable since the expectation of the global effects depends on the sample size configuration across the regions and specific effects $\hat{\alpha}_i$; while inference based on a random-effects model that does take into account between-region variability, maybe more generalizable and applicable to a global scale. There is a trade-off. The use of a random-effects model will require a much larger overall sample size for achieving the same power Quan et al. (2013), and the exchangeability among regions may also be questionable. With the random-effects model, the δ_{ij}'s are viewed as i.i.d. random variables from a common distribution, e.g., $\delta_0 \sim N\,(0, \Sigma)$. Then we have

$$\hat{\delta} - \delta_0 \approx N\left(0, \Sigma + \frac{\Omega_\delta}{n}\right),$$

where Ω_δ is the corresponding block of Ω^{-1} for δ.

12.2.5 Overall Treatment Effect and Sample Size

To obtain the overall treatment effect, let $\hat{\delta}_1$ and $\hat{\delta}_2$ be the estimated regional effects for both treatments, the estimated treatment effect is $\hat{\Delta} = \hat{\delta}_2 - \hat{\delta}_1$, and the asymptotic distribution of $\hat{\Delta} - \Delta_0$ can be derived based on model asymptotics (Yuan et al. 2021). Here $\Delta_0 = \delta_{20} - \delta_{10}$, δ_{20} and δ_{10} are the true effects of treatment 1 and 2 on the regions. Let n_1 and n_0 be the sample sizes in the two groups, $n = n_1 + n_0$. The asymptotic distribution of $\hat{\delta} - \delta_0$ has the form

$$\sqrt{n}\,(\hat{\Delta} - \Delta_0) \xrightarrow{D} N(0,\,\Omega)$$

for some Ω.

Quan et al. (2014) estimate the overall treatment difference effect over the regions by

$$\hat{\Delta} = \sum_{j=1}^{k} \frac{n_j}{n}(\hat{\delta}_{2j} - \hat{\delta}_{1j}).$$

In the fixed-effects model, let $\Delta_0 = \sum_{j=1}^{k} w_j \Delta_{0,j}$ be the true overall effect, and $w = (w_1, \dots, w_k)'$. Then the distribution of $\hat{\Delta}$ is approximately

$$\hat{\Delta} \sim N\!\left(\Delta_0,\, \frac{\sigma^2}{n}\right), \quad \sigma^2 = w'\Omega_0 w.$$

The required sample size n with power $1 - \beta$ to detect an overall treatment effect of α with significance level α is

$$n = \sigma^2 \frac{(z_\alpha + z_\beta)^2}{\alpha^2}.$$

Similarly, in the random-effects model, let $\Delta_j = \delta_{2j} - \delta_{1j}$, and $\Delta_j \sim N(\Delta_0, \tau^2)$, then approximately,

$$\hat{\Delta} \sim N\!\left(\Delta_0,\, \frac{\sigma^2}{n} + \tau^2 \sum_{j=1}^{k} w_j^2\right).$$

As in Quan et al. (2014), the required sample size with power $1 - \beta$ to detect an overall treatment effect of α with significance level α based on a one-sided test as the solution n of

$$\sum_{j=1}^{k} \frac{1}{\tau^2 + \sigma^2/(\tilde{n}w_j)} = \frac{(z_\alpha + z_\beta)^2}{\alpha^2}.$$

If $w_1 = \cdots = w_k$, then

$$\tilde{n} = \left(\frac{\alpha^2}{\sigma^2 (z_\alpha + z_\beta)^2} - \frac{\tau^2}{k\sigma^2} \right)^{-1}.$$

It is easy to see [4] $\tilde{n} \geq n$, with " = " only if $\tau^2 = 0$.

Extensive simulations have been performed to study the finite sample properties of the model in a setting with three covaraites and regions. When the true model departs from the logistic model, the estimates from the robust model have significantly smaller biases than those from the classical logistic model. Mean squared error (MSE = *Variance* + (*Bias*)^2) for the semiparametric model is also less than that of the logistic model. When the logistic model is true, the logistic model performs better with smaller average biases and greater power, as expected.

12.2.6 Model 2 Semiparametric Binary Model with a Nonparametric Link Function

We introduce another robust model recently developed for ordinal outcomes (Yuan, Duan and Tan (2021)) which includes binary response data as an important special case. To formulate the model for binary response case, let the observed data is $D_n = \{(y_i, x_i, z_i): i = 1, \ldots, n\}$ iid (y, x, z) from n independent individuals and k regions, the same as in Model 1 and see there for the description.

We specify the following semiparametric binary response model (Model 2)

$$P(y = 1 \mid x, z, F) = F(\beta'x + \delta'z), \tag{12.5}$$

where β is the regression coefficient, δ is the regional effect, and $F(\cdot)$ is an unknown distribution function. This is a single-index model, with the constraint $\|\beta\| = 1$ and $\delta_{11} = 0$ for model identifiability, where $F(\cdot)$ is an unknown distribution function. Thus it is much more flexible and robust than the parametric logistic model and Model 1.

The model parameters are estimated using the semiparametric maximum likelihood estimate with a shape constraint on F, which is monotone increasing. Again the Wald statistic is used to test the existence of regional treatment effects. Such a model belongs to the class of semiparametric or nonparametric models with shape constraints which have been studied by Kiefer and Wolfowitz (1976), Lo (1986), Bickel and Fan (1996), Stout (2008), Qin et al. (2014), and Yuan, Zhou, and Tan (2021), among others. Our goals are to estimate the regional effects of the treatments and test the null hypothesis of a homogeneous difference in treatment effects across the regions. One can analyze the data for each region separately, but the joint analysis, which uses the full data information, is better because there are common covariate effects among the regions. Denote $\theta = (\beta', \delta')'$, the log-likelihood for the observed data is

$$\ell(\theta, F \mid D_n) = \sum_{i=1}^{n} \{y_i \log F(\beta'x_i + \delta'z_i) + (1 - y_i)\log(1 - F(\beta'x_i + \delta'z_i))\}.$$

12.2.7 Model 2 Estimation

Let Θ be the range of θ and $\mathcal{F}$ be the collection of all distribution functions on R. The parameters are estimated by the maximum likelihood estimate $(\hat{\theta}, \hat{F})$,

$$(\hat{\theta}, \hat{F}) = \arg\max_{(\theta, F) \in (\Theta, F)} \ell(\theta, F \mid D_n). \tag{12.6}$$

The maximization in (12.6) can be carried out by the following iterative procedure. Given a starting value $\theta^{(0)}$ of θ, find $F^{(1)}(\cdot) \in \mathcal{F}$ as the maxima of $\ell(\theta^{(0)}, F \mid D_n)$, fix $F^{(1)}$, then find $\theta^{(1)} \in \Theta$ as the maxima of $\ell(\theta, F^{(1)} \mid D_n)$, and so on until the convergence of the sequence $\{(\theta^{(r)}, F^{(r)})\}$. Yuan, Duan and Tan[32][24] have shown the convergence of this procedure.

The maximization over F with monotone increasing constraint is non-standard. One way is to use the algorithm from Yuan, Duan and Tan (2021), as follows. Given $\theta^{(r)}$, let $w_{ij}^{(r)} = \beta^{(r)'}x_i + \delta^{(r)'}z_i$. Then

$$F^{(r+1)} = \arg\min_{F \in \mathcal{F}} \sum_{i=1}^{n} (F(w_{ij}^{(r)}) - y_i)^2.$$

The above-constrained minimization, which is subject to the monotonicity constraint on F, can be implemented with the pool-adjacent-violators algorithm (PAVA), using the R-package *isoreg* (see, e.g., Best and Chakravarti 1990, for more details).

The asymptotic behavior of $\hat{\theta}$ and $\hat{F}$ have been derived by Yuan, Duan and Tan (2021), where it is shown (without $\hat{\alpha}$), under suitable regularity conditions, that $\hat{\theta}$ and $\hat{F}$ are strongly consistent with the true parameters θ_0 and F_0 $(\|\hat{\theta} - \theta_0\| + \|\hat{F} - F_0\| = O_p(n^{-1/3}))$, $n^{1/3}(\hat{F}(t) - F_0(t))$ converges weakly to a random variable that follows Chernoff's distribution. However, it remains an open question on what the asymptotic distribution of $\hat{\theta}$ is. The same results hold here for binary outcomes under corresponding conditions. It is worth noting that

$\hat{F}$ is the nonparametric MLE of F, and any nonparametric MLE is a step function with knots at the observation points. Although $\hat{F}$ is not smooth, the estimates of β and δ are consistent, so the interpretability of these effects is valid.

To test the null hypothesis that the treatment difference is homogeneous across regions, namely, H_0: $\delta_{1s} - \delta_{2s} = C\,(s = 1, \ldots, k)$ for some constant C, vs. the alternative hypothesis H_1: the difference is not homogeneous, we can derive Wald test following the same procedure for Model 1 (see also Yuan, Wang and Tan 2018). The case for random effects and how to obtain the overall treatment effect is treated the same way as for Model 1.

Extensive simulation studies for Model 2 have also been performed to show the finite sample performance of the approach for a variety of F including standard normal, Beta, or exponential distributions for a given β and α. Then, we estimate the parameters θ from Model 2 for some different choices of θ_0, compare the corresponding estimates with the traditional logistic model, test the hypothesis of treatment vs control, i.e., both treatments have the same effect on each region and test the null hypothesis for consistency assessment, H_0 vs. the alternative hypothesis H_1. The estimates from robust model 2 have better overall performance than those from the traditional logistic model when the latter departs substantially from the true link. It is also shown that the estimated curves fit the true curves well, while the estimated logistic links can depart from the true curves significantly. However, when the logistic link is close to the true link, the logistic model performs as well, as expected. More importantly, the proposed model yields robustness in estimation which is appealing because we are interested in estimating regional treatment effects efficiently in MRCT studies and a misspecified model can have serious practical implications.

12.3 Application to an MRCT

Now, we illustrate the robust modeling approach with a real MRCT. The patient-level data of the trial is available publicly on Project Data Sphere, however, only in the control group, and for the treatment group, only group-level summary data is available. For the purpose of illustration in this article, we recreated the patient-level data for the treatment group based on the published marginal distributions of the outcome and covariates for the treatment group, dubbed the data semi-real data.

12.3.1 Metastatic Breast Cancer MRCT: The ROSE/TRIO-12 Study

This study (https://www.-projectdatasphere.org/projectdatasphere/Inthismulti-national/) is a randomized, double-blind, placebo-controlled phase III trial evaluating the addition of ramucirumab to first-line docetaxel chemotherapy in metastatic breast cancer patients from America, Europe, Australia and New Zealand, Asia, Middle East, and Africa. In this trial, 1,144 patients with human epidermal growth factor receptor 2 (HER2)-negative breast cancer who had not received cytotoxic chemotherapy were randomized at a 2:1 ratio to receive docetaxel 75 mg = m2 plus ramucirumab 10 mg = kg or docetaxel 75 mg= m2 plus placebo once every three weeks. Patients were stratified by previous taxane therapy, visceral metastasis, hormone receptor status, and geographic region (North or South America/Europe, Australia, or New Zealand/Asia, Middle East, or Africa). They were treated until disease progression, unacceptable toxicity, or other withdrawal criteria. The outcome of success is defined as complete and partial response in our example. Age, prior taxane therapy, visceral metastasis, hormone receptor status, and the number of metastatic sites were considered covariates. However, only the control group data in this study are available. We simulated the treatment group data based on the 10% absolute improvement in response to therapy, available covariate information for this group, and the estimated regression coefficients from the control group data using the logistic link. The estimates from both Models 1–2 and the logistic model are shown in Table 12.1 below. It is interesting to observe that the estimated λ is 0.132 with $sd = 0.041$, so an approximate 95% confidence interval (0.052, 0.212), suggesting it is significantly different from 0 and some departure from the conventional logistic model exists. To test treatment efficacy, if we set $(\delta_{21}, \delta_{22}, \delta_{23}) = (\delta_{11}, \delta_{12}, \delta_{13}) + (0.13, 0.13, 0.13)$, the Wald statistics of the two robust models is 15.5 and 14.4 with P-values < 0.001. Thus, based on the observed data, there is a significantly different treatment effect. For testing, if the treatment difference is consistent across regions, the Wald statistics are 1.67 and 0.15 (P-values > 0.53), suggesting no evidence against the null hypothesis of no regional difference. The logistic model gives similar results on consistency, namely, there is no regional difference in treatment improvement, however, the response rate is not significantly different between the treatment and control based on the logistic regression model ($P = 0.14$). The estimated $\hat{F}$ from robust model 2 is different from the logistic distribution (Figure 12.1). So both robust models offer additional advantages over the common logistic model.

12.4 Discussion and Conclusion

We have reviewed and introduced a robust estimate of regional and global treatment effects utilizing semiparametric regression models for MRCT with a binary primary endpoint. Our robust models include an extended logistic link model with a nonparametric term and one model with a nonparametrically specified link function. The method is robust against model assumptions. Our simulations show that the proposed models compare

TABLE 12.1

Parameter estimates for the breast cancer trial

Approaches	ROSE/TRIO-12 Breast Cancer Trial		
θ	$(\beta_1, \beta_2, \beta_3, \beta_4, \beta_5)$	$(\delta_{11}, \delta_{12}, \delta_{13}, \delta_{21}, \delta_{22}, \delta_{23})$	
Logistic	(0.0057, 0.19, −0.38, 0.0322, 0.694)	(−0.392, −0.463, −0.465, −0.27, −0.415, −0.409)	
[sd]	[0.006, 0.052, 0.144, 0.137, 0.152]	[0.244, 0.214, 0.288, 0.225, 0.342, 0.314]	
Test H_0 vs H_1	For treatment vs. control	Wald statistic = 3.22 P-value = 0.14	
Test H_0 vs H_1	For consistency assessment	Wald statistic = 0.428 P-value = 0.972	
Global treatment effect	$\hat{\delta}_0 = -0.097$ (Given $\delta_0 = -0.13$)	95% confidence interval: [−0.36, 0.04]	
Goodness of fit	MSE:0.238		
	$(\beta_1, \beta_2, \beta_3, \beta_4, \beta_5)$	$(\delta_{11}, \delta_{12}, \delta_{13}, \delta_{21}, \delta_{22}, \delta_{23})$	λ
Robust Model 1	(0.0057, 0.179, −0.28, 0.002, 0.577)	(−0.704, −0.863, −0.858, −0.21, −0.383, −0.379)	0.132
[sd]	[0.041, 0.0668, 0.150, 0.156, 0.166]	[0.438, 0.448, 0.446, 0.40, 0.451, 0.493]	(0.041)
Test H_0 vs H_1	For treatment vs. control	Wald statistic = 14.4 P-value < 0.001	
Test H_0 vs H_1	For consistency assessment	Wald statistic = 0.15 P-value = 0.98	
Global treatment effect	$\hat{\delta}_0 = -0.44$ (Given $\delta_0 = -0.13$)	95% confidence interval: [−0.49, 0.0134]	
Goodness of fit	MSE:0.238		
	$(\beta_1, \beta_2, \beta_3, \beta_4, \beta_5)$	$(\delta_{11}, \delta_{12}, \delta_{13}, \delta_{21}, \delta_{22}, \delta_{23})$	
Robust Model 2	(−0.0022, 0.0633, −0.122, 0.0292, 0.231)	(−0.427, −0.457, −0.417, −0.282, −0.414, −0.357)	
[sd]	[0.006, 0.051, 0.134, 0.096, 0.137]	[0.22, 0.199, 0.263, 0.211, 0.305, 0.283]	
Test H_0 vs H_1	For treatment vs. control	Wald statistic = 15.5 P-value < 0.001	
Test H_0 vs H_1	For consistency assessment	Wald statistic = 1.67 P-value = 0.543	
Global treatment effect	$\hat{\delta}_0 = -0.11$ (Given $\delta_0 = -0.13$)	95% confidence interval: [−0.23, 0.12]	
Goodness of fit	MSE:0.229		

$\delta_{2s} - \delta_{1s}$ is used as the index of the regional treatment effect; δ_0 = global treatment effect.

favorably to the commonly used logistic model, and the statistical test for treatment homogeneity among regions can be considerably more powerful than that based on the logistic model when the true link deviates from the logistic link function or there is a significant non-linear term. We applied the

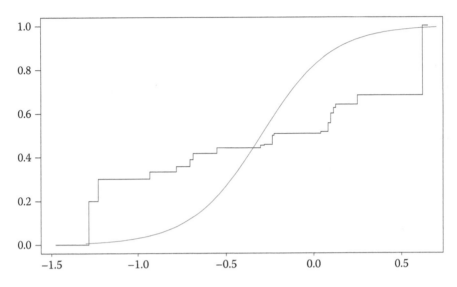

FIGURE 12.1
Estimated $\hat{F}$ vs. the logistic distribution in the breast cancer trial.

methods to the analysis of an MRCT for which partial real data is publicly available, and the robustness property of the model lends greater confidence to the regional treatment effect estimates and whether treatment differences among the multiple regions are consistent. Such analyses serve several purposes. They can be used (1) as a more robust model for treatment effect estimate; (2) as a sensitivity analysis; (3) to estimate parameters for the design of future MRCT. If one model is clearly better than the other, then the better model will be used as the final analysis model to determine treatment parameters. If the results from different models are similar, it would be a validation of the robustness of the simpler model. More robust estimates of the treat-effect sizes and variances can also be used to design the next MRCT. If an MRCT utilizes an adaptive design, the robust model may be applied to interim data following the adaptive procedure (say) a pre-specified group sequential boundary for assessing treatment effect and consistency. This may warrant further simulation studies on type I and II errors of the test statistic. The robust model can be utilized in practice in several ways. They can potentially be used for primary analysis as semi-parametric methods are gaining more recognition by a regulatory agency. In addition, they can be used for secondary and exploratory analysis that is needed to interpret trial results, or the sponsor may want to use the model to facilitate new MCRT protocol design and analysis. Our future research will develop model adequacy assessment measures, e.g., the Akaike information criterion, in the semiparametric model setting. In addition, it is known that even statistical tests based on parameter estimates from the common logistic regression may have type I errors deviating from the nominal 5% level, it may be worthwhile to perform further simulations under the specifics of a particular trial to confirm the type I error rate when using any non-linear models. We will then implement improvements in the R code for model estimation. Importantly, further applications of the approach to more MRCT data may reveal new insight on the regional treatment effects. The current R-codes for both models are available via the link: https://georgetown.box.com/s/ef5tzqv8mzokj4dkc764aaf3iw4njb6k

---

Acknowledgment

The authors thank the editors and reviewers for their constructive comments. Part of this work was the graduate research practicum project of the third author at Georgetown University.

References

Best, M.J., Chakravarti, N. 1990. Active set algorithms for isotonic regression; a unifying framework. *Mathematical Programming*; **47**: 425–439.

Bickel, P.J., Fan, J. 1996. Some problems on the estimation of unimodal densities. *Statistica Sinica*; **6**: 23–45.

Chen, J., Quan, H. (eds). 2016. *Multiregional Clinical Trials for Simultaneous Global New Drug Development*, CRC/Chapman Hall, Boca Raton, Florida.

Fedorov, V., Jones, B. The design of multicentre trials. 2005. *Statistical Methods in Medical Research*; **14**: 205–248.

Guo, H., Chen, J., Quan, H. 2016. Evaluation of local treatment effect by borrowing information from similar countries in multi-regional clinical trials. *Statistics in Medicine*; **35**: 671–684. doi: 10.1002/sim.6815.

Hung, H.M.J., Wang, S.J., O'Neill, R.T. 2010. Consideration of regional difference in design and analysis of multi-regional trials. *Pharmaceutical Statistics*; **9**: 173–178.

Kiefer, J., Wolfowitz, J. 1976. Asymptotic minimax estimation of concave and convex distribution functions. *Z. Wahrsch. Verw. Gebiete*; **34**: 73–85.

Lan, K.K.G., Pinheiro, J. 2012. Combined estimation of treatment effects under a discrete random effects model. *Statistics in Biosciences*; **14**: 235–244.

Lo, S.H. 1986. Estimation of a unimodal distribution function. *Annals of Statistics*; **14**: 1132–1138.

Qin, J., Garcia, T.P., Ma, Y., Tang, M.-X., Marder K., Wang, Y. 2014. Combining isotonic regerssion and EM algorithm to predict risk under monotonicity constraint. *Annals of Applied Statistics*; **8**: 1182–1208.

Quan, H., Li, M., Shih, J.W., Ouyang, S.P., Chen, J., Zhang, J., Zhao, P.L. 2013. Empirical shrinkage estimator for consistency assessment of treatment effects in multi-regional clinical trials. *Statistics in Medicine*; **32**: 1691–1706.

Quan, H., Mao, X., Chen, J., Shih, W.J., Quyang, S.P., Zhang, J., Zhao, P.L., Binkowitz, B. 2014. Multi-regional clinical trial design and consistency assessment of treatment effects. *Statistics in Medicine*; **33** (13): 2191–2205.

Senn, S.J. 1998. Some controversies in planning and analysing multi-centre trials. *Statistics in Medicine*; **17**: 1753–1765.

Stout, Q.F. 2008. Unimodal regression via prefix isotonic regression. *Computational Statistics and Data Analysis*; **53**: 289–297.

Wilks, S. S. 1938. The large-sample distribution of the likelihood ratio for testing composite hypotheses. *The Annals of Mathematical Statistics*; **9**: 60–62.

Yuan, A., Duan, C., Tan, M.T. 2021. Robust regression model for ordinal response. *Statistics and Its Interface*, 14:243–254. doi: 10.4310/20-SII631.

Yuan, A., Wang, S., Tan, M.T. 2018. Robust estimate of regional treatment effect in multi-regional randomized clinical trial in global drug development. *Statistics and Its Interface*; **11**: 129–139.

Yuan, A., Yang, C., Yu, S., Tan, M.T. 2021. Robust estimates of regional treatment effects in multiregional randomized clinical trials with semiparametric logistic model. *Pharmaceutical Statistics*, Published online 04 August 2021. https://doi.org/10.1002/pst.2157. 2021.

Yuan, A., Zhou, Y., Tan, M.T. 2021. Subgroup analysis with a nonparametric unimodal symmetric error distribution. *Communications in Statistics: Theory and Methods*, 50:17, 4000-4021, 2021. DOI: 10.1080/03610926.2019.1710754

13

Hierarchical Linear Models for Multi-Regional Clinical Trials

Seung-Ho Kang and Saemina Kim

13.1 Introduction

Recently, multi-regional clinical trials (MRCTs) have become popular in new drug development. MRCTs are conducted simultaneously across multiple geographical regions with a common protocol with the objective of world-scale development and approval of new drugs.

An important feature of MRCTs is that MRCTs data are naturally hierarchical in the sense that patients are nested within their own regions. This hierarchical structure makes the patients in the same region share some common intrinsic and extrinsic factors. This is an important potential concern of MRCTs, because these common factors may affect the treatment effect.

Recently, the ICH E17 guideline was issued to address various issues related to MRCTs (International Conference on Harmonization 2017). From a statistical point of view, an important issue is the development of appropriate statistical models for use in the planning and analysis of MRCT. MRCT is similar to meta-analysis in the sense that each region in MRCT corresponds to each study in meta-analysis and the primary analysis objective is to combine results from several regions (or studies). Therefore, meta-analysis models have been applied to MRCT. However, meta-analysis models have the following disadvantages.

1. As shown in Figure 13.1, MRCT data is structurally hierarchical, which means that the patient population consists of several regions and patients are nested within their own regions. An important concern with MRCT is that the treatment effect will vary from region to region because patients in the same region share similar

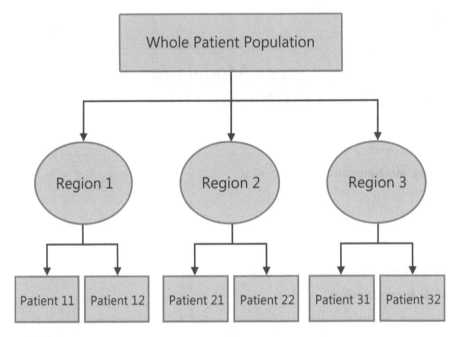

FIGURE 13.1
The hierarchical structure of multi-regional clinical trial data.

     intrinsic and extrinsic factors. Therefore, MRCT models should reflect this hierarchical structure properly, but the meta-analysis model does not.

2. In meta-analysis models, only regional summary values are used and the patient-level data are not used at all, although the patient-level data are available for the analysis of MRCTs. This will lead to the loss of information. Therefore, it is necessary to develop a statistical model that uses both patient-level data and region-level data.

3. In meta-analysis models, meta-regression analysis can be used to incorporate region-level covariates by using the mean values of the region-level covariates. However, it is not clear how to take into account patient-level covariates. We need to develop a new statistical model that patient-level data are adjusted clearly in patient levels.

In order to overcome these shortcomings, this chapter will address how to model MRCT data using the hierarchical linear model based on both patient-level data and region-level data.

13.2 Review of Statistical Models for MRCTs

In Section 13.2 we briefly review the statistical models for MRCTs which have been proposed so far. Let J represent the number of participating regions of MRCTs. Let Y_{ij} denote the continuous primary efficacy variable of the ith patient in the jth region. Using randomzaiton, patients are assigned to the test treatment group and placebo group with a 1:1 randomization ratio. For simplicity of presentation, let Y_{ij} denote the primary efficacy variable in the test treatment group in the jth region for $j = 1, 2, \cdots, J$ and it is assumed that

$$Y_{ij} \sim N(\mu_{Tj}, \sigma^2), \text{ for } i = 1, 2, \cdots, n_{Tj}.$$

Similarly, let Y_{ij} represent the primary efficacy variable in the placebo group in the jth region and it is assumed that

$$Y_{ij} \sim N(\mu_{Pj}, \sigma^2), \text{ for } i = n_{Tj} + 1, n_{Tj} + 2, \cdots, n_j.$$

The sample sizes of the test treatment group and the placebo group in the jth region are n_{Tj} and n_{Pj}, respectively, and the sample size of the jth region is $n_j = n_{Tj} + n_{Pj}$. The sample means of the primary efficacy variable in both the test treatment group and the placebo group in the jth region are denoted by

$$\bar{Y}_{Tj} = \frac{1}{n_{Tj}} \sum_{i=1}^{n_{Tj}} Y_{ij} \text{ and } \bar{Y}_{Pj} = \frac{1}{n_{Pj}} \sum_{i=n_{Tj}+1}^{n_j} Y_{ij}.$$

1. A fixed-effect model

   Let $\delta_j (=\mu_{Tj} - \mu_{Pj})$ represent the treatment effect in the jth region. Then a natural estimator of δ_j is the difference of two sample means obtained from the jth region. That is,

   $$\hat{\delta}_j = \bar{Y}_{Tj} - \bar{Y}_{Pj}.$$

   For fixed constants δ_j's, a fixed effect model assumes the following model for $\hat{\delta}_j$.

   $$\hat{\delta}_j = \delta_j + e_j, \text{ for } j = 1, 2, \cdots, J \tag{13.1}$$

where the error terms e_j's follow the normal distribution.

$$e_j \sim N\left(0, \ \sigma^2\left(\frac{1}{n_{Tj}} + \frac{1}{n_{Pj}}\right)\right).$$

Usually, it is assumed that $\delta_1 = \delta_2 = \ldots = \delta_J = \delta$. For a more detailed review of the fixed-effect model, please refer to Quan et al. (2013).

2. A continuous random effect model
   In a continuous random effect model, the true effect size is allowed to vary from region to region. Hung et al. (2010) proposed the following the continuous random effect model

$$\hat{\delta}_j = \delta_j + e_j, \ \text{ for } j = 1, 2, \ \cdots, J \tag{13.2}$$

where

$$\delta_j \sim N\left(\delta, \ \tau^2\right), \ e_j \sim N\left(0, \ \sigma^2\left(\frac{1}{n_{Tj}} + \frac{1}{n_{Pj}}\right)\right) \tag{13.3}$$

and τ^2 represents the between-region variance of the treatment effect.

3. A discrete random effect model
   In this model, the true regional treatment effects are treated as fixed parameters, not random variables that follow a distribution. On the other hand, the regional sample sizes are assumed to be random variables and follow a multinomial distribution (Lan and Pinheiro 2012). Liu et al. (2016) developed appropriate statistical procedures for MRCTs under this model. This model is not of interest here and will not be discussed further.

13.3 The Hierarchical Linear Model for MRCTs

In this section, we will build up a hierarchical linear model for MRCTs that employs both patient-level and region-level data. We will set up a level-1 model for patient-level data and a level-2 model for region-level data. First, Section 13.3.1 addresses the simplest hierarchical linear model when there are no patient-level covariates and no region-level covariates. Then, Section 13.3.2 deals with the hierarchical linear model, which includes patient-level covariates and region-level covariates. The hierarchical linear models described in Section 13.3 are also called the random coefficient models or meta-analysis using individual patient data.

13.3.1 When There Are No Patient-level Covariates and No Region-level Covariates

In this subsection we will consider the simplest case in which there are no patient-level covariates and no region-level covariates. The level-1 model includes only group indicator (X_{ij}) as follows.

$$Y_{ij} = \beta_{0j} + \beta_{1j} X_{ij} + r_{ij}, \quad r_{ij} \sim N(0, \sigma^2) \tag{13.4}$$

where Y_{ij} denotes the primary efficacy variable of the ith patient in the jth region and

$$X_{ij} = \begin{cases} 1 & \text{if test treatment } (i = 1, 2, \cdots, n_{Tj}) \\ 0 & \text{if placebo } (i = n_{Tj} + 1, n_{Tj} + 2, \cdots, n_j), \end{cases} \quad \text{for } j = 1, 2, \cdots, J \tag{13.5}$$

where $n_j = n_{Tj} + n_{Pj}$. In order to reflect that the value of the primary end-point may vary slightly from region to region due to intrinsic and extrinsic factors, the level-2 model assumes that only the slope β_{1j} includes a random variable (u_{1j}) and the intercept β_{0j} is a constant.

$$\beta_{0j} = \gamma_{00}, \ \beta_{1j} = \gamma_{10} + u_{1j}, \ u_{1j} \sim N(0, \ \tau^2), \ \text{for } j = 1, 2, \cdots, J. \tag{13.6}$$

Now we will describe the characteristics of the model in (13.4)–(13.6).

13.3.1.1 Relationship with the Fixed Effect Model

We consider the case of $\tau^2 = 0$ which is a special case of the model in (13.4)–(13.6). When $\tau^2 = 0$, the intercept (β_{0j}) and the slope (β_{1j}) are constants. As the primary response variable Y_{ij} does not depend on j, the treatment effect is constant regardless of regions. Then, the slope β_{1j} is estimated by the least square estimator. We can show easily that the least square estimator of the slope β_{1j} is the difference between the two sample means of the test treatment group and the placebo group in the jth region, because the independent variable X_{ij} is the indicator variable and takes on values of only zero or one,

$$\hat{\beta}_{1j} = \frac{S_{xy}}{S_{xx}} \equiv \frac{\sum_{i=1}^{n_j} (X_{ij} - \bar{X}_j)(Y_{ij} - \bar{Y}_j)}{\sum_{i=1}^{n_j} (X_{ij} - \bar{X}_j)^2} = \bar{Y}_{Tj} - \bar{Y}_{Pj} \tag{13.7}$$

where

$$\bar{X}_j = \frac{1}{n_j} \sum_{i=1}^{n_j} X_{ij}, \ \bar{Y}_j = \frac{1}{n_j} \sum_{i=1}^{n_j} Y_{ij}, \ \bar{Y}_{Tj} = \frac{1}{n_{Tj}} \sum_{i=1}^{n_{Tj}} Y_{ij}, \ \bar{Y}_{Pj} = \frac{1}{n_{Pj}} \sum_{i=n_{Tj}+1}^{n_j} Y_{ij}.$$

As a result, we can see that $\hat{\beta}_{1j}$ in (13.7) is equal to $\hat{\delta}_j$ in the fixed effect model in Section 13.1. In other words, $\bar{Y}_{Tj} - \bar{Y}_{Pj}$ is denoted as $\hat{\beta}_{1j}$ in this subsection and $\hat{\delta}_j$ in Section 13.1. For convenience, in this chapter, $\hat{\beta}_{1j}$ is called β-notation, and $\hat{\delta}_j$ is called δ-notation. Substituting (13.4) into (13.7) yields the following.

$$\hat{\beta}_{1j} = \bar{Y}_{Tj} - \bar{Y}_{Pj} \quad = \frac{1}{n_{Tj}} \sum_{i=1}^{n_{Tj}} (\beta_{0j} + \beta_{1j} + r_{ij}) - \frac{1}{n_{Pj}} \sum_{i=n_{Tj}+1}^{n_j} (\beta_{0j} + 0 + r_{ij})$$

$$= \beta_{1j} + \frac{1}{n_{Tj}} \sum_{i=1}^{n_{Tj}} r_{ij} - \frac{1}{n_{Pj}} \sum_{i=n_{Tj}+1}^{n_j} r_{ij} \quad \equiv \delta_j + e_j$$

by defining

$$\delta_j = \beta_{1j} \text{ and } e_j = \frac{1}{n_{Tj}} \sum_{i=1}^{n_{Tj}} r_{ij} - \frac{1}{n_{Pj}} \sum_{i=n_{Tj}+1}^{n_j} r_{ij}.$$

From (13.6), when $\tau^2 = 0$, the following relationship holds between β-notation and δ-notation.

$$\delta_j = \beta_{1j} = \gamma_{10}.$$

That is, the treatment effect is the same regardless of regions. Furthermore, the error term has the following distribution.

$$e_j = \frac{1}{n_{Tj}} \sum_{i=1}^{n_{Tj}} r_{ij} - \frac{1}{n_{Pj}} \sum_{i=n_{Tj}+1}^{n_j} r_{ij} \sim N\left(0, \ \sigma^2\left(\frac{1}{n_{Tj}} + \frac{1}{n_{Pj}}\right)\right).$$

Therefore, the models in (13.4)–(13.6) are more general models for which the fixed effect model in Section 13.1 is a special case.

13.3.1.2 Relationship with the Continuous Random Effect Model

Let us consider the relationship between the continuous random effect model in Section 13.1 and the model in (13.4)–(13.6). The distribution of the primary response variable of a patient in the test treatment group ($X_{ij} = 1$) is

$$Y_{ij} = \beta_{0j} + \beta_{1j} + r_{ij} \sim N(\beta_{0j} + \gamma_{10}, \tau^2 + \sigma^2).$$

The distribution of the primary response variable of a patient in the placebo group ($X_{ij} = 0$) is

$$Y_{ij} = \beta_{0j} + r_{ij} \sim N(\beta_{0j}, \sigma^2).$$

Then we can obtain the distribution of the estimator ($\hat{\delta}_j$) of the treatment effect in the jth region as follows.

$$\hat{\delta}_j = \frac{1}{n_{Tj}} \sum_{i=1}^{n_{Tj}} Y_{ij} - \frac{1}{n_{Pj}} \sum_{i=n_{Tj}+1}^{n_j} Y_{ij} \sim N\left(\gamma_{10}, \tau^2 + \sigma^2\left(\frac{1}{n_{Tj}} + \frac{1}{n_{Pj}}\right)\right). \quad (13.8)$$

where

$$Var(\hat{\delta}_j) = \frac{1}{n_{Tj}^2}\left(\sum_{i=1}^{n_{Tj}} Var(Y_{ij}) + 2\sum_{i,k=1\ i\ne k}^{n_{Tj}} Cov(Y_{ij}, Y_{kj})\right) + \frac{1}{n_{Pj}^2}\sum_{i=n_{Tj}+1}^{n_j} Var(Y_{ij})$$

$$= \frac{1}{n_{Tj}^2}\left[n_{Tj}(\tau^2 + \sigma^2) + 2\frac{n_{Tj}(n_{Tj}-1)}{2}\tau^2\right] + \frac{1}{n_{Pj}^2}n_{Pj}\sigma^2$$

$$= \tau^2 + \sigma^2\left(\frac{1}{n_{Tj}} + \frac{1}{n_{Pj}}\right).$$

Putting $\delta = \gamma_{10}$, we can see that the continuous random effect model in Section 13.1 is the same as the model in (13.4)–(13.6). The only difference is that the random effect model in Section 13.1 is based on the region-level summary values, while the models in (13.4)–(13.6) employ the patient-level data.

13.3.1.3 The Combined Model Is a Mixed Effect Model

By substituting equation (13.6) into (13.4), we obtain the following combined model.

$$Y_{ij} = \gamma_{00} + \gamma_{10}X_{ij} + u_{1j}X_{ij} + r_{ij}. \tag{13.9}$$

The model in (13.9) is a mixed-effect model because it includes both the fixed effects (γ_{00}, γ_{10}) and a random effect (u_{1j}). The model in (13.9) is different from the ordinary linear regression model because both u_{1j} and r_{ij} are random variables.

The distribution of the primary response variable of a patient in the test treatment group ($X_{ij} = 1$) is

$$Y_{ij} = \gamma_{00} + \gamma_{10} + u_{1j} + r_{ij} \sim N(\gamma_{00} + \gamma_{10},\ \tau^2 + \sigma^2).$$

Because patients in the test treatment group share u_{1j} in common, they are correlated. Their correlation coefficient is computed in Section 13.3.1.4. Hence, it is important to understand that the proposed hierarchical linear model is completely different from the regular regression model. Because the distribution of primary response variable of a patient in the placebo group ($X_{ij} = 0$) is given by

$$Y_{ij} = \gamma_{00} + r_{ij} \sim N(\gamma_{00},\ \sigma^2),$$

the treatment effect becomes $\gamma_{10}(=\gamma_{00} + \gamma_{10} - \gamma_{00})$, which is constant regardless of region. Therefore, the parameter γ_{10} represents the overall treatment effect.

This model assumes that the variance of the treatment group is greater than that of the placebo group. If the variance of the placebo group is larger, then we can code $X_{ij} = 1$ for the placebo group and the treatment effect becomes $-\gamma_{10}(=\gamma_{00} - (\gamma_{00} + \gamma_{10}))$.

13.3.1.4 The Correlation Coefficient Between Two Patients in the Same Region

The mixed-effect model in (13.9) has two random variables (u_{1j} and r_{ij}). The variance (τ^2) of the random effect (u_{1j}) denotes the between-region variability and the variance (σ^2) of the error term (r_{ij}) represents the within-region variability.

It is well known that a random effect produces a positive correlation coefficient between the two observations that have the same random effect. Such correlation is usually called the intra-class correlation coefficient, but it would be more appropriate to call it the intra-region correlation coefficient in the MRCT setting. We can compute the intra-region correlation coefficient as follows.

$$
\begin{aligned}
Var\,(Y_{ij}) \quad &= \quad Var\,[E\,(Y_{ij}\,|\,u_{1j})] + E\,[Var\,(Y_{ij}\,|\,u_{1j})] \\
&= \quad Var\,(\gamma_{00} + \gamma_{10}X_{ij} + u_{1j}X_{ij}) + E\,(\sigma^2) \\
&= \quad X_{ij}^2\tau^2 + \sigma^2 \\
Cov\,(Y_{ij},\,Y_{kj}) \quad &= \quad Cov\,(E\,[Y_{ij}\,|\,u_{1j}],\,E\,[Y_{kj}\,|\,u_{1j}]) + E\,[Cov\,(Y_{ij},\,Y_{kj}\,|\,u_{1j})] \\
&= \quad Cov\,(\gamma_{00} + \gamma_{10}X_{ij} + u_{1j}X_{ij},\,\gamma_{00} + \gamma_{10}X_{kj} + u_{1j}X_{kj}) + E\,[0] \\
&= \quad X_{ij}X_{kj}\tau^2
\end{aligned}
$$

$$
\begin{aligned}
Corr\,(Y_{ij},\,Y_{kj}) \quad &= \quad \frac{X_{ij}X_{kj}\tau^2}{[(X_{ij}^2\tau^2+\sigma^2)(X_{kj}^2\tau^2+\sigma^2)]^{1/2}} \ \text{for } i \neq k, \ j = 1,\,2,\cdots,J. \\
&= \quad \begin{cases} \tau^2/(\tau^2+\sigma^2), & \text{if two observations are from the treatment group} \\ 0, & \text{otherwise.} \end{cases}
\end{aligned}
$$

This is one of the most important results in this chapter. An important concern with MRCT is that intrinsic and extrinsic factors may affect the treatment effect. What statistical results do intrinsic and extrinsic factors produce in the mixed effect model in (13.9)? The answer to this question is as follows.

1. Patients in the test treatment group in the same region have a positive intra-region correlation coefficient. This is intuitively appealing because they share a common intrinsic and extrinsic factor and such common factor produces similar responses to the test treatment. A common intrinsic and (or) extrinsic factor in the mixed effect model in (13.9) is denoted by u_{1j}.

2. Although a positive intra-region correlation coefficient exists, the treatment effect of the mixed effect model in (13.9) is constant regardless of the region when there are no patient-level and region-level covariates.

The reason that there is no correlation between the two patients in the placebo group is just the coding scheme in (13.5). If we change the coding scheme as follows

$$
X_{ij} = \begin{cases} 1 & \text{if test treatment } (i = 1,\,2,\,\cdots,\,n_{Tj}) \\ -1 & \text{if placebo } (i = n_{Tj} + 1,\,n_{Tj} + 2,\cdots,n_j), \end{cases} \ \text{for } j = 1,\,2,\cdots,J.
$$

$$(13.10)$$

where $n_j = n_{Tj} + n_{Pj}$, then the same intra-region correlation coefficient exists in both the test treatment group and the placebo group:

$$Corr\,(Y_{ij},\,Y_{kj}) \;=\; \begin{cases} \tau^2/(\tau^2 + \sigma^2), & \text{if two observations are from same group} \\ -\tau^2/(\tau^2 + \sigma^2), & \text{if two observations are from different groups.} \end{cases}$$

On the other hand, this new coding scheme in (13.10) slightly changes the mean and variance of the distribution of $\hat{\delta}_j$, so that they are different from those in (13.3). Therefore, for simplicity of presentation, we will keep using the coding scheme in (13.5).

13.3.2 When There Are Patient-level Covariates and Region-level Covariates

Intrinsic and extrinsic factors may affect the treatment effect in MRCTs (International Conference on Harmonization 1998; International Conference on Harmonization 2017). There are two ways to incorporate intrinsic and extrinsic factors into the hierarchical linear models for MRCTs. The first one is the region-level error term (u_{ij}). Section 13.3.1.4 described that the region-level error term did not affect the overall treatment effect, although it produced a positive correlation coefficient between two patients in the test treatment group in the same region. The second ones are region-level covariates. In this subsection, we will look at how region-level covariates affect the overall treatment effect. To this end, it is necessary to first distinguish between patient-level covariates and region-level covariates.

Patient-level covariates are unique values for each individual patient, including the age, height, and weight of the patients. In other words, even if patients belong to the same region, they usually have a different value of patient-level covariates. On the other hand, if all patients in the same region have the same value, then such covariates are region-level covariates. Medical practice is an example of region-level covariates. For example, in the PLATO trial, the aspirin dosage influenced the treatment effect significantly (Carroll and Fleming 2013). If the aspirin dosage used was different for each patient and if such information was used, then the aspirin dosage will be a patient-level covariate. On the other hand, if there is only information on the average aspirin dosage used for each region and the average aspirin dosage is equally applied to all patients in the same region, the average aspirin dosage will be the region-level covariate.

In this section, for convenience of explanation, let us consider the case where there exists only one patient-level covariate (X_{2ij}) and only one region-level covariate (W_j).

13.3.2.1 *When Only the Intercept Includes a Region-level Covariate*

Both a treatment group indicator (X_{1ij}) and a patient-level covariate (X_{2ij}) are included in a level-1 model. For example, a patient-level covariate (X_{2ij}) can be age or blood pressure.

$$Y_{ij} = \beta_{0j} + \beta_{1j} X_{1ij} + \beta_{2j} X_{2ij} + r_{ij}, \quad r_{ij} \sim N(0, \sigma^2) \tag{13.11}$$

where

$$X_{1ij} = \begin{cases} 1 & \text{if test treatment } (i = 1, 2, \cdots, n_{Tj}) \\ 0 & \text{if placebo } (i = n_{Tj} + 1, n_{Tj} + 2, \cdots, n_j), \end{cases} \quad \text{for } j = 1, 2, \cdots, J.$$

A level-2 model assumes that a region-level covariate (W_j) is included only in the intercept, not in the slope.

$$\beta_{0j} = \gamma_{00} + \gamma_{01} W_j, \quad \beta_{1j} = \gamma_{10} + u_{1j}, \quad \beta_{2j} = \gamma_{20}, \quad u_{1j} \sim N(0, \tau^2). \tag{13.12}$$

We obtain the following combined model by substituting (13.12) to (13.11).

$$Y_{ij} = \gamma_{00} + \gamma_{01} W_j + \gamma_{10} X_{1ij} + \gamma_{20} X_{2ij} + u_{1j} X_{1ij} + r_{ij}.$$

The distribution of the primary response variable of a patient in the treatment group ($X_{ij} = 1$) is

$$Y_{ij} = \gamma_{00} + \gamma_{01} W_j + \gamma_{10} + \gamma_{20} X_{2ij} + u_{1j} + r_{ij}$$
$$\sim N(\gamma_{00} + \gamma_{01} W_j + \gamma_{10} + \gamma_{20} X_{2ij}, \ \tau^2 + \sigma^2). \tag{13.13}$$

The distribution of the primary response variable of a patient in the placebo ($X_{ij} = 0$) is

$$Y_{ij} = \gamma_{00} + \gamma_{01} W_j + \gamma_{20} X_{2ij} + r_{ij} \sim N(\gamma_{00} + \gamma_{01} W_j + \gamma_{20} X_{2ij}, \ \sigma^2). \tag{13.14}$$

It is important to note that the difference between two population means in (13.13) and (13.14) is γ_{10} and does not depend on j. Therefore, the treatment effect (γ_{10}) is constant regardless of regions.

The hierarchical linear model in (13.11) and (13.12) incorporates the intrinsic and extrinsic factors using the region-level error term (u_{1j}) and the region-level covariate (W_j). Although the intrinsic and extrinsic factors are fully reflected in the hierarchical linear model in these two ways, the overall treatment effect is constant across regions. Therefore, the hierarchical linear model in (13.11) and (13.12) is a very useful model that allows us to estimate the overall treatment effect while fully incorporating the intrinsic and extrinsic factors.

13.3.2.2 When the Slope Includes a Region-level Covariate

A level-1 model is the same as the model in (13.11). A level-2 model assumes that a region-level covariate (W_j) is included only in the slope, not in the intercept.

$$\beta_{0j} = \gamma_{00}, \; \beta_{1j} = \gamma_{10} + \gamma_{11}W_j + u_{1j}, \beta_{2j} = \gamma_{20}, \; u_{1j} \sim N(0, \; \tau^2). \quad (13.15)$$

Combining (13.11) and (13.15) leads to the following model.

$$Y_{ij} = \gamma_{00} + \gamma_{10}X_{1ij} + \gamma_{11}W_jX_{1ij} + \gamma_{20}X_{2ij} + u_{1j}X_{1ij} + r_{ij}. \quad (13.16)$$

The product term of the treatment indicator (X_{1ij}) and the region-level covariate (W_j) in the model (13.16) indicates an interaction between treatments and regions. That is, if a region-level covariate is included in the slope, then the treatment effect varies from region to region if $\gamma_{11} \neq 0$. In other words, the intrinsic and extrinsic factors expressed as regional covariates affect the overall treatment effect. It is important to test whether or not $\gamma_{11} = 0$. If $\gamma_{11} \neq 0$ and it is expected to be clinically meaningful in the design stage, it is not appropriate to employ MRCTs for new drug development. If $\gamma_{11} \neq 0$ and the value of γ_{11} is judged to be clinically meaningful in the analysis stage after execution of MRCTs, it is meaningless to estimate the overall treatment effect. In this case, the treatment effect can be estimated separately for each region through the model.

Therefore, the hierarchical linear model in (13.11) and (13.15) is a very useful model that allows us to investigate whether or not the intrinsic and (or) extrinsic factors expressed as region-level covariates affect the treatment effect.

13.3.2.3 The General Case

The hierarchical linear model described in Sections 13.3.2.1 and 13.3.2.2 can be extended to more general cases in order to include several patient-level covariates and region-level covariates (Raudenbush and Bryk 2002). The level-1 model with Q patient-level covariates can be described by

$$Y_j = X_j\boldsymbol{\beta}_j + r_j, \; r_j \sim N(0, \; \sigma^2I) \quad (13.17)$$

where Y_j is an n_j dimensional vector of the primary efficacy variables of the patients in the jth region, X_j is n_j by $(Q + 1)$ level-1 design matrix, β_j is a $(Q + 1)$ dimensional vector of unknown parameters, r_j is a n_j dimensional vector of random errors and I is n_j by n_j identity matrix. The level-1 model is the traditional multiple regression model.

The level-2 model assumes that β_j can be modeled as a linear model of F region-level covariates.

$$\beta_j = W_j \gamma + u_j, \ u_j \sim N(0, \ T) \tag{13.18}$$

where W_j is $(Q + 1)$ by F level-2 design matrix, γ is an F dimensional vector of fixed effects, u_j is a $(Q + 1)$ dimensional vector of level-2 errors or random effects, and T is an arbitrary $(Q + 1)$ by $(Q + 1)$ variance-covariance matrix.

The following combined model can be obtained by substituting equation (13.18) into (13.17).

$$Y_j = X_j W_j \gamma + X_j u_j + r_j. \tag{13.19}$$

The model in (13.19) is a well-known linear mixed-effects model, and the statistical inference for the fixed effects γ and variance components T have been studied extensively (Demidenko 2005; McCulloch et al. 2008). Specifically, statistical inference for the fixed effects γ is usually based on the asymptotic normality of the maximum likelihood estimators. Because the overall treatment effect and the interaction between treatments and regions are elements of the fixed effects γ, statistical inference for these two parameters can be conducted using the asymptotic normality of the maximum likelihood estimators.

13.4 Testing the Overall Treatment Effect

In this section, we consider only the hierarchical linear model without patient and regional level covariates in (13.4) and (13.6) for simplicity of explanation. The hypotheses for the overall treatment is given by

$$H_0: \gamma_{10} = 0 \text{ versus } H_1: \gamma_{10} \neq 0.$$

When the hierarchical linear model includes either patient-level covariates or region-level covariates, the statistical inference can be conducted based on the maximum likelihood estimator, as mentioned in Section 13.3.2.3. In this section, we will examine the type I error rates of the following three test methods.

13.4.1 Use of the Sample Ratio as Weights When the True Model Is the Hierarchical Model

We consider the maximum likelihood estimator of the overall treatment effect (γ_{10})

$$\hat{\delta}_M = \sum_{j=1}^{J} \frac{n_j}{N} \hat{\delta}_j$$

where $N = \sum_{j=1}^{J} n_j$ denotes total sample size of overall regions. This estimator is a weighted average of $\hat{\delta}_j$'s where the sample ratios (n_j/N) are used as weights. After some algebra, we can obtain the distribution of $\hat{\delta}_M$

$$\hat{\delta}_M \sim N\left(\gamma_{10}, \frac{1}{N^2} \sum_{j=1}^{J} n_j^2\left(\tau^2 + \sigma^2\left(\frac{1}{n_{Tj}} + \frac{1}{n_{Pj}}\right)\right)\right),$$

because $\hat{\delta}_j$'s follow the normal distribution from (13.8) and $\hat{\delta}_M$ is a linear combination of $\hat{\delta}_j$'s. By Slutsky's theorem, the following test statistic (S_r) converges in distribution to the standard normal distribution under the null hypothesis as $n_j \to \infty$ for all $j = 1, 2, \cdots, J$.

$$S_r = \frac{\hat{\delta}_M}{\sqrt{\frac{1}{N^2} \sum_{j=1}^{J} n_j^2\left(\hat{\tau}^2 + \hat{\sigma}^2\left(\frac{1}{n_{Tj}} + \frac{1}{n_{Pj}}\right)\right)}}$$

where $\hat{\tau}^2$ and $\hat{\sigma}^2$ are some consistent estimators of τ^2 and σ^2, respectively.

However, the asymptotic distribution of the test statistic (S_r) may not be accurate due to the following reasons.

i. In order for $\hat{\tau}^2$ to be a consistent estimator of τ^2, we need the number of regions (J). However, the number of regions (J) may not be large enough in most MRCTs.

ii. Quan et al. (2014) and Sidik and Jonkman (2007) showed that many estimators of τ^2 underestimated τ^2, which makes the type I error inflated. Therefore, it is very important to choose an accurate estimator of τ^2.

In this study, we have conducted simulation studies on the empirical type I error rates for the following three kinds of estimators of τ^2.

a. The restricted maximum likelihood estimator (REML)

b. The empirical Bayes estimator

c. Model error variance estimator with variance component (MVvc) type estimator

For more information on these three estimators, see Sidik and Jonkman (2007).

13.4.2 Use of the Sample Ratio as Weightings and Incorrectly Assuming $\tau^2 = 0$ In spite of $\tau^2 >> 0$

In this sub-section, we investigate the empirical type I error rates for testing the overall treatment effect when the fixed effect model is incorrectly assumed $(\tau^2 = 0)$, although the true model is the hierarchical linear model $(\tau^2 > 0)$. Let S_f denote the test statistic when the fixed effect model is incorrectly assumed. In other words, the test statistic (S_f) is the same as S_r except incorrectly assuming $\tau^2 = 0$ in spite of $\tau^2 > 0$. The specific form of the test statistics (S_f) is given as follows.

$$S_f = \frac{\hat{\delta}_M}{\sqrt{\frac{1}{N^2} \sum_{j=1}^{J} n_j^2 \hat{\sigma}^2 \left(\frac{1}{n_{Tj}} + \frac{1}{n_{Pj}} \right)}}$$

Regardless of the value of J, there are many consistent estimators of σ^2 such as MLE (maximum likelihood estimator) and REML, as long as $n_j \to \infty$ for all $j = 1, 2, \cdots, J$. Therefore, even if the value of J is small, by Slutsky's theorem, the test statistic (S_f) converges in distribution to the standard normal distribution under the null hypothesis as $n_j \to \infty$ for all $j = 1, 2, \cdots, J$.

13.4.3 Use of Inverse-variance Weight of $\hat{\delta}_j$

The way of constructing the minimum variance unbiased estimator among linear combinations of $\hat{\delta}_j$'s is to use the reciprocal of the variance (Δ_j) of $\hat{\delta}_j$ as weights because $\hat{\delta}_j$'s are unbiased estimators of the overall treatment effect (γ_{10}). However, an estimator of Δ_j is used in real practice, because Δ_j includes unknown parameters. The following estimator of the overall treatment effect (γ_{10}) is obtained.

$$\hat{\delta}_L = \frac{\sum_{j=1}^{J} \hat{\Delta}_j^{-1} \hat{\delta}_j}{\sum_{k=1}^{J} \hat{\Delta}_k^{-1}}$$

where

$$\hat{\Delta}_j = \hat{\tau}^2 + \hat{\sigma}^2 \left(\frac{1}{n_{Tj}} + \frac{1}{n_{Pj}} \right).$$

Because it is extremely difficult to find the exact distribution of $\hat{\delta}_L$, we need to find a limiting distribution of $\hat{\delta}_L$. For this purpose, we need to assume not only $n_j \to \infty$ for all $j = 1, 2, \cdots, J$, but also $J \to \infty$. This is because $\hat{\tau}^2$ should be a consistent estimator of τ^2. Under these two assumptions, we have

$$\hat{\Delta}_j \xrightarrow{p} \tau^2 \text{ and } \hat{\delta}_j \xrightarrow{d} N(\gamma_{10}, \tau^2).$$

Finally, we obtain

$$\sqrt{J} (\hat{\delta}_L - \gamma_{10}) \xrightarrow{d} N(0, \tau^2) \text{ as } n_j \to \infty \text{ for all } j = 1, 2, \cdots, J \text{ and } J \to \infty.$$

Based on this limiting distribution we can construct the following new test statistics (S_w).

$$S_w = \frac{\hat{\delta}_L}{\sqrt{\hat{\tau}^2/J}}.$$

The distribution of the test statistic (S_w) may not be close to the standard normal distribution because the number of regions (J) is small in most MRCTs. Simulation studies in Section 13.4 show that the empirical type I error rates are inflated in many cases.

13.5 Simulation Studies

The empirical type I error rates of S_r, S_f, and S_w maybe not be close to the nominal level because the value of J is small and the estimation of τ^2 is not accurate. Because we want to know which of the two causes affects the empirical type I error rates, we will consider the following two additional statistics in this study.

$$S_r^0 = \frac{\hat{\delta}_M}{\sqrt{\frac{1}{N^2} \Sigma_{j=1}^J n_j^2 \left(\tau^2 + \sigma^2 \left(\frac{1}{n_{T_j}} + \frac{1}{n_{P_j}}\right)\right)}} \quad S_w^0 = \frac{\hat{\delta}_L}{\sqrt{\tau^2/J}}$$

The denominators of these two statistics include unknown parameters (σ^2, τ^2), not estimators. Therefore, these two statistics cannot be test statistics in a strict sense. However, we will also investigate these two statistics in order to examine the effect of the small value of J, regardless of the accuracy of the estimation of τ^2 and σ^2.

Tables 13.1 and 13.2 show the empirical type I error rates for the equal allocation cases and the unequal allocation cases, respectively. In each case, 2000 simulations were conducted and each treatment group was allocated with an equal sample size. The REML estimators of τ^2 and σ^2 were computed by PROC MIXED and the empirical Bayes estimators were computed by PROC NLMIXED in SAS. The MVvc was computed directly using the closed formula in Sidik and Jonkman (2007). When we estimated the values of τ and σ using PROC MIXED and PROC NLMIXED, zero was rarely

TABLE 13.1

The empirical type I error rates in cases of equal sample sizes $\alpha = 2.5\%$ method-d=estimation method of τ^2

(j, n_j)	(τ, σ)	Method	S_r	S_r^0	S_f	S_w	S_w^0
(3,600)	(2,10)	REML	10.85	2.60	22.85	15.62	3.60
		EB	2.95	2.60	22.85	4.65	3.60
		MVvc	8.75	2.60	22.85	15.25	3.60
(3,600)	(1,10)	REML	6.90	2.20	11.55	16.33	7.05
		EB	5.41	2.20	11.57	9.78	7.05
		MVvc	6.15	2.20	11.55	22.60	7.05
(3,600)	(0.5,10)	REML	3.40	2.65	4.70	17.26	16.75
		EB	3.70	2.65	4.75	9.97	16.75
		MVvc	3.25	2.65	4.70	28.20	16.75
(5,400)	(2,10)	REML	8.45	2.80	19.45	14.88	4.40
		EB	1.55	2.80	19.51	3.08	4.40
		MVvc	5.85	2.80	19.45	11.35	4.40
(5,400)	(1,10)	REML	5.50	3.00	8.60	19.22	8.45
		EB	3.70	3.00	8.50	9.96	8.45
		MVvc	4.25	3.00	8.60	21.00	8.45
(5,400)	(0.5,10)	REML	3.15	2.80	3.95	21.33	20.20
		EB	3.05	2.80	3.91	11.02	20.20
		MVvc	2.60	2.80	3.95	27.80	20.20

TABLE 13.2

The empirical type I error rates in cases of unequal sample sizes allocation = sample sizes allocated to each region, A=(1000,600,200) B=(600,600,400,200,200), method=estimation method of τ^2, α = 2.5%

J	Allocation	(τ,σ)	Method	S_r	S_r^0	S_f	S_w	S_w^0
3	A	(2,10)	REML	11.05	2.80	25.85	15.98	4.20
			EB	3.10	2.80	25.81	3.45	4.20
			MVvc	7.80	2.80	25.85	15.70	4.20
3	A	(1,10)	REML	7.10	2.55	13.20	15.88	7.65
			EB	5.65	2.55	13.26	7.91	7.65
			MVvc	6.20	2.55	13.20	22.00	7.65
3	A	(0.5,10)	REML	3.85	2.75	5.60	17.53	16.75
			EB	4.31	2.75	5.71	7.77	16.75
			MVvc	3.40	2.75	5.60	26.85	16.75
5	B	(2,10)	REML	8.75	2.60	20.65	14.26	4.55
			EB	1.80	2.60	20.70	2.85	4.55
			MVvc	5.65	2.60	20.65	11.30	4.55
5	B	(1,10)	REML	5.75	2.55	10.35	19.85	9.25
			EB	4.25	2.55	10.30	10.23	9.25
			MVvc	4.70	2.55	10.35	20.75	9.25
5	B	(0.5,10)	REML	3.45	2.80	4.40	21.66	19.05
			EB	3.00	2.80	4.30	10.43	19.05
			MVvc	2.95	2.80	4.40	27.30	19.05

obtained as the estimated value. The frequency of zero values increased with smaller τ. When $\hat{\tau} = 0$, the test statistic of S_w is not defined. We calculated the empirical type I error rate by removing all such cases.

Tables 13.1 and 13.2 show us the following results.

i. The empirical type I error rates of S_r^0 are close to 2.5%. This implies that the empirical type I error rates of S_r can be close to 2.5% even when the value of J is either 3 or 5, as long as the variance of $\hat{\delta}_M$ can be estimated accurately.

ii. The empirical type I error rates of S_r in which τ^2 is estimated by the empirical Bayes estimator is closer to the nominal level than for the REML and MVvc methods. However, the performance of S_r with the empirical Bayes estimator is not very satisfactory because its empirical type I error rates are greater than the nominal level in some cases. Further research is needed on a new estimation method that can estimate τ^2 more accurately when the number of regions has a value as small as 3 and 5.

iii. The empirical type I error rates of S_f are much higher than the nominal level in many cases. For example, when $(J, n_j) = (3,600)$ and $\sigma = 10$, and the empirical Bayes estimator is used for the estimation of τ^2, the empirical type I error rates of S_f are 4.75%, 11.57%, and 22.85% at $\tau = 0.5$, 1.0, and 2.0, respectively. Furthermore, the empirical type I error rate increases as does the value of τ. That is, the type I error rate is inflated if the positive between-region variability ($\tau^2 > 0$) is ignored.

iv. The empirical type I error rates of S_w^0 are much higher than the nominal level in many cases. It implies that the type I error rate of S_w^0 is inflated when the value of J is either 3 or 5, regardless of the estimation method of τ^2. Because the performance of S_w^0 is poor, we do not even need to discuss S_w anymore.

13.6 Discussion

Hierarchical linear models for MRCTs proposed in this paper have the following advantages and features.

1. As seen in Figure 13.1 the data from MRCTs are naturally hierarchical. The hierarchical linear models can incorporate this hierarchical structure.

2. An important feature of this hierarchical structure is that the patients in the same region share some common intrinsic and extrinsic factors. This is an important potential concern of MRCTs, because these common factors may affect the treatment effect.

3. There are two ways to incorporate intrinsic and extrinsic factors into the hierarchical linear models for MRCTs. The first one is the region-level error term (u_{ij}) in (13.6). The second ones are region-level covariates (W_j) introduced in Section 13.3.2.

   a. The region-level error term
      Section 13.3.1.4 showed that the region-level error term (u_{ij}) produced a positive correlation coefficient between two patients in the test treatment group in the same region. This is intuitively appealing because they share a common intrinsic and extrinsic factor and such common factor produces similar responses to the test treatment. Nevertheless, Section 13.3.1.4 also described that the region-level error term did not affect the overall treatment effect if there are no region-level covariates.

b. The region-level covariates
    If region-level covariates are included only in the intercept, the treatment effect is constant across region. Hence, the intrinsic and extrinsic factors expressed as region-level covariates do not affect the treatment effect as shown in Section 13.3.2.1. On the other hand, if region-level covariates are included only in the slope, the treatment effect may vary from region to region if the value of γ_{11} is not equal to zero. Therefore, the hierarchical linear model in Section 13.3.2.2 allows us to investigate whether or not the intrinsic and (or) extrinsic factors expressed as region-level covariates affect the treatment effect.

4. The hierarchical linear models include the fixed effect model and the continuous random effect model in Section 13.2 as special cases. The advantage of the hierarchical linear model is that it can include patient-level data while including the existing models as special cases. Therefore, hierarchical linear models open up a way to develop more general models.

5. The hierarchical linear models include patient-level covariates in the level-1 model and region-level covariates in the level-2 model, respectively. Section 13.3.2.2 showed that the region-level covariates may make the treatment effect vary from region to region, while the patient-level covariates do not. This can clearly indicate that patient-level covariates and region-level covariates play different roles for modeling MRCTs data and facilitate clear communication between statisticians and clinicians.

6. The hierarchical linear model proposed in this study divides observed variations into intra-regional variation and inter-regional variation. The intra-regional variability represents the inter-patient variability due to, e.g., age and personal health status and the inter-regional variation represent between-regional variability due to region-specific characteristics. In other words, the hierarchical linear model represents MRCT data as clustered data. This is appealing in the sense that the patients in the same region share some common intrinsic and extrinsic factors.

7. So far, many methods such as single imputation, multiple imputations, MMRM (mixed model for repeated measurements), and pattern mixture models have been proposed and studied for dealing with missing values (Little and Rubin 2019). All of these methods were based on patient-level data. Because the proposed hierarchical linear model in this study is based on patient-level data, we can directly apply these methods. On the other hand, because the fixed effect model and the continuous random effect

model in Section 13.2 are based solely on region-level summary data, it is not clear how to handle missing values.

8. We have investigated statistical methods for testing the overall treatment effect in Section 13.4. After demonstrating the efficacy of a test treatment in all participating regions, the second objective of MRCTs is to examine the consistency of the treatment effect across regions. Quan et al. (2013) proposed a way of assessing the consistency of treatment effects across regions based on the empirical shrinkage estimator for individual regions. Their empirical shrinkage estimator is a weighted average of $\hat{\delta}_j$ and $\hat{\delta}_M$, which are based on the continuous random-effect model in Section 13.2. Because the hierarchical linear model proposed in this paper has the same $\hat{\delta}_j$ and $\hat{\delta}_M$, the consistency of treatment effects can be evaluated using the method of Quan et al. (2013) when there are no patient-level covariates and no region-level covariates. The shrinkage estimator of $\boldsymbol{\beta}_j$ is given by (Raudenbush and Bryk 2002, p 49)

$$\hat{\boldsymbol{\beta}}_j^* = \hat{\boldsymbol{\Lambda}}_j \hat{\boldsymbol{\beta}}_j + (\boldsymbol{I} - \hat{\boldsymbol{\Lambda}}_j) \boldsymbol{W}_j \hat{\boldsymbol{\gamma}}$$

where

$$\hat{\boldsymbol{\Lambda}}_j = \hat{\boldsymbol{T}} (\hat{\boldsymbol{T}} + \hat{\sigma}^2 (\boldsymbol{X}_j^t \boldsymbol{X}_j)^{-1})^{-1}.$$

9. An important future study is to develop statistical procedures for assessing the consistency of treatment effects across regions based on the shrinkage estimator when either patient-level covariates or region-level covariates exist.

10. This chapter deals with two-level hierarchical linear models that consist of patient-level models and region-level models. We will be able to extend two-level hierarchical linear models to three-level hierarchical linear models. Possible examples of three-level hierarchical linear models are (region, nation, patient), (pooled region, region, patient), (region, patient, repeated measures within patients). Research on this issue is ongoing.

11. Recently, Park and Kang (2021a) extended the hierarchical linear models to hierarchical generalized linear models so that the response variables can follow the exponential family, such as the Binomial distribution and the Poisson distribution. And Park and Kang (2021b) studied the statistical properties of the random slope hierarchical linear model for MRCTs.

References

Carroll, K.J., and Fleming, T.R. 2013. Statistical evaluation and analysis of regional interactions: the PLATO trial case study. *Statistics in Biopharmaceutical Research* 5:91–101.

Demidenko, E. 2005. Mixed Models: Theory and Applications. Hoboken, New Jersey: Wiley.

Hung, H.J., Wang, S.J., and O'Neill, R.T. 2010. Consideration of regional difference in design and analysis of multi-regional trials. *Pharmaceutical Statistics* 9:173–178.

International Conference on Harmonization. 1998. Tripartite guidance E5, ethnic factors in the acceptability of foreign data.

International Conference on Harmonization. 2017. General principles for planning and design of multi-regional clinical trials.

Lan, K.G., and Pinheiro, J. 2012. Combined estimation of treatment effects under a discrete random effects model. *Statistics in Biosciences* 4:235–244.

Little, R.J.A., and Rubin, D.B. 2019. Statistical Analysis with Missing Data, 3rd edn. Hoboken, New Jersey: Wiley.

Liu, J.T., Tsou, H.H., Gordon Lan, K.K., Chen, C.T., Lai, Y.H., Chang, W.J., Tzeng, C.S., and Hsiao, C.F. 2016. Assessing the consistency of the treatment effect under the discrete random effects model in multiregional clinical trials. *Statistics in Medicine* 35:2301–2314.

McCulloch, C.E., Searle, S.R., and Neuhaus, J.M. 2008. Generalized, Linear, and Mixed Models, 2nd edn. Hoboken, New Jersey: Wiley.

Park, J. and Kang, S.H. 2021a. Hierarchical generalized linear models for multi-regional clinical trials. *Statistics in Biopharmaceutical Research*. 10.1080/19466315 .2020.1862702

Park, C. and Kang, S.H. 2021b. Random Intercept Hierarchical Linear Model for Multi-regional Clinical Trials. Submitted.

Quan, H., Li, M., Shih, W.J., Ouyang, S.P., Chen, J., Zhang, J., and Zhao, P.L. 2013. Empirical shrinkage estimator for consistency assessment of treatment effects in multi-regional clinical trials. *Statistics in Medicine* 32:1691–1706.

Quan, H., Mao, X., Chen, J., Shih, W.J., Ouyang, S.P., Zhang, J., Zhao, P.L., and Binkowitz, B. 2014. Multi-regional clinical trial design and consistency assessment of treatment effects. *Statistics in Medicine* 33:2191–2205.

Raudenbush, S.W., and Bryk, A.S. 2002. Hierarchical Linear Models: Applications and Data Analysis Methods, 2nd edn. Thousand Oaks: SAGE Publications.

Sidik, K., and Jonkman, J.N. 2007. A comparison of heterogeneity variance estimators in combining results of studies. *Statistics in Medicine* 26:1964–1981.

14

Local Treatment Effect Estimation by Borrowing Information from Similar Regions in Multi-Regional Clinical Trials

Hua Guo, Joshua Chen, and Hui Quan

14.1 Introduction

Multiregional clinical trials (MRCTs) enable simultaneous submission of marketing authorization applications and allow to evaluate the potential heterogeneity of treatment effects across regions or subpopulations due to differences in intrinsic and extrinsic factors. As specified in ICH E17 guideline (ICH E5, 1998; ICH E17, 2018), the primary reason for performing MRCT is to evaluate the overall treatment effect based on the overall population; in addition, the guideline explicitly specifies that the Statistical Analysis Plan (SAP) should describe statistical methods for estimating and reporting treatment effects and measures of their uncertainty for individual regions. It is impossible to have a sufficient sample size to obtain the local significance of regional treatment effect as this is against the purpose of MRCT. If the sample size in a region is small, the estimation of the local treatment effect may need to borrow information from the other regions based on similarity in intrinsic or extrinsic factors. ICH E17 guideline states that "If the sample size in a region is so small that the estimates of effect will likely be unreliable, the use of other methods should be considered, including the search for options for additional pooling of regions based on commonalities, or borrowing information from other regions or pooled regions using an appropriate statistical model."

Empirical shrinkage estimates described by Quan et al. (2013) may be considered to obtain estimates for individual countries that improve efficiency by incorporating data from the other countries. This method treats all other countries equally thus ignoring similarity to the country of interest.

In this chapter, the focus will be to lay out methods for estimating country-specific treatment effects and borrow more information from similar countries and less from dissimilar countries. We firstly review fixed and random effect models for estimating local regional treatment effects. Then we describe a statistical framework of borrowing information from the other regions based on a tree structure, defined by the similarity between regions (Guo et al., 2016). Tree structures can be constructed from either continuous or categorical similarity scale. One example of a continuous similarity scale is the HDI recommended by the PhRMA MRCT working group (Tanaka et al., 2011; United Nations Development Program). HDI is a useful composite measure that takes into account numerous extrinsic factors on a national basis, defined as a function of adult literacy, gross domestic product, and educational levels. On the other hand, if a limited number of regions with members of countries in each region are pre-defined, information can be borrowed from countries in the same region based on the tree constructed from the categorical similarity scale. A clinical example is provided to illustrate the proposed methods.

14.2 Method

14.2.1 Fixed Effects Models

We assume that the endpoint follows a normal distribution. Let β_i indicate the true treatment effect for country i, and denote the number of countries in a multi-regional trial by I. Then the estimates of treatment effect for country i follows

$$d_i \mid \beta_i \sim N\left(\beta_i, \, v_i\right), \text{ for } i = 1, \, \cdots, \, I, \qquad (14.1)$$

where $v_i = \frac{2\sigma^2}{N_i}$ is the corresponding standard error, σ^2 is the variance of the endpoint, and N_i is the sample size for each treatment group in country i.

For the fixed effects model, β_is are fixed parameters. A commonly used estimate of the overall treatment effect $\hat{r}$ is a weighted average of individual d_is

$$\hat{r} = \sum_{i=1}^{I} w_i d_i,$$

where weight $w_i = \frac{N_i}{\sum_{i=1}^{I} N_i}$. The estimate of treatment effect $\hat{\beta}_i$ for individual country i utilizes data from country i only and ignores information from the other countries. When the data are unbalanced across the I countries, the sample size for country i might be small which results in that d_i might be unreliably associated with large variability.

14.2.2 Star-Tree Random Effects Models

In the random effect model proposed by Hung et al. (2010), β_is are random variables and are assumed independently and identically follow a normal distribution

$$\beta_i | \gamma, \tau \sim N(\gamma, \tau). \tag{14.2}$$

This model is defined as a star-tree random effect model as shown in Figure 14.1. Each β_i is assumed to be exchangeable and the model ignores the relationship between countries. For example, treatment effects for the United States (US) and Canada might be more similar by sharing common extrinsic factors than treatment effects in Africa. The random effect model does not incorporate the relationship among countries, instead, it assumes individual true treatment effects are from the same parent distribution. Assume γ, τ, and σ are known the posterior estimate of β_i is in the form of

$$\tilde{\beta}_i | \gamma, \tau, \sigma^2 = f_i d_i + (1 - f_i)\gamma, \text{ with } f_i = \tau/(\tau + v_i), \tag{14.3}$$

$$\text{var}(\tilde{\beta}_i) = \tau(1 - f_i)$$

Thus, this estimator borrows information from the other countries through shrinking towards the overall treatment effect γ. Quan et al. (2013) discuss the application of a similar model to obtain shrinkage estimates to quantify regional treatment effects allowing γ to be estimated.

In terms of the other estimating methods, there are three approaches to obtain the estimates of β_i when γ, τ and σ are unknown. The first is based on full maximum likelihood (ML) estimation of γ, τ and σ^2 and empirical Bayes (EB) estimation of β_i; the second is based on restricted maximum likelihood (REML) estimates of τ and σ^2 and EB estimation of γ and β_i; the third is to use a fully Bayesian approach to ensure inference is based on the joint distribution of all unknowns given only the data. When the number of units I is large, EB-ML and EB-REML work well. However, when I is small and especially when the data are unbalanced, i.e., with a very small sample size for some units, there are distinct advantages in using a fully Bayesian

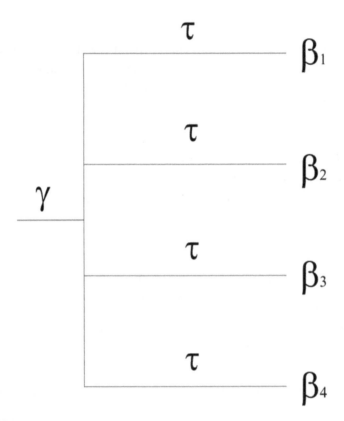

FIGURE 14.1
A star tree with edge length of τ to connect four children (β_1, β_2, β_3, β_4) and the parent root γ for the traditional random-effects model $\beta_i \mid \gamma$, $\tau \sim N(\gamma, \tau)$.

approach. Inference about any unknown completely takes into account uncertainty about the other unknowns as recommended by Raudenbush and Bryk (2002, pages 399–435).

14.2.3 Tree-Based Method with a Continuous Similarity Scale

In this section, we lay out a general statistical framework in which the similarity among regions (sample units) is described on a continuous scale. We first construct a relationship tree based on the continuous similarity scale. Then we allow local treatment effects to be random effects and to follow the Gaussian process $[\beta(t), \ t \geq 0]$ along the constructed tree to incorporate tree relationship into the modeling. Thereby we borrow more information through shrinking towards the common parent in estimating the local treatment effects for closely related countries than for distantly related countries. The PhRMA MRCT group proposes to use HDI as one

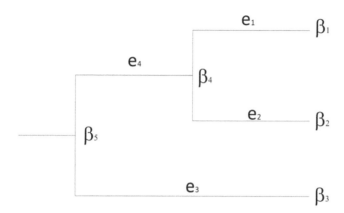

FIGURE 14.2
An example tree using hierarchical clustering method with average linkage.

example of a continuous similarity scale (Tanaka et al., 2011, United Nations Development Program). The other types of continuous similarity scores can be used to construct trees as well when applicable.

We illustrate the proposed model using a simple example with three sample units. Suppose there are three regions where unit 1 and unit 2 are neighbors with a closer relationship relative to unit 3 as shown in Figure 14.2. Branches lengths are provided along the branches (edges) in the tree. True treatment effects are $\beta_{\text{tip}} = (\beta_1, \beta_2, \beta_3)'$, and β_1 and β_1 are neighbors sharing a parent β_4; β_3 *and* β_4 have a common parent, the root β_5.

The raw estimate of treatment effects, $\mathbf{d} = (d_1, d_2, d_3)'$, given true treatment effects, follows

$$\left. \begin{pmatrix} d_1 \\ d_2 \\ d_3 \end{pmatrix} \right| \begin{pmatrix} \beta_1 \\ \beta_2 \\ \beta_3 \end{pmatrix} \sim N\left(\begin{pmatrix} \beta_1 \\ \beta_2 \\ \beta_3 \end{pmatrix}, \mathbf{V} \right), \tag{14.4}$$

$$\text{with } \mathbf{V} = \begin{bmatrix} v_1 & 0 & 0 \\ 0 & v_2 & 0 \\ 0 & 0 & v_3 \end{bmatrix}.$$

Further, assume β_1 and β_2 given the parent β_4 follow

$$\left. \begin{pmatrix} \beta_1 \\ \beta_2 \end{pmatrix} \right| \beta_4 \sim N\left(\begin{pmatrix} \beta_4 \\ \beta_4 \end{pmatrix}, \lambda \begin{bmatrix} e_1 & 0 \\ 0 & e_2 \end{bmatrix} \right), \tag{14.5}$$

and

$$\begin{pmatrix} \beta_3 \\ \beta_4 \end{pmatrix} \Bigg| \beta_5 \sim N\left(\begin{pmatrix} \beta_5 \\ \beta_5 \end{pmatrix}, \lambda \begin{bmatrix} e_3 & 0 \\ 0 & e_4 \end{bmatrix} \right). \tag{14.6}$$

Thus

$$\begin{pmatrix} \beta_1 \\ \beta_2 \\ \beta_3 \end{pmatrix} \Bigg| \beta_5 \sim N\left(\begin{pmatrix} \beta_5 \\ \beta_5 \\ \beta_5 \end{pmatrix}, \lambda T \right), \tag{14.7}$$

$$\text{with } T = \begin{bmatrix} e_1 + e_4 & e_4 & 0 \\ e_4 & e_2 + e_4 & 0 \\ 0 & 0 & e_3 \end{bmatrix}$$

Here, only β_5 is a fixed parameter; β_1, β_2, β_3 and β_4 are random effects.

We restrict an equal length from root to each tip. Therefore, $e_1 = e_2$, and $e_3 = e_1 + e_4$. The variance is proportional to branch length e_i with a scale parameter λ. To exam prior covariance matrix T for random effects β_{tip}, correlation of β_1 and β_2 given β_5 is $\frac{e_4}{e_4 + e_1}$, but correlation among β_1 and β_3 given β_5 is 0. The tree constructed in this way ensures children who share a parent are more correlated than children without sharing a common parent in T. When all three children share a common parent (i.e., $e_4 = 0$), the model becomes a conventional random effect model. The general framework for the model is described in the following subsections as proposed by Guo et al. (2016).

14.2.3.1 Representing the Relationship Among Sample Units in a Tree

The relationship among the sample units is described using a rooted tree $G = (V, \mathcal{E})$ with vertex-set V and edge-set $\mathcal{E}$, which is a directed graph containing no cycles but with branches connected. All vertices, except one called the "root," connect via an edge to exactly one parent vertex, restricting $|V| = |\mathcal{E}| - 1$. We index vertices and edges such that vertex i is incident to its parent vertex $pa(i)$ via edge i. The vertex-set V of a tree relating I sampling units consists of I vertices generally called tips. For a bifurcating tree (any parent node can give rise to only two children), the tips relate to each other through $I - 2$ internal vertices and one root vertex. Connecting the vertices are edges that make up $\mathcal{E}$ with known edge weights $e_1, \cdots, e_{2I-2}$ for a bifurcating tree, regularly called branch lengths.

To fully use the continuous HDI information, we use hierarchical clustering techniques to construct a rooted ultrametricity tree to characterize the relationship between sample units. After the construction, node-set $\mathcal{V}$ and edge-set $\mathcal{E}$ are both available using the HDI information.

14.2.3.2 Brownian Diffusion on Trees

Brownian diffusion is a continuous-time Markov process with continuous sample paths. To apply the process along with tree $\mathcal{G}$, we view the diffusion as acting on the random effects $\boldsymbol{\beta}$ along the edges. Along an edge, diffusion occurs as a stationary independent increment with a mean 0 and a variance scaled by the edge weight. Further, given the realization of the process at a parent vertex, diffusion along the descendent edges is independent. We consider normally distributed increments to characterize the diffusion process.

To make the model explicit, let $\boldsymbol{\beta} = (\beta_1, \cdots, \beta_{I+J}, \beta_{root})$ where the first I terms correspond to the random effects for the sampling units $\boldsymbol{\beta}_{tip}$, the last term represents the root vertex, and there are J internal nodes. Here, the only β_{root} is a parameter and all the other β_i s are random effects with

$$\beta_i \mid \beta_{pa(i)} \sim N(\beta_{pa(i)}, \lambda e_i), \tag{14.8}$$

where $i = 1, \cdots, I + J$, $pa(i)$ is the parent node of node i and λ is a positive number. Therefore, we posit that random tip effects β_is follow a Brownian diffusion process (BDP) over the tree $\mathcal{G}$, and denote the process as

$$\boldsymbol{\beta}_{tip} = (\beta_1, \cdots, \beta_I) \sim BDP(\mathcal{G}, \beta_{root}, \lambda). \tag{14.9}$$

The joint distribution of the proposed model for a given tree in a Bayesian framework can be written as

$$\begin{aligned} P(\mathbf{D}, \boldsymbol{\beta}_{tip}, \Theta, \Phi) &= P(\Theta)P(\mathbf{D} \mid \boldsymbol{\beta}_{tip}, \Theta)P(\Phi)P(\boldsymbol{\beta}_{tip} \mid \Phi) \\ &= P(\Theta)P(\mathbf{D} \mid \boldsymbol{\beta}_{tip}, \Theta)P(\beta_{root})P(\lambda)P(\boldsymbol{\beta}_{tip} \mid \beta_{root}, \lambda), \end{aligned} \tag{14.10}$$

where

$$P(\boldsymbol{\beta}_{tip} \mid \Phi) = P(\boldsymbol{\beta}_{tip} \mid \beta_{root}, \lambda) = \prod_{i=1}^{I+J} P(\beta_i \mid \beta_{pa(i)}, \lambda),$$

$\mathbf{D}$ denotes the observed data. There are two parts for the joint distribution: 1) $P(\mathbf{D} \mid \boldsymbol{\beta}_{tip}, \Theta)$ describes how the observed data $\mathbf{D}$ relate with $\boldsymbol{\beta}_{tip}$, probably through, e.g., ANCOVA, ANOVA or other models, and Θ is the collection of parameters for modeling the observed data. 2) $P(\boldsymbol{\beta}_{tip} \mid \Phi)$ describes the relationship among $\beta_i s$., and $\Phi = \{\beta_{\text{root}}, \lambda\}$ is a collection of ancillary parameters for modeling β_{tip}.

A rooted tree graph **G** is used to describe the relationships across the sampling units. Units with similar scores are classified into the same level of the tree and share a common parent. By allowing local treatment effects to be random effects and following a BDP along the tree, (1) the estimates of descendent child nodes shrink towards a common parent as shown at the beginning of Section 14.2.3. The child borrows more "information" from the neighbors sharing the same parent; (2) in our model construction, we ensure the children sharing the same parent are more correlated. Through both approaches, we get more similar estimates for children sharing the same parent.

This framework is a generalization of the comparative method, contrasts method, popular in evolutionary biology, and recent repeated measurement extensions for normally distributed observations (Guo et al., 2007).

We used the tree structure to capture the prior information to model the relationships between sample units. A tree provides a more intuitive description of prior information and a layout of relationships among sample units than a complicated covariance matrix in the case of a large number of regions. The BDP model could be easily extended to multiple dimension random effect vectors along the tree by replacing the scale constant λ with a positive definite scale matrix Ω; however, the covariance matrix in such a situation will be too complicated to write out for multiple-dimensional random effects.

14.2.4 Two-Level, Multi-Fork Tree Model for Categorical Similarity

In this section, we extend the BDP model from a continuous similarity scale to a categorical scale. One example of a categorical scale is to define geographic regions with a few country members. A two-level model can be proposed to incorporate the membership information into a tree to obtain the treatment effect estimate of a country by borrowing more information from members in the same region. In such a model, a country is a level 1 unit that is located within a certain Level 2 unit, such as a region with a few countries as members.

We denote the treatment effect from country i in region r by β_{ir}. At level 1, the random effect β_{ir}, is drawn mutually independent from the same normal distribution with a common mean $\beta_{region(r)}$ and a variance t_1 in the form of

$$\beta_{ir} \sim N\left(\beta_{region(r)}, t_1\right), \tag{14.11}$$

where $i = 1, \cdots, I_r$, and I_r is the number of members in region r.

At level 2, the treatment effect for region r, $\beta_{region(r)}$, mutually independently follows a normal distribution with an overall mean β_{root} and a variance t_2

$$\beta_{region(r)} \sim N(\beta_{root}, \ t_2). \tag{14.12}$$

To make the model more flexible, one can further relax the model by letting each region r to have its own variance $t_{region(r)}$

$$\beta_{ir} \sim N(\beta_{region(r)}, \ t_{region(r)}) \tag{14.13}$$

However, it is difficult to get an accurate estimate of $t_{region(r)}$ when the number of units in region r is not large enough. For region r with only one member, only the region-level model is available and described as $\beta_r \sim N(\beta_{root}, \ t_2)$.

The proposed two-level model could be viewed as a BDP over a two-level, multi-fork tree without a drifting factor. In contrast to the tree for the continuous similarity with known edge lengths, the edge lengths in the tree for a two-level model are unknown parameters and should be estimated from data because there is no prior information for branch lengths. Only membership is available as the prior information. The estimated branch lengths are t_1 or $t_{region(r)}$ (the within-region and between-unit variance) at level 1 and t_2 (the between-region variance) at level 2.

The local estimates of treatment effects borrow more information from the members in the same region by shrinking towards a common parent. Given the β_{root}, the members within the same region share a common covariance t_2, and the members from different regions have covariance 0. This results that the treatment effect for a sample unit β_{ir} has a larger correlation with those of the members in the same region group relative to members from the other regions.

14.2.5 Implementation

We use Bayesian inference to fit the data. The advantage of Bayesian inference is that it takes account of the uncertainty of all these parameters. We use Open BUGS (Lunn et al., 2009) to construct Markov chain Monte Carlo (MCMC) chains that generate random samples from model posterior distributions. Based on the posterior distribution of β_{tip}, we produce estimates $\hat{\beta}_{tip}$ of treatment effects for individual units. The convergence for multiple chains can be assessed using Gelman-Rubin scale reduction factors that compare variation in the sampled parameter values within and between chains with values under 1.1 indicating convergence (Gelman et al., 2013).

14.3 Trial Example

We illustrate the application of the BDP model for both continuous similarity scale HDI and categorical similarity scale using the same diabetes clinical trial example (Guo et al., 2016). The example evaluates one diabetic drug vs placebo in A1C change from baseline at Week 24 in patients with type 2 Diabetes Mellitus (T2DM). A total of 340 patients from 18 countries were included in the analysis population with varied sample sizes n_i for country i with $i = 1, \cdots, 18$.

The primary efficacy endpoint Y changed from baseline in Hemoglobin A1C (A1C) at week 24. An analysis of covariance (ANCOVA) model was used to estimate the treatment effect, adjusting for baseline A1C and pharmacotherapy status at screening (on or not on an anti-hyperglycemic agent). Let X_1 indicate intercept term, X_2 as treatment indicator, X_3 as baseline A1C, X_4 as prior pharmacotherapy status (binary variable). Let treatment effect β_i be a random effect, diffusing along the tree through BDP as described in Section 14.2.3. ANCOVA model then takes the form of

$$y_{ij} = x1_{ij}\alpha_1 + x2_{ij}\beta_i + x3_{ij}\alpha_2 + x4_{ij}\alpha_3 + \varepsilon$$

Where $\varepsilon \sim N(0, \sigma^2)$, α_1, α_2 and α_3 are fixed effects. This model is analogous with the ANCOVA model with a country-by-treatment interaction term (i.e., traditional subgroup analysis) in that it estimates the treatment effects for individual countries; the improvement over the traditional subgroup analysis is that it allows treatment effects for closely related countries to be strongly correlated by allowing Brownian diffusion over the relationship tree either based on a continuous similarity scale tree or categorical similarity scale as shown below.

1. As one example for a continuous similarity scale, the similarity in HDI among countries is available (Tanaka et al., 2011) and provided by the country in the second and third panels in Figure 14.3. Therefore, we first constructed a tree using the hierarchical clustering method with arithmetic mean linkage. A relationship tree using HDI is depicted in Figure 14.3 left panel. This algorithm constructs a rooted tree based on a pairwise similarity matrix from a HDI distance matrix. At each step, the nearest two clusters are combined into a higher-level cluster. The distance between any two clusters A and B is taken to be the average of all distances between pairs of subjects "x" in A and "y" in B, i.e., the mean distance between elements of each cluster. Then random effects will be in the form of

$$(\beta_1, \cdots, \beta_I) \sim BDP(\mathcal{G}, \beta_{\text{root}}, \lambda).$$

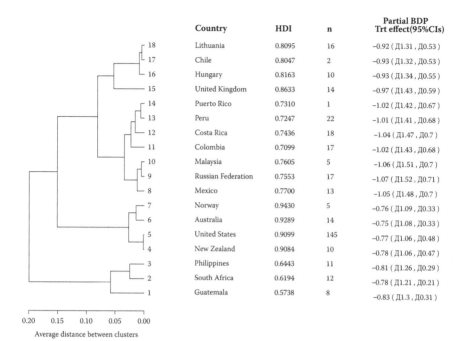

FIGURE 14.3
A constructed hierarchical tree based on human development (HDI) index from 18 countries (the left three panels) and the treatment-effect estimates by country using a partial BDP model along the constructed HDI tree (the rightmost panel).

We name this model as a partial random-effect BDP model. A partial random-effect BDP model could be further extended to a full random effect BDP model by letting the effects of confounding covariates be random effects instead of fixed effects and follow BDP over the tree.

2. A two-level multi-fork tree model was used to fit data from 18 countries in 5 regions of the same clinical trial described in Section 14.2.4. The membership of each region is listed in Table 14.1. The random effects will follow Equations 14.12 and 14.13.

3. For comparison, we evaluated the star-tree random-effect model in the example by letting β_is independently and identically follow a normal distribution

$$\beta_i \sim N(\beta_{root}, \tau^2).$$

We use Bayesian inference to fit the data. The non-informative priors are used for α_1, α_2, α_3, β_{root}, λ and τ.

In Table 14.1, countries were grouped into regions on a categorical scale using regional information as prior information instead of using a continuous scale (e.g., HDI) to cluster countries. The top panel in Table 14.1

TABLE 14.1

Patient accounting by country and summary of results in a change from baseline in A1C (%) at Week 24 using two-levelmulti-fork tree model compared with Star-tree model

Region	Country	n_i	Traditional subgroup analysis Mean (95% CI)	Star-treeRandom-effect Model Mean (95% CI)	Two-levelMulti-fork tree Model Mean (95% CI)
US	United States	145	−0.69(−1.00, −0.38)	−0.76(−1.04 , −0.47)	−0.74(−1.03, −0.44)
Latin	Guatemala	8	−0.93(−1.95, 0.08)	−0.92(−1.41, −0.45)	−0.96(−1.48, −0.43)
	Mexico	13	−1.10(−1.86, 0.35)	−0.96(−1.44, −0.54)	−0.99(−1.49, −0.53)
	Colombia	17	−1.01(−1.81, −0.21)	−0.93(−1.41, −0.50)	−0.97(−1.47, −0.49)
	Costa Rica	18	−1.48(−2.21, −0.74)	−1.06(−1.61, −0.64)	−1.09(−1.65, −0.64)
	Peru	22	−0.85(−1.63, −0.09)	−0.89(−1.34, −0.45)	−0.93(−1.41, −0.44)
	Puerto Rico	1	−0.68(−2.91, 1.55)	−0.90(−1.47, −0.36)	−0.95(−1.54, −0.31)
	Chile	2	−1.15(−3.38, 1.07)	−0.92(−1.50, −0.40)	−0.97(−1.57, −0.36)
EU	Norway	5	−0.53(−2.11, 1.05)	−0.88(−1.41, −0.34)	−0.88(−1.59, −0.01)
	Russian Federation	17	−1.66(−2.39, −0.94)	−1.11(−1.7, −0.67)	−1.25(−1.96, −0.7)
	United Kingdom	14	−1.18(−2.04, −0.33)	−0.97(−1.48, −0.53)	−1.03(−1.66, −0.47)
	Hungary	10	−1.22(−2.24, −0.21)	−0.96(−1.50, −0.50)	−1.03(−1.71, −0.42)
	Lithuania	16	−0.53(−1.29, 0.24)	−0.81(−1.24, −0.33)	−0.79(−1.34, −0.12)
Asia	Philippines	11	−1.11(−2.24, 0.01)	−0.94(−1.48, −0.47)	−0.91(−1.62, −0.29)
	Malaysia	5	−0.83(−2.38, 0.73)	−0.91(−1.45, −0.38)	−0.84(−1.58, −0.1)
	New Zealand	10	−1.29(−2.21, −0.38)	−0.99(−1.52, −0.55)	−0.97(−1.68, −0.61)
	Australia	14	−0.41(−1.17, 0.35)	−0.79(−1.21, −0.27)	−0.69(−1.22, −0.05)
Africa	South Africa	12	−0.08(−1.09, 0.92)	−0.77(−1.23, −0.18)	−0.69(−1.18, 0.05)
Region Effect					
Latin	–	81	–	–	−0.96(−1.36, −0.59)
EU		62	–	–	−0.94(−1.40, −0.52)
Asia		40	–	–	−0.84(−1.29, −0.40)
Overall		340	−0.86(−1.10, −0.62)*	−0.92(−1.21, −0.63)	−0.83(−1.22, −0.43)

* The overall treatment effect is estimated based on a fixed–effect model.

provides the estimates for individual countries based on traditional sub-group analysis, star-tree random-effect model, and two-level multi-fork tree model. Treatment effect estimates for regions with multiple members using a two-level multi-fork tree model are provided in the second panel of Table 14.1. The fourth panel in Figure 14.3 shows the estimations of treatment effect based on the partial random-effect BDP model over the HDI tree.

Treatment effects of individual countries in the two-level tree model shrink towards the regional effect with narrower confidence intervals relative to those in the traditional subgroup analysis model.

Compared with the traditional subgroup model, the estimates of local country treatment effects in star-tree, two-level multi-fork tree, and partial BDP models have narrower confidence intervals.

There are three observations when comparing results from the traditional subgroup model and the partial BDP model.

1. There are four larger clusters based on the constructed HDI tree: cluster 1 (Lithuania, Chile, Hungary, UK), cluster 2 (Puerto Rico, Peru, Costa Rica, Colombia, Malaysia, Russian Federation, and Mexico), cluster 3 (US, New Zealand, Norway, and Australia), cluster 4 (Philippines, South Africa, Guatemala).

2. The estimates of local country treatment effects appear similar within the same cluster. For example, the US and New Zealand are closely related in the HDI tree, the treatment effect estimates for both countries are similar; it is not the case for the star-tree random effect model, the estimates and 95% CIs are −0.76% (−1.04%, −0.47%) and −0.99% (−1.52%, −0.55%) for the US and New Zealand, respectively.

3. For the country with a larger sample size, such as the US, the estimate of treatment effect using a partial random effect BDP model is similar to that in the star tree random-effect model; for the country with a smaller sample size, such as New Zealand, Australia, or Norway, the estimates of treatment effects borrow more information from the neighborhoods defined by the tree.

By incorporating tree information and borrowing information from the neighborhood defined by a tree, the point estimates of treatment effects in the partial random effect model shrink together; the confidence intervals tend to be narrower compared with the star-tree random effect.

When comparing the estimates of local country treatment effects between star-tree and two-level multi-fork tree, we observe that the estimates of country treatment effects within the same region tend to shrink towards the regional treatment effect, especially for countries with small sample sizes, such as Malaysia, Chile, etc. This aligns with our expectation that the point estimates of treatment effects borrow information from the neighborhood defined by the two-level multi-fork tree.

14.4 Discussion

In this chapter, we summarize methods for estimating local treatment effects in an MRCT, with a focus on borrowing information from the neighborhoods. The neighborhood is defined by a tree built from the similarity score on a continuous scale or a categorical scale. By letting treatment effects from sample units following a BDP along the tree, we demonstrated that the local treatment effect estimate borrows more information from units that are similar but less from units that are different. A unit with a smaller sample size also borrows more information from the others than a unit with a larger sample size because the prior process $P(\beta_{tip} | \beta_{root}, \lambda)$ contributes more to the inference of the local treatment effect.

HDI is recommended from the PhRMA MRCT working group (Tanaka et al., 2011) as one useful composite continuous similarity score that takes into account numerous extrinsic factors on a national basis. Geographic region is chosen as one example of the categorical similarity score. Other approaches, either using different tree-building methods or based on other similarity scales relying on intrinsic or extrinsic factors, may be used in the proposed methods. Regardless, a similarity scale that determines how much information to borrow from each country should be pre-specified before data unblinding.

To check model misspecification by evaluating the impact of changes to the tree on the estimation of treatment effects, we simplified the detailed bifork tree in Figure 14.3 to a simple 4-cluster tree. Results derived from these two trees are similar. This suggests that slight modification on the tree will not substantially affect the estimation of country treatment effects. This phenomenon offers some simplicity in practice. Once a continuous similarity score is selected, one can construct a hierarchical tree without struggling much to define regions and still get robust country treatment effects.

The idea depicted here can be easily generalized to non-linear models. As examples for illustration, we can first derive country-level log odds ratios for a logistic regression model or the country-level log hazard ratios for survival analysis. We then apply the tree model described in Equation 14.9 to these country-level estimates of treatment effects.

Our objective is to provide one approach to estimate the country-specific treatment effect for each local country with information from the country of interest and borrow more information from similar countries and less from dissimilar countries. The proposed method is able to estimate the treatment effect for the local country and overall treatment effect simultaneously. The method belongs to random-effects models. As discussed by others (Quan et al., 2013), compared to the fixed effects model, the random-effects model taking into account between-country variability requires a relatively larger sample size for the overall treatment effect evaluation but provides much more generalizable trial results. One may still use fixed-effects to estimate the overall treatment effect with a reasonable overall sample size, and then to use the proposed method to estimate the country-specific treatment effect, especially for those countries with a small sample size by borrowing information from the similar neighborhood defined by intrinsic or extrinsic factors. Further theoretical and computational comparisons among these models as well as the interpretations of the corresponding trial results are worth further research.

References

Gelman A., Carlin J.B., Stern H.S., Dunson D.B., Vehtari A., and Rubin D.B. 2013. *Bayesian Data Analysis*. Chapman and Hall, New York.

Guo H., Weiss R.E., Gu X., and Suchard M.A. 2007. Time squared: Repeated measures on phylogenies. *Molecular Biology and Evolution* 24(2): 352–362.

Guo H., Chen J., and Quan H. 2016. Evaluation of local treatment effect by borrowing information from similar countries in multi-regional clinical trials. *Statistics in Medicine* 35: 671–684.

Hung H.M.J., Wang S.J., and O'Neill R.T. 2010. Consideration of regional difference in design and analysis of multi-regional trials. *Pharmaceutical Statistics* 9: 173–178.

ICH International Conference on Harmonization Tripartite Guidance E5: Ethnic Factor in the Acceptability of Foreign Data. The US Federal Register. 1998; 83: 31790–31796.

ICH International Conference on Harmonization Guidance E17 in 2018: General Principles for Planning and Design of Multi-Regional Clinical Trials. 2018.

Lunn D., Spiegelhalter D., Thomas A., and Best N. 2009. The BUGS project: Evolution, critique and future directions (with discussion). *Statistics in Medicine* 28: 3049–3082.

Quan H., Li M., and Shih J.W., et al. 2013. Empirical shrinkage estimator for consistency assessment of treatment effects in multi-regional clinical trials. *Statistics in Medicine* 32: 1691–1706.

Raudenbush S.W. and Bryk A.S. 2002. *Hierarchical Linear Models (Second Edition)*. Sage Publications, Thousand Oaks.

Tanaka Y., Mak C., Burger B., et al. 2011. Points to consider in defining region for a multiregional clinical trial: Defining region work stream in PhRMA MRCT key issue team. *Drug Information Journal* 45: 575–585.

United Nations Development Program. International human development indicators. http://hdr.undp.org/en/statistics/.

15

Global Drug Development: Multi-Regional Clinical Trials (MRCTs) – China's Pursuit

Weichung J. Shih, Tai Xie, and Kun He

15.1 Introduction

15.1.1 Multi-regional or Multi-national?

First, let us put the title in the spotlight: is it "Multi-regional" or "Multinational"? There are actually different situations for each term. "Multinational" is a more appropriate term when clinical trials involve only a few countries, each with sizeable participating subjects. On the other hand, "multiregional" is more inclusive and appropriate when trials recruit more groups of countries, where member countries in each group having similar cultural backgrounds, similar practices in treating patients or sharing same regulatory agencies; see more discussion on this aspect in Wittes (2016).

No matter which situation is the case, MRCT is one global trial because all members of the investigative research "team" will share one "master" protocol. The "master" protocol defines the method to be used for classifying participants by country, by groups of countries, by geographical proximity, or some other system, so that some pooling is possible later, if necessary.

The following chart is an example of a real global trial. The Asia Pacific (APAC) region grouped Australia, S. Korea, and Thailand; the East Europe (EU) region grouped France, Germany, Hungary, Italy, Netherlands, and Spain; the EMMEA region grouped Russia, Turkey, and Poland; the Latin America region has only Mexico in this trial, and North America grouped United States (USA) and Canada. For each region, the chart shows the final number of sites, the total number of patients screened, and randomized. (Figure 15.1)

DOI: 10.1201/9781003109785-15

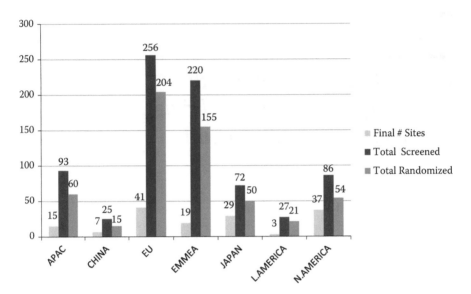

FIGURE 15.1
Region, country, and patient distributions of an example of a real global trial.

15.1.2 MRCTs: Bilateral Opportunities for China

The International Council for Harmonization (ICH) met in Montreal, Canada from May 27 to June 1, 2017. Among other decisions, the ICH Assembly approved the China Food and Drug Administration (CFDA) as a new Regulatory member and Pharmaceutical Inspection Cooperation Scheme (PIC/S) as a new Observer (www.ich.org). (Note: CFDA has now been restructured to become known as The National Medical Products Administration or NMPA). With this new membership, a new global environment is created, and MRCTs provide bilateral opportunities for China in the following way:

For Chinese international pharma companies, MRCTs mean a broad avenue for them to conduct clinical trials globally (i.e., "go to the world" business model), thereby for them to strategically develop worldwide market applications with international partners much faster. Notable examples include BeiGene Ltd. and Hengrui Medicine. For example, it now takes only 60 working days for China to approve clinical trials, compared to waiting for several years before. This rapid pace makes it possible to include China in Phases 2 and 3 worldwide. In addition, US regulators will accept Chinese data if global quality standards are met. Increasingly, Chinese firms are looking to hold IND in pre-IND meetings with the US-FDA and Chinese-NMPA to ensure that clinical programs are fully harmonized in these two major markets.

For global international companies, MRCTs under ICH standards mean a new era for them to include Chinese medical institutions and facilities as collaborators in their global trials. An example is the speed of patient recruitment. In areas where trials in the US have difficulty recruiting patients, including oncology, NASH, chronic diseases, and many rare diseases, China has a large number of untreated patients concentrated in major cities' best medical centers and hospitals. For example, the table below shows the number of PD-1 /PD-L1 trials and the number of newly diagnosed patients in patients with non-small cell lung cancer (NSCLC) in the US and China each year. Not surprisingly, in China, the speed and direct cost of patient recruitment look more attractive. The bilateral gap is narrowing as innovative Chinese companies and more internationally influential pharmaceutic companies begin to take advantage of China's appeal. The potential impact on trial time and costs provides a compelling reason to rethink the balance between the US/EU and China research centers. (Table 15.1)

In summary, advantages of MRCTs include increasing the developmental efficiency of medical therapies, promoting local regional (Chinese) clinical research, providing local regulatory authorities (NMPA) a large body of the data including Chinese patients studied under the same standard to evaluate the medical product, benefiting Chinese patients to access the drug around the same times as patients of other countries.

Because of these advantages, including China in MRCTs is a rising trend since NMPA became a regular member of ICH. The question we discuss in this article is as follows: what are the pertinent issues with MRCTs, and current common statistical approaches? We need to first briefly review the recent ICH guidance E-17 regarding MRCTs.

TABLE 15.1

Comparison of China-US non-small cell lung cancer (NSCLC) trials with anti-PD1/ PD-L1 treatment

	China	**US**
Number of trials[1]	48	114
Potential patients newly diagnosed (thousand)	780[2] (annually)	234[3] (2018)
Recruitment rate (patients per month)[4]	0.4–0.6	0.05–0.1
Cost per subject (Direct cost phase III trial)[4]	USD 25,000	~ USD 69,000

1 Clinicaltrial.gov Trial started: 01/01/2013–01/04/2019.
2 Feng et al. Current cancer situation in China – Cancer Communications (2019) 39:22; https://doi.org/10.1186/s40880-019-0368-6 (accessed on 9/23/2020).
3 American Cancer Society: Key Statistics for Lung Cancer. https://cancer.org/cancer/non-small-cell-lung-cancer/about/key-statistics.html (accessed on 9/23/2020).
4 PhRMA: Biopharmaceutical Industry-Sponsored Clinical Trials: Impact on State Economies, 2015.

15.2 ICH E-17: 7 Basic Principles of MRCT

There are seven principles of MRCT as follows:

1. Strategic use of MRCTs, properly designed and executed according to E-17.
2. Intrinsic and extrinsic factors identified early.
3. MRCTs planned under the assumption that the treatment effect applies to the entire target population. Strategic allocation of the sample size.
4. Pre-specified pooling of regions or subpopulations.
5. A single primary analysis approach planned.
6. Ensure high quality of study design according to ICH E6 in all regions.
7. Efficient communication at the planning stage.

The middle three items (3) – (5) are especially pertinent to statistical considerations in the design and analysis of an MRCT. They cover the topics of treatment effect and sample size.

15.2.1 Treatment Effect

Let us first discuss the principle: "MRCTs planned under the assumption that the *treatment effect* applies to the entire target population" under the first half of (3). There are actually two main aims of MRCT in terms of the treatment effect. The primary aim is to show the overall (pooled) treatment effect. The other is to assess region-specific effects to satisfy individual region's requirements when the overall effect is shown. This is not trivial as one would think, because the definition of the overall treatment, denoted as θ, is model dependent. For a fixed-effect model, it is a weighted average of the (fixed) individual treatment effects of the participating regions. Weights are proportions of the sample sizes. Hence, the overall treatment effect is trial specific. For a random-effect model, the individual treatment effects are random, with θ as their parent mean. Their pros and cons are as follows:

The fixed-effects model requires a smaller overall sample size, but the results may be less generalizable than the random-effects model. On the other hand, the assumption of exchangeability of the regional effects θ_i's in a random-effects model is hard to justify, depending on covariates adjustment (Quan et al., 2017). The fixed-effects model, adjusting for key covariates (regional or subject levels) is more realistic, and is currently applied to most MRCTs.

15.2.2 Sample Size

The second half of (3) stated the principle of "strategic allocation of the sample size." It is regarding the sample size contribution and requirement of the participating regions (e.g., China). We should recognize first that the sample size in an MRCT does not necessarily reflect the disease prevalence, as other social-culture, economic, regulatory, and/or business factors also influence the patient's accrue rates among regions. Statistical methods for sample size determination are interrelated to two issues: (a) How to analyze the data to show the overall effect, and (b) how to utilize the whole data to assess individual region effect. The first "how to" is answered in principle by using the fixed-effects model. The current common approach to the second "how to" is by using "consistency" assessments. An MRCT needs to have enough *power* for showing the overall treatment effect. In addition, it also needs to have sufficient probability for showing consistency. The probability for showing consistency is termed "assurance probability" (to distinguish it from "power" for the overall treatment effect).

We focus on the "consistency" assessment in the following, and shall see that the discussion will involve the principle (4) on "pre-specified pooling of regions or subpopulations" as well.

15.2.3 Consistency Assessments

The central approach of sample size determination for MRCTs is based on the concept of "consistency," as an extension from the design and analysis of bridging studies (Shih, 2001) in ICH-E5. As laid out in Shih and Quan (2013), there are two kinds of "consistency" in MRCTs: Consistency Across Regions (CAR) and Consistency for Region of Interest (C-ROI).

15.2.3.1 Consistency Across Regions: CAR

CAR is similarity or homogeneity of treatment effects across regions, represented by $\{\theta_i, i = 1,..., K\}$. There are two main methods: Treatment-by-region interaction test including quantitative or qualitative interactions, and simultaneous consistency assessment where each and every region is considered. Notice that the assessment of CAR is for the purpose of making an appropriate inference and interpretation regarding the overall treatment effect.

Examples of simultaneous consistency assessment for CAR are:

- Japanese Pharmaceutical Medical Device Agency (JPMDA): no observed qualitative treatment-by-region interaction:

  $\hat{\theta}_i > 0$, for all $i = 1,.., K$

- Quan's (2010) generalization and more stringent:

$\hat{\theta}_i > \lambda\widehat{\theta}$, for all $i =1,...,$ K, where λ is a pre-specified fraction of treatment effect preservation, e.g., $\lambda=1/K$.

For the simultaneous consistency assessment, the number of regions K should not be large in order to have enough patients from individual regions to satisfy a reasonable assurance probability. For example, if there are K = 3 regions with identical true treatment effect in a study designed with a 90% power for a significant overall treatment effect and 80% assurance probability of satisfying JPMDA's consistency criterion, then the smallest region must contribute at least 15% of all patients in the study (see Quan et al., 2010). With K = 4, then the assurance probability of showing consistency decreases to ~70%.

15.2.3.2 Consistency for Region of Interest: C-ROI

C-ROI is consistency between a specifically targeted region θ_T (i.e., a particular θ_i) and θ. When only a specific region of interest (ROI) is the concern (e.g., China), we need C-ROI, not CAR. C-ROI has been considered for bridging studies prior to the MRCT era (Shih, 2001). It relates to the above Principles (3) "strategic allocation of the sample size" and (4) "pre-specified pooling of regions or subpopulations".

Examples of C-ROI are listed in the following: For some threshold value 0 < λ, $\lambda' < 1$

- JPMDA: $\hat{\theta}_T \geq \lambda\widehat{\theta}$ (>0) for a specific λ ($\lambda > 0.5$ is a common practice)
- $\lambda \leq \hat{\theta}_T/\widehat{\theta} \leq 1/\lambda'$
- $\hat{\theta}_T \geq \left(\frac{1}{\lambda}\right)\min(\hat{\theta}_i, \quad i = 1, \quad ..K, \quad i \neq T)$
- $P_p(\hat{\theta}_T \mid [\hat{\theta}_i, i = 1, ...,K, i \neq T]) \geq r$-$th$ quantile of the distribution of $\{P_p(\hat{\theta}_j \mid [\hat{\theta}_i, i = 1,...,K, i \neq j]); j = 1, ..K, j \neq T\}$, where $P_p(y \mid z)$ denotes the predictive probability of y given z.

More discussion of the above examples was given in Shih (2016). Currently, the most common practice is using the JPMDA criterion with $\lambda = 0.5$.

As we alluded to previously, an MRCT needs to have enough power for showing the overall treatment effect, as well as sufficient assurance probability for showing consistency. In notation, let A = {Positive overall effect} and P(A) = power, B = {C-ROI shown for region T} and P(B) = assurance probability. The total sample size N is usually calculated to meet power = P(A). Hence, a question is raised: should the allocation of region T be calculated to meet P(A, B), P(B), or P (B|A)?

Quan et al. (2010) showed that P(A∩B) ≈ P(A)P(B) with the JPMDA criterion and under the condition $\theta_T = \theta$. Therefore, we may simply consider using P(A) and P(B) separately, and ultimately the successful regional registration probability P(A∩B), as the product of the power and the assurance probability. With this setting, Quan et al. (2010) derived a closed-form solution for sample size allocation with the JPMDA criterion when assuming $\theta_T = \theta$. The proportion of patients from Region T is simply

$$f_T = \frac{z_{\beta'}^2}{(z_\alpha + z_\beta)^2 (1 - \lambda)^2 + z_{\beta'}^2 (2\lambda - \lambda^2)} \tag{15.1}$$

where z_p is the upper p-tile of the standard normal distribution, the overall sample size is for $1 - \beta$ overall power via a one-sided test at significance level α, and $1 - \beta'$ is the desired *assurance probability* for consistency in region T. For instance, if $\lambda = 0.5$, $1 - \beta = 0.9$, $\alpha = 0.025$ (one-sided) and $1 - \beta' = 0.8$, then $f_T = 22.4\%$. In such a case, when there are 5 or more regions/nations, it is then impossible to satisfy all their demand simultaneously. If $\lambda = 0.7$, $1 - \beta = 0.9$ and $1 - \beta' = 0.8$, then $f_T = 44.5\%$. In such a case, there can only be 2 regions/nations to satisfy their demand simultaneously. This demonstrates that an increase in λ has a big impact on f_T, and we must consider the number of regions/nations carefully in an MRCT.

Another interesting C-ROI criterion together with a positive overall effect was proposed by Ikeda and Bretz (2010) to satisfy any one of the following:

- Significant overall effect $\widehat{\theta}$ and $\hat{\theta}_T \geq \lambda\widehat{\theta}$, or
- Significant overall effect $\widehat{\theta}$ and a positive trending regional effect $\hat{\theta}_T$ (e.g., $\hat{\theta}_T > \theta*$), or
- Significant regional effect $\hat{\theta}_T$ at a reduced level (e.g., 0.25 or other level in agreement with the local regulatory agency)

15.3 Operation of MRCT with C-ROI and Two-stage Designs

The operational aspect of MRCT with consistency requirement for a specific ROI is similar to the "Basket Trial" concept. That is, there is one "master protocol" with sub-protocols for each specific region when necessary. The sub-protocol is to satisfy the specific requirement from the ROI such as the consistency criterion (e.g., choice of λ), permitted rescue or concomitant therapies, safety monitoring process, etc. subject to negotiation and agreement with the local IRB and regulatory authority.

A common situation is that countries participate an MRCT at various time schedules, some earlier and some later, due to different regulatory reviews and other conditions. See Figure 15.2 for a real MRCT example, where China activated after all other countries have already activated. Furthermore, some countries may have regulatory-mandate on minimal sample size (depending on diseases). The impact on both the power for overall effect and the assurance

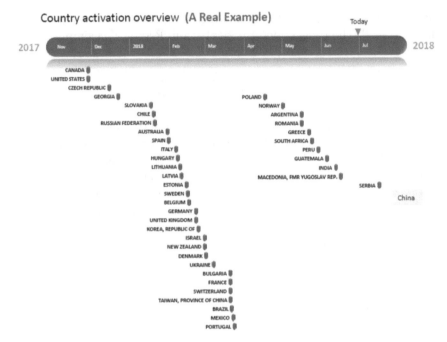

FIGURE 15.2
Staggered trial activations by countries in an MRCT.

probability for C-ROI needs to be considered. Usually, two-stage design is more suitable to handle these situations, as discussed in Luo et al. (2010). Let us discuss two-stage designs for two different situations illustrated by Figure 15.3.

15.3.1 For Regions Without a Mandate Minimum Sample Size

Using Figure 15.3 as an illustration, we suppose that the main stage for the overall analysis is locked when N = 900 is reached according to the power calculation in an MRCT design. Korea, e.g., is the specific country for the C-ROI analysis. Suppose that Korea activated the MRCT later than the majority of other countries and that its regulatory does not have a mandate for a minimum sample size for this trial but requires to satisfy its consistency requirement. Then, without prolonging the time for the analysis of the overall treatment effect, the extension of C-ROI analysis for Korea to the second stage is at an as-needed basis.

More specifically, recall A = {Positive overall effect} and B = {C-ROI shown for region K}. The closed-form solution in Eq. (15.1) of sample size allocation to the country was to satisfy P(*A*) and P(B), and ultimately needed to satisfy P(A∩B) for the specific region K at a desirable level. Since P(A∩B) < P(B), we may need to increase the sample size for region K.

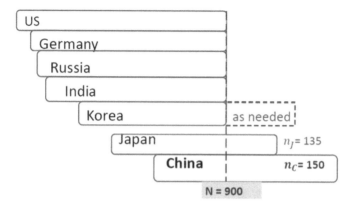

Two-stage design:
- Lock for overall analysis when N=900 for the main stage
- Extended stage for specific region with regulatory mandate minimum or as needed

FIGURE 15.3
Illustration of two-stage design in MRCT with staggered country activation.

Without prolonging the trial duration for the overall assessment, Luo et al. (2010) proposed a 2-stage adaptive design. First, if A∩B is already met, i.e., the overall effect is positive and C-ROI for region K is established at the main stage, then there is no need for extension of additional sample size for region K. However, if A is met, but not B, then we could meet B in an extension just for region K only by performing a "sample size re-estimation" using the main stage information, $(\hat{\theta}_K, \hat{\theta})$, where $\hat{\theta}_K$ is the observed treatment effect for region K and $\hat{\theta}$ is the observed overall treatment effect at the main stage. For the latter case, as A has been shown, the overall effect will not be revisited, and no multiple assessments for the overall effect. (The estimate of the overall effect may be updated later when the extension of region K is completed.) The question is: how many additional subjects are needed in the supplemental cohort for the specific region K? This can be accomplished by setting a desirable conditional assurance probability $P(B_X \mid \hat{\theta}_K, \hat{\theta}) = 1 - \beta_{2s}$ in the region-specific sub-protocol, where B_X = {C-ROI shown for region K in the extension stage including the supplemental cohort}, and enrolling additional $N_{k,s}$ subjects from region K to satisfy this conditional assurance probability. Notice that, from the inequality,

$$P(A \cap B) \le P((A \cap B) \cup (A \cap B_X)) \le P(A)$$

the power is increased by the extension of the specific region K (the first inequality), and the type I error rate is controlled by the overall analysis type-I error rate (second inequality). The detailed formula for the sample size of the supplemental cohort $N_{k,s}$ is given by Luo et al. (2010).

15.3.2 For Region with a Mandate Minimum Sample Size but Late Participation

Continuing Figure 15.3 as an illustration, some countries, e.g., China, activated the MRCT later than the majority of other countries, and assume that its regulatory has a mandate for minimum sample size (e.g., $n_c = 150$) for this trial as well as a consistency requirement. Then, without prolonging the time for the analysis of the overall treatment effect, the extension of C-ROI analysis for China to the second stage is necessary. The additional sample size for China can be accomplished by the same way as in the Korea case mentioned in the previous section, i.e., calculating the additional $m_{c,s}$ needed to satisfy a desirable conditional assurance probability $P(B_X \mid \hat{\theta}_C, \hat{\theta})$ that is pre-specified in the region-specific sub-protocol, where B_X= {C-ROI shown for region C in the extension stage including the supplemental cohort}, $\hat{\theta}$ is the observed overall treatment effect and $\hat{\theta}_C$ is the observed regional treatment effect from m_c patients in China at the main stage. With the mandate minimum sample size, we then take the maximum of mandate minimum sample size n_c and $m_c + m_{c,s}$ as the total number of patients to enroll from region C.

15.3.3 Numerical Example

An MRCT is conducted with the change of HbA1C at 12 months as the primary endpoint. The specific ROI is China. The protocol assumes SD = 0.013 and θ = 0.005. Hence, the total N = 286 is needed (1:1 ratio) for testing the overall effect with power = 90% and alpha = 0.05 (2-sided) in Stage 1.

Suppose that the JPMDA C-ROI criterion with λ=0.5 is used and assume $\theta_C = \theta$. If we plan f_C = 20%, then m_c = 286*0.2 = 58 subjects from China. From Eq. (15.1), where $T = C$, we obtain the assurance probability $P(B) = 1 - \beta' = 0.784$. Hence, $P(A \cap B) \approx P(A)P(B) \approx 71\%$.

For desirable $P(A \cap B) = 80\%$, then $f_C \geq 40\%$, which may not be feasible at Stage 1 to reach due to the deadline of filing overall to other regions and late entry of China to MRCT. Hence, adopting the two-stage design strategy is more suitable for the situation.

Go with the plan to set f_C=20% at stage 1 for the overall effect and to file NDA for other regions, while knowing that $P(A \cap B) < 80\%$ for China. Suppose that the observe $\hat{\theta}$ = 0.0044 (and $p < 0.0043$, demonstrating significant overall effect) and $\hat{\theta}_C$ = 0.002 (<0.0044/2, indicating the JPMDA C-ROI criterion with λ=0.5 not met) at stage 1, amend the local study to extend to Stage 2.

Suppose we set the conditional assurance probability $P(B_X \mid \hat{\theta}_C, \hat{\theta})$ = $1 - \beta_{2s}$ = 80% and obtain $m_{c,s}$ = 76 (formula Eq. (18) of Luo et al. 2010).

At stage 2, we check the JPMDA C-ROI criterion (λ=0.5) with $m_c + m_{c,s}$ = 58+76 = 134 Chinese subjects for China. If the NMPA mandates a minimum of n_c = 150 subjects from China, the additional 76 is still not enough and at least additional 92 subjects are needed for China.

On the other hand, suppose we set the conditional assurance probability $P(B_X \mid \hat{\theta}_C, \hat{\theta})$ = $1 - \beta_{2s}$ = 90%, then $m_{c,s}$ = 134. At stage 2, we check the JPMDA C-ROI criterion (λ= 0.5) with $m_c + m_{c,s}$ = 58+134 = 192 (>150 mandate minimum) subjects for China.

15.4 Final Remark–A Bridging Study Experience with China

This chapter is based on our presentation at the 2018 International Chinese Statistical Association (ICSA) China Conference in Qingdao City. We focused on China as the region of special interest in this article. As we see from the above discussions, there is increased complexity of design and conduct in the MRCTs. As pointed out in Shih (2016), the bridging study strategy according to ICH E-5 guideline is still a viable alternative for global drug development. Historically, the concept of consistency was originated from the bridging strategy. Yathindranath et al. (2014) reported a recent trend that drug makers tend to utilize more of the bridging study strategy as their first option for registration in certain regions. In a sense, the bridging study strategy can be viewed as a special scenario of the two-stage MRCT design. Since China joined ICH as a regular member in 2017, when the E-17 guideline on MRCT was published in the meantime, it did not have any experience with the previous E-5 guideline involving bridging studies. Then, how would China's NMPA handle a bridging study for global drug reviews? We present a recent experience in the following.

A new drug was developed to treat polycythemia vera (PV), a clonal stem cell malignancy that requires life-long treatment following diagnosis, to reduce the risk of arterial and venous thromboses, progression to myelofibrosis and acute myeloid leukemia, and early death. The new drug was approved by the EMA in 2018 based on global data including a pivotal long-term (over 3 years) multi-national randomized phase III trial. The manufacturer was seeking regulatory approval(s) for marketing the drug in China (and other Asian Pacific countries) in 2020. NMPA requested to conduct a local study in China. After reviewing the data (which supported the EMA's approval) and having thorough discussions, NMPA agreed that the local trial may be a single arm with a short-term follow-up. What the

TABLE 15.2

Sample size calculation for the example in
Section 15.4

Sample Size n	$P(\hat{r} = k/n > 0.231 \mid r = 0.312)$
24	0.80745
25	0.83963
26	0.74739
27	0.78480
28	0.81790
29	0.84687
30	0.87201
31	0.79789
32	0.82776
33	0.85407
34	0.87704
35	0.80987
36	0.83704
37	0.86107
38	0.88216
39	0.82089
40	0.84574
41	0.86780
42	0.88725
43	0.83105
44	0.85390
45	0.87424
46	0.89223
47	0.84047
48	0.86155
49	0.88037
50	0.89707

sample size should be and how to assess consistency were the major statistical questions to consider.

The Chinese study protocol adopted complete hematologic response rate
(CHR) at 26 weeks as the primary efficacy endpoint. Based on the results of
the pivotal multinational Phase III trial, the estimated CHR at 26-week was
31.2% and the lower bound of the 95% confidence interval was 23.1% for the
test drug. The consistency criterion was that the observed CHR in China's
local study needs to exceed the observed lower bound, i.e., $\hat{r} = k/n > 0.231$.
The assurance probability for this consistency was set to be at least
80%. Assuming the true CHR in China would be the same as what was

observed in the pivotal study, the sample size n was calculated to satisfy $P(\hat{r} = k/n > 0.231 \mid r = 0.312) \geq 80\%$.

Using the normal approximation $\hat{r} \sim N\left(r, \frac{r(1-r)}{n}\right)$, $n \geq \frac{r(1-r)Z_{0.8}^2}{(r-0.231)^2} = 24$. This matches well with $P(\hat{r} = k/n > 0.231 \mid r = 0.312) = P(k > n \times 0.231 \mid r = 0.312) = \sum_{k=n\times0.231}^{n}\binom{n}{k}r^k(1-r)^{n-k} = 0.807$ for $n = 24$. However, considering the discrete nature of binomial distribution of $\hat{r}$ with small sample size, a more detailed calculation was performed in Table 15.2. As shown, n would be conservatively chosen to be at least 36 to guarantee the assurance probability above 81%.

References

American Cancer Society: Key Statistics for Lung Cancer. https://cancer.org/cancer/non-small-cell-lung-cancer/about/key-statistics.html (accessed on 9/23/2020).

European Medicines Agency. ICH guideline E17 on general principles for planning and design of multi-regional clinical trials. December 18, 2017. https://www.ema.europa.eu/en/ich-guideline-e17-general-principles-planning-design-multi-regional-clinical-trials (accessed on 9/23/2020).

Feng RM et al. Current cancer situation in China: good or bad news from the 2018 Global Cancer Statistics? *Cancer Communications* 2019; 39: 22. 10.1186/s40880-019-0368-6 (accessed on 8/15/2021).

Ikeda K and Bretz F. Sample size and proportion of Japanese patients in multi-regional trials. *Pharmaceutical Statistics* 2010; 9:207–216.

Luo X, Shih WJ, Ouyang SP and DeLap RJ. An optimal adaptive design to address local regulations in global clinical trials. *Pharmaceutical Statistics* 2010; 9:179–189.

PhRMA: Biopharmaceutical industry-sponsored clinical trials: Impact on state economies, 2015. http://phrma-docs.phrma.org/sites/default/files/pdf/biopharmaceutical-industry-sponsored-clinical-trials-impact-on-state-economies.pdf (accessed on 9/23/2020).

Quan H, Zhao PL, Zhang J, Roessner M and Aizawa K. Sample size considerations for Japanese patients in a multi-regional trial based on MHLW Guidance. *Pharmaceutical Statistics* 2010; 9:100–112.

Quan H, Li M, Chen J, Gallo P, Binkowitz B, Ibia E, Tanaka Y, Ouyang SP, Luo X, Li G, Menjoge S, Talerico S and Ikeda K. Assessment of consistency of treatment effects in multiregional clinical trials. *Drug information Journal* 2010; 44:617–632.

Quan H, Mao X, Tanaka Y, Chen J, Zhang J, Zhao PL, Binkowitz B, Li G, Ouyang SP and Chang M. Example-based illustrations of design, conduct, analysis and result interpretation of multi-regional clinical trials. *Contemporary Clinical Trials* 2017; 58: 13–22.

Shih WJ. Clinical trials for drug registrations in Asian-Pacific countries: Proposal for a new paradigm from a statistical perspective. *Controlled Clinical Trials* 2001; 22:357–366.

Shih WJ and Quan H. Consistency in bridging studies and global multiregional trials. In *Design and Analysis of Bridging Studies* 2013, edited by JP Liu, SC Chow and CF Hsiao, CRC Press, Boca Raton, FL.

Shih WJ. Bridging studies versus multiregional trials. In *Multiregional Clinical Trials for Simultaneous Global New Drug Development* 2016, edited by J Chen and H Quan, CRC Press, Boca Raton, FL.

Wittes J. Independent data monitoring committees in multiregional clinical trials. In *Multiregional Clinical Trials for Simultaneous Global New Drug Development* 2016, edited by J Chen and H Quan, CRC Press, Boca Raton, FL.

Yathindranath S, Kureish A, Singh A. Evolution of the clinical trial landscape in Asia Pacific. *Open Access Journal of Clinical Trials* 2014; 6:75–84.

16

Statistical Considerations in Design, Execution, and Analysis of Multiregional Clinical Trials: Consistency Evaluation and Adaptive Trials

Lanju Zhang and Weining Z. Robieson

16.1 Introduction

A multiregional clinical trial (MRCT) is a single trial conducted across multiple regions. The regions can be considered in the geographical sense but more appropriately in the regulatory sense. For example, countries in the European Union (EU) are typically considered as one region. Due to intrinsic and extrinsic factors (ICH E5), a drug may perform differently from region to region. Traditionally, a drug first gets approved in one region or a few regions based on the trials conducted in the region(s), and then expanded to other regions through bridging studies. This sequential approach certainly delays patient access to efficacious drugs in later regions. An MRCT can overcome this deficiency by investigating a drug in multiple regions simultaneously.

Multiregional trials have historically been used as a quick way to recruit participants with rare diseases or in special populations (like children or the elderly) or for large-scale studies (such as vaccine safety and effectiveness). MRCTs are becoming the preferred choice for investigating new medications in today's global market. MRCTs may enable simultaneous submission of marketing authorization applications and support regulatory decision-making in multiple regions, allowing earlier access to new drugs worldwide.

The between-region variability is a challenge for MRCTs. In this chapter, we first discuss the criteria for regional consistency evaluation. As adaptive

DOI: 10.1201/9781003109785-16

designs are increasingly used in MRCTs, we then discuss the impact of between-region variability on adaptive MRCTs. Specifically, the chapter is organized as follows. In Section 16.2, we emphasize the importance of randomization stratification in MRCTs. In Section 16.3, we propose a new approach to consistency evaluation in MRCTs and compare it to other approaches through simulation. In Section 16.4, we discuss the challenges of regional variability on the design, analysis, and monitoring of adaptive MRCTs and make recommendations to minimize its impact. In Section 16.5, sample size consideration is briefly discussed. Section 16.6 provides an approach for MRCT extension to a region in which an insufficient number of patients have been enrolled from the global trial. We conclude in Section 16.7.

16.2 Randomization Stratification in MRCTs

As we will discuss in later sections, the region is a factor as a basis for consistency evaluation in MRCTs. To reduce bias from treatment imbalance within regions, it is important to stratify the randomization by region. This is mentioned in ICH E17, but may not be done routinely by many MRCTs. For example, guselkumab's two Phase 3 global trials (Deodhar et al. 2020; Mease et al. 2020) for psoriatic arthritis stratified randomization by two other factors, but not by site, region, or country; its two Phase 3 global trials for psoriasis (Blauvelt et al. 2017; Reich et al. 2017) mentioned stratified analysis by investigation sites but didn't mention whether randomization was stratified by sites. All these trials are MRCTs. Randomization stratification by region should be emphasized for MRCT trial design and reported in the study report as a good practice.

One concern of including region in stratification is that stratifying randomization by too many factors may lead to imbalance due to increased incomplete strata. This can be mitigated by block randomization. Recently, Cui et al. (2020) suggested intensive stratification of randomization for subgroup analysis. According to them, stratification should include as many factors as possible. Take the guselkumab trial (Mease et al. 2020) as an example. The trial randomized 741 patients to three arms with two stratification factors, each having two levels. If taking randomization block size 3, the number of strata, according to Kernan et al. (1999), can be determined by total sample size divided by 4 times the block size, i.e., 740/3/4 = 61.7. Because the two factors considered by the trial resulted in 2×2 = 4 strata, another factor with 15 levels could still be included. This additional factor might well be region so that the necessary subgroup analysis by region could be subject to less bias from treatment imbalance in the regions.

16.3 Considerations of Consistency in MRCT

Because the region has many of the same features as other factors, e.g., sex and age, that divide the patient population into subgroups, we start our discussion with general subgroup problems in clinical trials.

16.3.1 Subgroup Problems in Clinical Trials

16.3.1.1 Limitation of Evidence Evaluation Based on Mean Difference for Drug Approval

Drug approval requires substantial evidence from adequate and well-controlled trial(s) to support the claim of the effectiveness of the new drug. In many situations, two independent trials are preferred. This calls for high statistical rigor on trial design, execution, and analysis, e.g., randomization, blinding, statistical analysis plan including control of the type I error rate, and statistically significant and clinically meaningful results.

On the basis of randomization, a population model is usually used for statistical analyses, assuming trial patients are a random sample from a homogeneous population, sometimes after adjustment of baseline covariates (Chapter 4 of Rosenberger and Lachin 2016). Statistical inference is typically to compare the mean difference between patients who are treated with the investigational drug and those who are treated with the control.

A statistically significant mean difference cannot guarantee all patients in the target population will benefit from the investigation drug. In Figure 16.1, panel a shows very little overlap of the densities of two means when the sample size equals 234, determined to have 90% power, a mean difference of 0.3, 2-sided type I error rate 0.05, and standard deviation of 1. However, at the individual level (sample size is 1 per arm) in panel d, there is little separation between the two densities. Therefore, a portion of the indicated patient population may not benefit much from the drug, even if substantial evidence has been established based on the population mean for drug approval.

16.3.1.2 Subgroup Analysis in Clinical Trials

This helps to understand the issues of subgroup analysis in clinical trials. In Figure 16.1, as sample sizes decrease from panels a to d, the overlap of mean densities of the two treatment groups increases. This implies that the

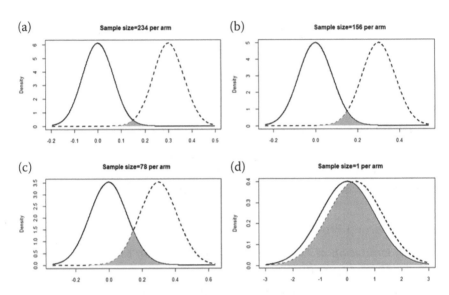

FIGURE 16.1
Overlap of densities of means of the drug (dashed line) and control (solid line) groups with a mean difference of 0.3, the standard deviation of 1, and different sample sizes.

treatment differences in smaller subgroups can have a higher chance of being different from the overall effect as in panel a and could even be in the opposite direction. Figure 16.2 depicts the probability of observing consistent subgroup treatment differences (all > 0) versus the number of

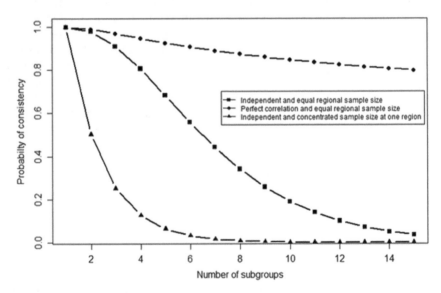

FIGURE 16.2
Probability of consistent subgroup difference with 2-sided $\alpha = 0.05$ and $\beta = 0.1$.

subgroups assuming the same true treatment difference in all these groups. When subgroup treatment differences are independent, this probability is lowest when the total sample size is concentrated to a subgroup, as shown in a triangled curve in Figure 16.2 where 0.00001 of the total sample size is allocated to all but one subgroup and the remaining to that one subgroup; and this probability is highest when the total sample size is equally distributed among all subgroups (Li et al. 2007), as shown in the squared curve in Figure 16.2. Correlation of subgroup treatment differences may be introduced when they are estimated from the same model or based on shrinkage estimator (Quan et al. 2013). A positive correlation will increase the probability of consistency. The dotted curve in Figure 16.2 depicts the probability with perfect correlation among subgroup treatment differences and equally distributed sample sizes. In all scenarios, the probability decreases as the number of subgroups increases. However, sample size distribution is critical. For example, this probability quickly drops below 20% when there are four subgroups with sample sizes concentrated to one subgroup (triangled curve) while the probability is still about 20% when there are ten subgroups with equally distributed sample sizes (squared curve).

In both Figures 16.1 and 16.2, a homogeneous population is assumed. In clinical trials, the patient population is not always homogeneous; their baseline characteristics, e.g., age, sex, disease severity, and medical history, are often different. These factors, and many others and even unobserved ones, can affect treatment responses, and accordingly the treatment differences. The heterogeneity of treatment differences due to these factors may further decrease the probability of consistency. For this reason, it is clearly cautioned in ICH E9 that subgroup analyses are exploratory in nature and their interpretation should be made in this context, although It is stipulated that subgroup analysis based on these factors should be routinely conducted.

16.3.2 Consistency Criteria and Evaluation in an MRCT

16.3.2.1 Overall Consistency

Region naturally is a subgroup factor. All the problems discussed in the previous section apply to subgroups defined by region (Kawai et al. 2007). In other words, treatment effect consistency across all regions should be evaluated in MRCTs. This is called overall consistency.

Several criteria have been proposed for overall consistency evaluation (Chen et al. 2010). The most popular one is Method 2 (Ministry of Health Labor and Welfare MHLW of Japan 2007), already mentioned in Section 16.3.1.2 in a subgroup analysis setting. It requires observed treatment differences in all regions to be in the same direction (>0) or above the same threshold (Quan et al. 2013). One problem with this criterion is that the probability of consistency quickly drops as the number of regions increases, even when the true underlying treatment effect is the same for all regions. For example, in Figure 16.2 even with six regions, the probability of consistency drops below 60% under equal sample size allocation and can drop much lower than 60% when sample sizes are not equally allocated. Gail and Simon's (1985) Q-test formalized this approach into a hypothesis test with the null hypothesis of mean treatment differences of all regions in the same direction. Region and treatment effect interaction tests can also be used. The testing approaches usually take the null hypothesis as consistency or homogeneity of treatment effect and failure to reject null confers consistency. This kind of hypothesis set up is not appropriate because a failure of rejection may be due to lack of power. To clearly describe different probabilities, we simply call consistency as negative and inconsistency as positive. Then we can evaluate the false positive rate and false-negative rate under different situations.

We propose another approach for overall consistency evaluation. We consider a meta-analysis of data from different regions and use outlier detection by Viechtbauer and Cheung (2010). If there is not any outlier, then overall consistency is established and vice versa.

In the following, we run simulations to compare the performance of these methods. In the simulation, we take the random-effect model as in Quan et al. (2013). Let r be the number of regions, X_{ij} and Y_{ik} be the response (the larger the better) of subject j in control group and subject k in the treatment group, respectively, in region i, and

$$X_{ij} \sim N(\mu_{iX}, \ \sigma^2) \text{ and } X_{ik} \sim N(\mu_{iY}, \ \sigma^2), \ i = 1, \ ..., \ r.$$

Let $\delta_i = \mu_{iY} - \mu_{iX}$, and assume the treatment differences from all regions follow an independent normal distribution,

$$\delta_i \sim N(\delta, \ \tau^2).$$

Given δ, σ and type I error rate α, determine sample size per arm N' to have $(1 - \beta)$ power as follows,

$$N' = \frac{2\sigma^2(Z_\alpha + Z_\beta)^2}{\delta^2}. \tag{16.1}$$

The formula does not take random effects into account. For simulation purposes, we increase N' by 20% to account for the heterogeneity of treatment differences to get $N = 1.2N'$ per arm. In practice, one can use a formula in Hung et al. (2010) to determine sample size incorporating between-region variability.

Three approaches are considered. The first is the outlier detection approach based on a meta-analysis. As recommended by Viechtbauer and Cheung (2010), we use studentized residuals to detect outliers. If there exists a residual whose absolute value exceeds a threshold, we will say treatment differences are not consistent. The second approach is the interaction test. We use F-test by comparing residuals of the full model that includes treatment, region, and region and treatment interaction term with a restricted model that includes treatment and region only. The third approach is Method 2 (Ministry of Health Labor and Welfare MHLW of Japan 2007), requiring observed treatment differences all > 0.

Gail and Simon (1985)'s approach was also considered but it understandably led to much higher positive rates than Method 2 under all scenarios no matter how we tuned the thresholds based on formula (A1) in their paper. Therefore, we will not report its results here.

To specify simulation settings, we assume $\sigma = 1$, $\delta = 0.25$, $\alpha = 0.025$ (1-sided), $\beta = 0.1$, $r = 4$, 7, 10, $\tau = 0.031$, 0.062, 0.25. Despite a random effect model, we assume treatment difference in Region 1 can differ from other regions systematically by $\delta_{10} = E(\delta_1) - \delta = 0$, -0.3, -0.5, -1, so that we can evaluate the false positive rate when $\delta_{10} = 0$ and the false-negative rate when $\delta_{10} \neq 0$.

The simulated positive rates are displayed in Table 16.1 for different combinations of parameters of r, τ, δ_{10}, and when the total sample size is evenly distributed among regions. To control the false positive rate to be around 0.05 when $r = 4$, we choose a threshold of 0.8 in meta-analysis outlier approach and p-value threshold 0.05 for F-test in the interaction approach (also see Table 16.2 later). In addition, the power of the global test by pooling all regions is also shown. The conditional positive rates, the probability of inconsistency when the global test of treatment difference is significant, are shown in the last three columns of Table 16.1. All simulations had 4000 replicates.

From Table 16.1, we can see from column six that again Method 2 can have a very high false-positive rate when $\delta_{10} = 0$, which increases significantly as the number of regions r or between-region variability τ increase. From columns five and seven we can see that positive rates of both the Meta outlier approach and the Interaction test approach increase as Region 1 difference increases and do not change much as the number of region r increases. We think this is one of the advantages of using these two approaches. However, the Interaction test approach positive rates are more sensitive to between-trial variability than Meta outlier approach. The last three columns show that the conditional positive rates displayed a similar pattern.

Since sample size distribution can also affect consistency evaluation (Figure 16.2), we run another simulation assuming sample size distribution is concentrated in Region 1 or Region r. More specifically, in Table 16.2 when $nd = 1$ the first $(r - 1)$ regions have 5% of N and the last

TABLE 16.1

Positive rates, global power, and conditional positive rates of three approaches: meta-analysis outlier (Meta), Method 2 (M2), and interaction test (IT). Sample size N variation is due to rounding to keep an integer sample size for each region

r	τ	δ_{10}	Overall N per Arm	Positive Rate			Global Power	Conditional Positive Rate		
				Meta	M2	IT		Meta	M2	IT
4	0.03	0	404	0.00	0.14	0.06	0.94	0.00	0.11	0.06
		-0.3	404	0.00	0.68	0.33	0.70	0.00	0.58	0.33
		-0.5	404	0.04	0.96	0.73	0.41	0.04	0.92	0.73
		-1	404	0.88	1.00	1.00	0.03	0.93	1.00	1.00
	0.06	0	404	0.00	0.20	0.09	0.93	0.00	0.15	0.09
		-0.3	404	0.00	0.69	0.36	0.69	0.00	0.58	0.37
		-0.5	404	0.05	0.96	0.73	0.43	0.05	0.91	0.75
		-1	404	0.86	1.00	1.00	0.04	0.84	1.00	1.00
	0.25	0	404	0.06	0.57	0.59	0.80	0.06	0.46	0.60
		-0.3	404	0.11	0.79	0.71	0.61	0.11	0.67	0.71
		-0.5	404	0.23	0.89	0.81	0.47	0.22	0.78	0.81
		-1	404	0.74	1.00	0.98	0.18	0.71	0.98	0.98
7	0.03	0	406	0.00	0.50	0.06	0.94	0.00	0.47	0.06
		-0.3	406	0.01	0.78	0.16	0.84	0.01	0.74	0.16
		-0.5	406	0.08	0.95	0.42	0.72	0.08	0.93	0.43
		-1	406	0.84	1.00	0.98	0.34	0.83	1.00	0.98
	0.06	0	406	0.00	0.54	0.08	0.93	0.00	0.50	0.08
		-0.3	406	0.01	0.78	0.21	0.82	0.01	0.74	0.21
		-0.5	406	0.08	0.95	0.44	0.71	0.08	0.93	0.44
		-1	406	0.83	1.00	0.97	0.33	0.82	1.00	0.97
	0.25	0	406	0.12	0.81	0.61	0.83	0.12	0.77	0.61
		-0.3	406	0.15	0.89	0.66	0.72	0.15	0.85	0.66
		-0.5	406	0.27	0.95	0.78	0.64	0.26	0.92	0.78
		-1	406	0.77	1.00	0.97	0.39	0.77	1.00	0.97
10	0.03	0	410	0.01	0.75	0.06	0.95	0.01	0.74	0.06
		-0.3	410	0.02	0.88	0.12	0.87	0.02	0.86	0.12
		-0.5	410	0.11	0.96	0.27	0.82	0.11	0.95	0.27
		-1	410	0.80	1.00	0.88	0.56	0.80	1.00	0.88
	0.06	0	410	0.01	0.76	0.07	0.94	0.01	0.74	0.07
		-0.3	410	0.03	0.89	0.14	0.88	0.03	0.87	0.14
		-0.5	410	0.12	0.97	0.31	0.80	0.12	0.96	0.31
		-1	410	0.80	1.00	0.88	0.57	0.80	1.00	0.87
	0.25	0	410	0.20	0.92	0.59	0.86	0.20	0.91	0.59
		-0.3	410	0.25	0.95	0.64	0.78	0.25	0.94	0.64
		-0.5	410	0.36	0.97	0.75	0.72	0.36	0.96	0.75
		-1	410	0.78	1.00	0.95	0.55	0.78	1.00	0.95

Meta = meta-analysis outlier; M2 = Ministry of Health Labor and Welfare of Japan Method 2; IT = interaction test.

TABLE 16.2

Positive rates, global power, and conditional positive rates of three approaches, meta-analysis outlier (Meta), Method 2 (M2), and interaction test (IT) with r=7 regions

nd	τ	δ_{10}	Overall N per Arm	Positive Rate Meta	M2	IT	Global Power	Conditional Positive Rate Meta	M2	IT
1	0.03	0	403	0.09	0.76	0.06	0.94	0.09	0.75	0.06
		-0.2	403	0.11	0.84	0.07	0.92	0.11	0.83	0.07
		-0.4	403	0.19	0.91	0.12	0.89	0.19	0.90	0.12
		-0.6	403	0.34	0.96	0.24	0.87	0.35	0.96	0.25
		-0.8	403	0.53	0.99	0.41	0.84	0.54	0.99	0.41
	0.06	0	403	0.10	0.77	0.07	0.91	0.09	0.75	0.07
		-0.2	403	0.12	0.82	0.09	0.89	0.12	0.81	0.09
		-0.4	403	0.20	0.90	0.15	0.88	0.20	0.89	0.15
		-0.6	403	0.34	0.95	0.26	0.83	0.34	0.94	0.26
		-0.8	403	0.55	0.99	0.43	0.81	0.54	0.99	0.43
	0.25	0	403	0.33	0.87	0.39	0.73	0.32	0.83	0.36
		-0.2	403	0.35	0.90	0.42	0.70	0.34	0.87	0.40
		-0.4	403	0.40	0.94	0.46	0.70	0.40	0.92	0.46
		-0.6	403	0.51	0.96	0.55	0.68	0.52	0.95	0.56
		-0.8	403	0.66	0.98	0.67	0.65	0.68	0.98	0.70
2	0.03	0	403	0.08	0.76	0.05	0.93	0.08	0.75	0.05
		-0.1	403	0.10	0.78	0.07	0.71	0.10	0.72	0.07
		-0.2	403	0.12	0.83	0.14	0.34	0.12	0.64	0.12
		-0.3	403	0.15	0.93	0.26	0.09	0.17	0.58	0.25
		-0.4	403	0.19	0.99	0.45	0.01	0.23	0.65	0.38
	0.06	0	403	0.10	0.77	0.07	0.91	0.10	0.76	0.07
		-0.1	403	0.11	0.79	0.09	0.69	0.10	0.73	0.08
		-0.2	403	0.14	0.84	0.15	0.35	0.13	0.67	0.12
		-0.3	403	0.16	0.93	0.28	0.12	0.15	0.62	0.24
		-0.4	403	0.19	0.98	0.46	0.02	0.08	0.53	0.33
	0.25	0	403	0.32	0.86	0.39	0.73	0.32	0.82	0.36
		-0.1	403	0.32	0.89	0.39	0.60	0.30	0.82	0.32
		-0.2	403	0.36	0.91	0.45	0.45	0.33	0.83	0.33
		-0.3	403	0.37	0.93	0.54	0.30	0.30	0.79	0.32
		-0.4	403	0.42	0.95	0.61	0.19	0.30	0.78	0.33

Meta = meta-analysis outlier; M2 = Ministry of Health Labor and Welfare of Japan Method 2; IT = interaction test.

region has size $N[1 - 0.05(r - 1)]$ so the sample size is concentrated in the last region; when $nd = 2$ the last $(r - 1)$ regions have 5% of N and the first region has size $N[1 - 0.05(r - 1)]$ so the sample size is concentrated in the first region.

We can see from Table 16.2 that when the sample size is concentrated in the last region and Region 1 treatment difference increases, positive rates of the Meta outlier approach are higher than that of the interaction test approach, which means Meta outlier approach is more powerful in detecting true inconsistency. This difference diminishes when between-region variability increases. On the other hand, when the sample size is concentrated in Region 1 and Region 1 difference increases, positive rates of interaction tests are much higher than that of the Meta outlier approach. This is due to the large sample size in Region 1 magnifies the impact of Region 1 difference on the interaction test.

Overall, the Meta outlier approach is a reasonable approach to identify a region with treatment effects different from other regions. Extensive simulations should be conducted to determine a good threshold that will produce reasonable positive rates in different situations.

If an overall regional inconsistency is identified, further review of intrinsic and extrinsic factors should be conducted to understand the outlying region.

16.3.2.2 Region-Specific Consistency

There is one distinction of the region from other subgroup factors. For other factors, as discussed in the previous section, analysis is exploratory in nature and so is its interpretation. However, a region sometimes corresponds to a regulatory body and the regulatory body must make a regulatory decision on the drug, using the information from the subgroup as well as the whole trial.

As discussed in ICH E17, region-specific consistency of treatment effect should be evaluated for regional regulatory review. There are many criteria for region-specific consistency assessment. The most popular one is Method 1 (MHLW), requiring the observed region-specific treatment difference to be larger than, say, 50% of the observed global treatment difference. Although this approach can be used for sample size calculation by requiring the criterion holds with a probability of 80%, the inference is only based on the observed treatment difference. Chen and Wang (2016) proposed a modified Fisher's least difference to compare each region to all other regions, controlling the overall type I error rate when such region-specific assessment is made to all regions. Quan et al. (2013) proposed a shrinkage estimator of region-specific treatment effect combining region-specific data and global data.

In our opinion, multiregional clinical trials are not designed for region-specific inference. We agree that it is important to examine region-specific data in the backdrop of whole trial data, but such examination should be a "review issue" and not based on a hypothesis test in the MRCT setting. An example can be found in Section 16.4.1 (MERIT-HF study).

16.4 Statistical Considerations in Adaptive MRCT

Both adaptive designs and designs involving multiple geographic regions are becoming increasingly common in clinical trials in recent years. There are many advantages to both designs.

The United States (US) Food and Drug Administration (FDA) Adaptive Design for Clinical Trials of Drugs and Biologics guidance defines adaptive design as "a clinical trial design that allows for prospectively planned modifications to one or more aspects of the design based on accumulating data from subjects in the trial." Common adaptive designs include sample size re-estimation, group sequential design, dropping inferior treatment group(s), and seamless "combined-phase" designs. The types of adaptations that can be made include stopping the trial for futility or overwhelming efficacy and modifications to sample size, patient population, treatment arms, or patient allocation ratios.

Adaptive designs can make clinical trials more flexible by conducting interim analysis utilizing accumulating data in the trial to modify the trial's course in accordance with pre-specified rules. Trials with an adaptive design are often more efficient, informative, and ethical than trials with a traditional fixed design since they often require fewer participants and thus reduce the timeline and cost (Pallmann et al. 2018). Interim analyses provide the opportunity to reduce trial participants' exposure to an ineffective compound; minimize trial costs in cases of dropping an ineffective dose or futility stopping of entire trial; and accelerate the overall development program by making decisions at earlier time points, e.g., prepare for next phase of trial or expand manufacturing at large scale. For the last scenario (accelerating the overall development program), even though the interim analysis may not necessarily change the conduct of the current study, nonetheless the decisions being made before final results are available have major consequences, and the considerations discussed in this section apply to these studies as well.

Both adaptive trial and MRCT are complex in terms of trial design, planning, and execution. Each has its unique set of challenges. When the features of these two types of designs are combined in a single trial, special care should be taken to ensure that the trial is designed to achieve the objectives and yield results that are interpretable.

16.4.1 Examples of Adaptive MRCTs

Below are a couple of examples of MRCTs that were stopped after an interim analysis but some regional variations in treatment effect were later found (Li et al. 2020).

MERIT-HF Study

The MERIT-HF study (MERIT-HF Study Group 1999) evaluated the effect of metoprolol CR/XL on congestive heart failure (CHF) compared to placebo. It was conducted in 13 European countries and in the US. Primary endpoints were as follows: (1) all-cause mortality; (2) all-cause mortality + all-cause hospitalization. An α-level of 0.05 (two-sided) was allocated to these endpoints as 0.04 and 0.01, respectively. The trial utilized a group sequential design with predetermined interim analyses when 25%, 50%, and 75% of expected total deaths had occurred. The trial was terminated for a statistically significant reduction in all-cause mortality after the second pre-planned interim analysis (50% information fraction). The hazard ratio (HR) for all-cause mortality was 0.66 (nominal $p < 0.0001$), and the HR for the mortality-hospitalization composite was 0.81 ($p=0.00012$). Results were consistent across 12 predefined subgroups, which did not include region or country.

During the US FDA's review of the New Drug Application (NDA) (FDA 2000), the statistical reviewer conducted a subgroup analysis by region (US vs. Europe) and noted a strong suggestion of a treatment-by-region interaction ($p=0.006$) for all-cause mortality: in Europe, HR=0.55 ($p=0.0001$), while in the US, HR=1.05 ($p=0.80$). For the mortality-hospitalization composite, effects were similar (0.84 vs. 0.81) in both regions.

FDA conducted extensive exploratory analyses to explore the poorer US effect of the first primary endpoint (FDA 2000). No plausible covariates stood out to explain the US mortality result. FDA interpreted that the absence of observed benefit in the US was perhaps due to chance, but was more likely caused by inter-country differences in gender distribution of randomized patients, cause of deaths in CHF, or other demographic or medical practice differences.

Ultimately, FDA reviewers emphasized that the overall efficacy had been established by the pre-specified primary analysis in the overall population, and the US patient population had not been intended to be used to evaluate the overall efficacy (FDA 2000). This is consistent with ICH E17 that the primary reason for performing MRCTs is to evaluate the overall treatment effect based on data from subjects in all regions. In 2009, FDA approved metoprolol for the treatment of CHF based on the MERIT-HF study, but regional differences were described in the product label (FDA 2009).

About 9 years elapsed between the MERIT-HF NDA and FDA approval of metoprolol, mainly due to the suspected inconsistency issues. FDA stated that "Nonetheless, subgroup analyses can be difficult to interpret and it is not known whether these represent true differences or chance effects." (Figure 16.3)

HOPE Study

The Heart Outcomes Prevention Evaluation (HOPE) trial was a double-blind, placebo-controlled, randomized study to evaluate the effects of

All Patients Randomized

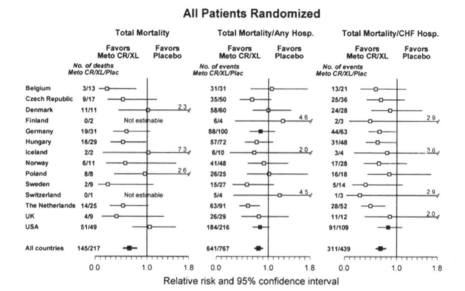

FIGURE 16.3

Relative risk and 95% confidence interval in MERIT-HF trial (Reprinted with permission from Wedel H., DeMets D., Deedwania P., et al. Challenges of subgroup analyses in multinational clinical trials: experiences from the MERIT-HF trial. *Am Heart J* 2001;142(3):502–511.)

ramipril for preventing cardiovascular (CV) events in patients at high risk (Yusuf et al. 2000; Arnold et al. 2003). A total of 9297 high-risk patients with evidence of vascular disease or diabetes plus one other CV risk factor, and not known to have a low ejection fraction or heart failure, were randomly assigned to receive ramipril (10 mg once per day orally) or matching placebo for a mean of five years. The primary endpoint was time to a composite of myocardial infarction (MI), stroke, or death from CV causes.

Four formal interim analyses were planned. The statistical monitoring boundary indicating that ramipril had a beneficial effect was a difference in the primary outcome of 4 standard deviations (SD) between groups during the first half of the study and of 3 SD during the second half. The respective boundaries indicating that ramipril had a harmful effect were 3 SD and 2 SD. The trial was stopped at an interim analysis based on a recommendation from its Data Monitoring Committee (DMC) due to clear evidence of benefit for ramipril (crossing of monitoring boundaries in two consecutive reviews) (Arnold et al. 2003). A primary event occurred in 14.0% of ramipril patients and 17.8% of placebo patients, a 22% risk reduction (HR=0.78, 95% CI: 0.70–0.84, $p < 0.001$). The results were also significant for each component of the composite endpoint. Some subpopulations had been pre-defined in the protocol based upon, e.g., presence or absence of diabetes, CV disease, hypertension, microalbuminuria;

also, gender, and age. The effect of ramipril on the primary endpoint was consistent across all the subpopulations.

This trial had been conducted in 4 regions and 19 countries from Europe and the Americas (Arnold et al. 2013): Canada (59% of total enrollment), the US (9%), Europe (14 countries totaling 21%), and Latin America (3 countries totaling 11%). Yusuf and Wittes (2016) described considerable country variations in treatment effects. Canada, with the highest enrollment, had almost the same observed effect as the overall estimate (RR=0.78). Countries with low enrollment showed much larger effect variations; some yielded outcomes favoring placebo over ramipril. This variation, however, may just be due to the randomness resulting from the small country sample sizes and thus should not be over-interpreted, as pointed out by the authors. Had regional effects been included in the protocol as a predefined subpopulation, a prior assessment of the likelihood of a qualitative treatment-by-region interaction (i.e., a directional treatment difference across regions) could have been provided. Li et al. (2020) suggested that the DMC charter can advise a monitoring committee to look closely at the pattern of regional results before making a decision to halt a trial early when evidence of efficacy is lacking in some regions.

16.4.2 Differences in Regulatory and Ethics Committee Approval Processes of Study Protocols

Countries have different processes for approving clinical trial protocols. In the US, an application to initiate the first clinical trial of a new medication is made by a company (sponsor) by submitting an Investigational New Drug (IND) application. The FDA requires a 30-day review period for the IND. After this 30-day hold, the sponsor company can initiate its first Phase 1 clinical trial in any or all of the 50 states. If all is well, the sponsor will not hear back from the FDA. This is referred to as the "no news is good news" response from the FDA. All subsequent clinical trials or substantial amendments of ongoing trials will require the sponsor to submit an update to the initial IND to the FDA (Pierro 2018).

In the EU, the sponsor cannot initiate clinical trials until it receives approval for the Clinical Trial Application (CTA), even if the 30-day period has elapsed. The harmonized CTA authorization process consists of 2 parts: Part I of joint assessment coordinated by the Reference Member State (RMS) which takes up to 45 days (and possible extension of up to 31 days) and Part II of national assessment by each Member State Concerned (MSC) which takes up to 45 days (and possible extension of up to 31 days) (Broich 2018).

Besides regulatory agency approval, there is a requirement of Institutional Review Board (IRB) or ethics committee (EC) approval as well. The process and timelines for approval various greatly from region to region, and for different types of study sites. Sites in Latin America (average 16.1 months) and Eastern Europe (average 14.7 months) had longer cycle times than sites

"First Patient-In" Cycle Time by Region

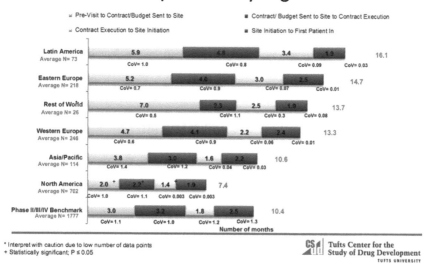

FIGURE 16.4
"First patient-In" cycle time (Months) by region (Reprinted with permission from Getz K.A., Lamberti M. J., Chakravarthy R., Assessing Practices & Inefficiencies with Site Selection, Study Start-Up, and Site Activation, Tufts Center for the Study of Drug Development, Tufts University School of Medicine, August 4, 2016, *Applied Clinical Trials*.)

in other regions, and North American sites (7.4 months) took the least amount of time to first patient-in (Getz et al. 2016). (Figure 16.4)

In aducanumab Phase 3 global clinical trials, implementing a protocol amendment across 20 countries, hundreds of sites, and multiple ethics committees took a long time. Patient consents to the protocol amendment took place over more than 18 months (FDA Advisory Committee Meeting November 6, 2020, Biogen prerecorded presentation transcripts).

These regulatory and IRB/EC timelines play important roles in MRCTs execution. In adaptive MRCTs, the variation in time to protocol approval and site initiation are critical elements that should be considered in the study design stage for sample size, interim analysis timing, and interim decision criteria.

16.4.3 Statistical Considerations in Design Stage of an Adaptive MRCT

Many computer simulations are conducted during the planning stage of an adaptive trial to establish the operating characteristics of the trial. The operating characteristics should include type I and type II errors, the chance of producing erroneous conclusions, and the reliability of treatment effect estimates.

These simulations will evaluate the operating characteristics of the trial under many variations of the possible scenarios:

- Treatment effect profiles of the investigational, active control, and placebo control groups. Many dose-response effect size scenarios should be included.
- Variance-covariance matrix including correlation between visits for longitudinal data
- Number of patients in each treatment group
- Enrollment rate
- Dropout pattern
- Number of interims and interim analysis timing

The number of interim analyses, the timing of each interim analysis as well as adaptation decision criteria should be tweaked for optimal operating characteristics considering all scenarios. The decision criteria should be robust under variations of the above-mentioned parameters.

Regions in which a trial is conducted may naturally differ in aspects of ethnicity, culture, patient population, and local medical practice. While we may not expect these differences to have a major impact on treatment effects, we should remain open to this possibility due to the critical implications for interpretation of how, where, and under what circumstances treatment is most beneficial (Gallo et al. 2011). MRCT is generally conducted when there is a belief in homogeneity of effect across regions (ICH E17). Sometimes the knowledge is not fully gained from prior trials. Heterogeneity could be observed during the prior trials or the trial under design either because true differences exist or due to chance as demonstrated in Section 16.3.1.2. This makes adaptation difficult. The treatment effect profiles for the simulation could include some variations of regional effect to reflect the uncertainty regarding the region homogeneity so the impact at interim analyses could be evaluated with simulation results.

It has been observed in many trials across a range of indications that the variability increases as the number of sites and countries increases. If the trial parameters were based on results from single-country or single-region trials, the range of variability assumptions to be used in the simulations should be widened.

Often, the enrollment rate considered in simulations is flat rates across the trial's enrollment period, e.g., ten patients/week. However, most trialists know that the enrollment rate is almost never flat during a trial. There is typically a ramp-up period when the enrollment rate rapidly increases to a peak enrollment rate where it remains relatively stable.

Due to the long lead-in time of some countries and regions, it is possible that when the information fraction predetermined for an interim analysis is met, study sites in some countries have not even been initiated or started enrolling patients. The lag in country enrollment is an important element that should be taken into account during trial simulation when determining the timing of interim analyses. The differences in start-up time and inconsistent enrollment rates could mean that the contribution of each country or region to the overall subject population may change over time and the differences in country contributions may be associated with differences in the baseline demographic characteristics.

A fundamental assumption of interim analyses is that available data predict future data, i.e., there is no or little temporal heterogeneity. The effects of temporal heterogeneity may not be of consequence for trials without adaptive features; however, it may have a meaningful impact on study designs that employ adaptive elements. The difference in country lead-in time could be a source of temporal heterogeneity. The study team should consider whether enrollment in countries that are initiated first needs to be slowed down to decrease temporal heterogeneity caused by varying proportions of regional enrollment over the duration of the trial. Regardless, analysis of country- and region-level data at interim analyses should be pre-specified in the DMC charter for broader information.

With adaptive features like dropping a dose, there could be too few patients from a certain region to make the full decision and it cannot be recovered.

The study team needs to weigh the design burden with the potential benefit when determining the adaptive features of an MRCT. Besides time taken to conduct simulations which is part of any adaptive trials, the additional design burden of an adaptive MRCT also includes the time required to obtain and coordinate feedbacks from multiple regulatory agencies and operation challenges.

16.4.4 Statistical Considerations in Executing Interim Analyses of an Adaptive MRCT

16.4.4.1 Blinded Study Monitoring by Study Team

Appropriate site selection and training always play an important role in the execution of a successful trial, but it is even more critical in an adaptive MRCT to ensure a consistent setting throughout the trial and to increase the probability of success.

Blinded trial monitoring during a study is an essential component for ensuring high quality in trial conduct and data integrity. In adaptive MRCTs, real-time monitoring of potential issues that could lead to regional and temporal heterogeneity is critically important. Systematic deviation from the protocol within a region should be corrected promptly. Missing data rates and patterns should also be evaluated as differences across regions could be a flag for a data quality issue needing further investigation.

Disparity across regions in adverse event rates could suggest an un-suspected ethnically sensitive population or region-specific safety concern that could influence efficacy outcomes (Gallo et al. 2011).

The study team should have active oversight of country contribution and performance during trial conduct and carefully consider how many parti-cipants each country contributes to the dataset. Blinded monitoring of the primary and secondary endpoints included in the decision criteria should be performed to detect any possible country and region variations as well as outliers that may influence the decision criteria. If necessary, additional simulations could be performed based on new assumptions derived from accumulating blinded data to potentially modify the interim timing and decision criteria. If the study initiation in certain countries is delayed and the country/region will not have an expected representation in the interim analysis, the decision should be made as soon as possible whether an in-terim analysis should be delayed or canceled. Such modifications to the adaptive features of the design after the trial has been initiated do not violate the principle that the adaptation needs to be prospectively defined because "prospective" means that the adaptation is planned and details specified before any comparative analyses of accumulating trial data are conducted (FDA Adaptive Design guidance). Nonetheless, in most cases, changes to the adaption algorithm may require protocol amendment and revision to the DMC charter.

16.4.4.2 Informing and Preparing the DMC and Sponsor Review Committee (SRC) Prior to the First Interim Analysis

For many trials, the study team documents the interim analysis decision criteria in the DMC charter and relies on the DMC to make their re-commendation following the pre-set rules. However, one needs to under-stand that even the most comprehensive simulations performed pre-trial cover only a subset of all possible scenarios, and unforeseen situations often come up after the trial starts.

The interactions between the study team and the DMC prior to the first interim analysis should be far beyond a kickoff meeting and the finalization of the DMC charter. Due to the complexity in the design and execution of such trials, collaborations between the trial statistician and the DMC sta-tistician during the design or trial initiation stages are crucial so that the DMC statistician has a thorough understanding of the adaptation elements and operating characteristics. To make the most informative decision, the DMC statistician and other DMC members need to understand how the simulations were performed, the range of assumptions they cover, how the decision criteria were chosen, and which compromises may have been made when determining the decision criteria. This will ensure the trial is carried out according to plan and the DMC could intervene in the event that any of the design assumptions is violated.

Sometimes the DMC mechanism involves a sponsor review committee (SRC) to make the final decision for the fate of the trial based on DMC recommendations. The SRC typically consists of a small group of sponsor senior members who are not directly involved in the conduct of the trial. In such a case, detailed trial design parameters should also be communicated to the SRC before the first interim analysis.

16.4.4.3 Unblinded Evaluation by the DMC

At each interim analysis, the DMC statistician should provide the other DMC members with an assessment of how well the study dataset conforms to underlying simulation assumptions. The DMC statistician needs to caution the DMC that the data may be uninterpretable if the interim dataset deviates greatly from these assumptions, and potentially even suggest to DMC that no analysis be performed and no decision be made if the dataset deviates greatly from assumptions.

For trials that may be terminated early because a substantial benefit has been observed, however, consideration may still need to be given to the adequacy of data with regard to other issues such as safety, duration of benefit, outcomes in important subgroups, and important secondary endpoints (FDA Guidance for Clinical Trial Sponsors: Establishment and Operation of Clinical Trial Data Monitoring Committees). Primary efficacy data should be complemented by a careful assessment of the consistency of trial results beyond the primary variable(s), including results in important subgroups, and the adequacy of the safety database. A discussion is needed as to whether all the requisite information can be provided if the study is stopped at interim analysis (EMA CHMP reflection paper 2007).

It has been well established that region and country is an important subgroup that should be taken into account at interim analysis.

Differences in treatment effects are commonly observed across countries and regions during an interim analysis, either due to true underlying patient characteristics, culture background and standard of care, or just an artifact of noise due to the smaller sample size of the interim dataset. If the pooled results of the primary and key secondary endpoints meet the pre-defined decision criteria for success or futility, the DMC statistician should be vigilant in detecting potential region variation. If the treatment effect is dominated by data from a particular region while the opposite trend is observed in other regions, the DMC should carefully evaluate whether the decision criteria should be followed to declare the end of the trial for success despite such variation, because it may cause the drug to be not approvable in the countries where the effect was not observed. If the trial is stopped for success while the effect is not shown in one or more regions, the regulatory agencies in affected regions/countries may not approve the drug due to lack of effect. This may render future studies in the region not feasible due to the small population. The chance to develop the drug in that region could be lost.

If there is an SRC that is part of the DMC mechanism, the information should also be conveyed to the SRC to facilitate their final decision-making.

Interim monitoring of unblinded data may also offer opportunities to identify and mitigate inconsistency. The DMC needs to decide what information to communicate to the Steering Committee to make proper decisions, while at the same time maintaining study integrity. This requires careful and timely communication between the DMC and other parties (Li et al. 2020).

16.5 Sample Size Considerations in MRCT

ICH E17 has an extensive discussion on sample size consideration. Here we point out two important steps. One is the sample size for the MRCT. Since treatment effect heterogeneity is not avoidable, sample size determined based on Formula (16.1) in Section 16.3.2.1 should be adjusted. One approach is to use the formula given by Hung et al. An empirical approach is to increase the sample size calculated using (16.1) by, say, 20% as we did in the simulation. For adaptive MRCTs, sample size should be determined based on extensive simulations.

The second step is sample size distribution among different regions. From Figure 16.2 we see that equal distribution can reduce the false positive rate based on Method 2. However, equal distribution may extend enrollment time because different regions may start enrollment at different times and with different enrollment rates. A good strategy should take into account all the following factors, known treatment effect heterogeneity, projected enrollment start time and rates, minimum sample size requirement of regional regulatory agencies. For an adaptive MRCT, the regional sample size distributions at planned interim analyses should be considered.

16.6 Extension of MRCT with a Local Trial

In some situations, a particular region may only enroll very limited subjects in an MRCT due to regional enrollment delays or slow enrollment rates. More subjects may need to enroll in a separate trial for approval in this region and regulatory review is based on statistical inference. One approach is to use a bridging study for establishing equivalence between this region and other regions. Instead, Zhou et al. (2017) proposed an "interpretation-centric" approach to design the regional trial taking all available data in MRCT into account. To illustrate, suppose there are N subjects per arm in the MRCT and n_1 subjects per arm in Region 1 of interest. It is decided that n_1 is not enough for regulatory approval and a local trial in Region 1 is needed. With Region 1's regulatory input, if there had been p (percent) of Region 1 subjects in the MRCT ($Np > n_1$) the MRCT then would have met the sample size requirement for regulatory approval in Region 1. Then we want to design a local trial of sample size subjects per arm such that a significant result will be shown based on the following weighted estimator

$$\hat{\delta} = p\hat{\delta}_1 + (1 - p)\hat{\delta}_o$$

where $\hat{\delta}_1$ is the treatment effect estimate in Region 1 based on $(n_1 + m)$ subjects of Region 1 and $\hat{\delta}_o$ is the treatment effect estimate based on all other regions in the MRCT. Sample size m can be determined to have adequate power with the formula given in Zhou et al. (2017).

The design of the local trial is conducted from the MRCT perspective. The sample size is determined as to how many more patients from the target region could have been enrolled in the MRCT such that the regulatory sample size requirement for the region is met and a significant result for the region can be achieved by borrowing data from other regions in the MRCT. This is the same rationale of shrinkage estimator by Quan et al. To give an example, suppose $N = 250$ is needed in an MRCT with $n_1 = 10$, meaning Region 1 only accounting for 4% of the total sample size. The regulatory agency in Region 1 determined that $p = 30\%$ is required for approval. It is determined $m = 36$ per arm is needed for a local trial to have 80% power with 1-sided $\alpha = 0.025$. For details, please refer to Zhou et al. (2017).

16.7 Conclusions and Discussions

Region is an important subgroup factor in MRCTs. Subgroup analysis by region is not only a requirement of ICH E9, but also one in ICH E17. It not only shares the same issues of subgroup analysis based on other factors, but also has its unique connotation because a region may correspond to a regulatory body. This means that we do not only need to evaluate the overall consistency of treatment effect of all regions, but also region-specific consistency. In this chapter, we reviewed approaches for these two types of consistency evaluation and proposed a new approach, outlier based on meta-analysis, for overall consistency evaluation. Simulation showed that its performance is very appealing with respect to the number of regions and between-region variability, compared to Method 2 (MHLW) and interaction test. An appropriate threshold for outlier detection should be selected to ensure appropriate false positive and negative rates.

Region consistency may become more problematic in adaptive MRCTs when the interim analysis is conducted at a fraction of the total sample size. If a regional inconsistency is observed at an interim analysis, the trial could potentially be allowed to continue even though the stopping rule was met on the overall population. Because sample size distribution can affect consistency evaluation, the study team needs to take into consideration at the design stage how the potential different sample size distributions at interim analyses and study end may impact the consistency evaluation. For example, equal distribution can reduce the false positive rate based on Method 2, but equal distribution may be impossible to achieve at interim analyses due to varying site activation times at different regions.

Adaptive design places major responsibilities on the study team, DMC, and SRC to carry out the design intent of the trial. The burden on the study team, DMC, and SRC for an adaptive MRCT is even greater. It takes careful planning and meticulous execution to conduct a successful adaptive MRCT.

References

Arnold J.M., Yusuf S., Young J. et al. Prevention of heart failure in patients in the Heart Outcomes Prevention Evaluation (HOPE) study. *Circulation*. 2003; 107(9): 1284–1290.

Blauvelt A., Papp K.A., Griffiths C.E.M. et al. Efficacy and safety of guselkumab, an anti-interleukin-23 monoclonal antibody, compared with adalimumab for the continuous treatment of patients with moderate to severe psoriasis: results from the phase III, double-blinded, placebo- and active comparator-controlled VOYAGE 1 Trial. *J Am Acad Dermatol*. 2017; 76: 405–417.

Broich K. CT authorization in the EU: present and future. 09 March 2018. https://www.ema.europa.eu/en/documents/presentation/presentation-module-5-clinical-trials-european-union_en.pdf

Chen J., Quan H., Binkowitz, B. et al. Assessing consistent treatment effect in a multi-regional clinical trial: a systematic review. *Pharm Stat*. 2010; 9: 242–253.

Chen J. and Wang H. Multiregional clinical trials: assessing consistency of treatment effect. In *Multiregional clinical trials for simultaneous global new drug development*. Edited by Chen J. and Quan H. 2016 , 41–52. Chapman and Hall/CRC.

Cui L., Xu T., and Zhang L. Issues related to subgroup analysis and use of intensive stratification. In *Design and analysis of subgroups with biopharmaceutical applications*. Edited by Ting N., Cappelleri J.C., Ho S. and Chen D.-G. 2020, 1–17. Springer.

Deodhar A., Helliwell P.S., Boehncke W.-H. et al. Guselkumab in paitents with active psoriatic arthritis who were biologic-naïve or had previously received TNFa inhibitor treatment (DISCOVER-1): a double-blind, randomized, place-controlled phase trial. *Lancet*. 2020; 395: 1115–1125.

European Medicines Agency, Committee for Medicinal Products for Human Use (CHMP), Reflection Paper on Methodological Issues in Confirmatory Clinical

Trials Planned with an Adaptive Design, London, 18 October 2007 Doc. Ref. CHMP/EWP/2459/02.

FDA. Medical Review(s) for Toprol-XL (metoprolol succinate). https://www.accessdata.fda.gov/drugsatfda_docs/nda/2000/N-19–962S013_Toprol_Medr.pdf. 2000.

FDA Toprol package insert. https://www.accessdata.fda.gov/drugsatfda_docs/label/2009/019962s038lbl.pdf. 2009.

FDA. Meeting of the Peripheral and Central Nervous System Drugs Advisory Committee Meeting. November 6, 2020. Biogen Pre-Recorded Presentation Transcripts. https://www.fda.gov/media/143507/download

Gail M, Simon R. Testing for qualitative interaction between treatment effects and patient subsets. *Biometrics*. 1985; 41: 361–372.

Gallo P., Chen J., Quan H. et al. Consistency of treatment effect across regions in multiregional clinical trials, Part 2: monitoring, reporting, and interpretation. *Drug Inf J*. 2011; 45: 603.

Getz K.A., Lamberti M.J., Chakravarthy R., Assessing practices & inefficiencies with site selection, study start-up, and site activation, Tufts center for the study of drug development, Tufts University School of Medicine. *Appl Clin Trials*. 2016. Downloaded from https://www.appliedclinicaltrialsonline.com/view/limited-boosts-study-start

Hung H.M.J., Wang S.J., and O'Neill R.T. Consideration of regional difference in design and analysis of multi-regional trials. *Pharm Stat*. 2010; 9:173–178.

Kawai N., Chuang-Stein C., Komiyama O., and Li Y. An approach to rationalize partitioning sample size into individual regions in a multiregional trial. *Drug Inf J*. 2007; 42:139–147.

Kernan W., Viscoli C., Makuch R., Brass L., and Horwitz R. Stratified randomization for clinical trials. *J Clin Epidemiol*. 1999; 52: 19–26.

Li Z., Chuang-Stein C., and Hoseyni C. The probability of observing negative subgroup results when the treatment effect is positive and homogeneous across all subgroups. *Drug Inform J*. 2007; 41: 47–56.

Li G., Quan H., Lan G. et al. Lessons Learned from multi-regional trials with signals of treatment effect heterogeneity. *Ther Innov Regul Sci*. 2020; 54: 21–31.

Mease P.J., Rahman P., Gottlieb A.B. et al. Guselkumab in biologic-naïve patients with active psoriatic arthritis (DISCOVER-2): a double-blind, randomized, placebo-controlled phase 3 trial. *Lancet*. 2020;395: 1126–1136.

MERIT-HF Study Group. Effect of metoprolol CR/XL in chronic heart failure: metoprolol CR/XL randomized intervention trial in congestive heart failure (MERIT-HF). *Lancet*. 1999; 353: 2001–2007.

Ministry of Health Labor and Welfare (MHLW) of Japan. Basic concepts for joint international clinical trials. September 28, 2007.

Pallmann P., Bedding A.W., Choodari-Oskooei, B. et al. Adaptive designs in clinical trials: why use them, and how to run and report them. *BMC Med*. 2018; 16: 29.

Pierro M. Initiating multinational clinical trials: major differences between the U.S. And EU. Guest Column August 23, 2018. https://www.clinicalleader.com/doc/initiating-multinational-clinical-trials-major-differences-between-the-u-s-and-eu-0001

Quan H., Li M., Shih W.J. et al. Empirical shrinkage estimator for consistency assessment of treatment effects in multi-regional clinical trials. *Stat Med*. 2013; 32: 1691–1706.

Reich K., Armstrong A.W., Foley P. et al. Efficacy and safety of guselkumab, an anti-interleukin-23 monoclonal antibody, compared with adalimumab for the continuous treatment of patients with moderate to severe psoriasis: results from the phase III, double-blinded, placebo- and active comparator-controlled VOYAGE 2 Trial. *J Am Acad Dermatol*. 2017, 76: 418–431.

Rosenberger W.F. and Lachin J.M. *Randomization in clinical trials: Theory and practice,* 2nd edition. 2016 Wiley, New Jersey.

Viechtbauer W. and Cheung M.W.L. Outlier and influence diagnostics for meta-analysis. *Rese Synth Methods*. 2010; 1: 112–125.

Wedel H., DeMets D., Deedwania P. et al. Challenges of subgroup analyses in multinational clinical trials: experiences from the MERIT-HF trial. *Am Heart J*. 2001; 142(3): 502–511.

Yusuf S. and Wittes J. Interpreting geographic variations in results of randomized controlled trials. *N Engl J Med*. 2016; 375(23): 2263–2271.

Yusuf S., Sleight P.E., Pogue J.F., Bosch J., Davies R., and Dagenais G.. Effects of an angiotensin-converting-enzyme inhibitor, amipril, on cardiovascular events in high-risk patients. *N Engl J Med*. 2000; 342(3): 145–153.

Zhou Y., Cui L., Yang B., Zhang L., and Shen F. Regional efficacy assessment in multiregional clinical development. *J Biopharm Stat*. 2017; 27: 673–682.

17

Multiple Endpoints in Multiregional Clinical Trials

Toshimitsu Hamasaki, Yuh-Jenn Wu, and Chin-Fu Hsiao

17.1 Multiple Endpoints

Recently, multiregional clinical trials (MRCTs), which involve recruiting participants from many countries and regions worldwide under the same protocol, have been widely conducted by global pharmaceutical companies. The objective of such trials is to accelerate the development of a new treatment and shorten its approval time in key markets. Most recent approaches for designing and evaluating MRCTs have focused on one primary endpoint. In some therapeutic areas, the clinical efficacy of a new treatment may be characterized by several possibly correlated endpoints because there are two or more different features that are critically important to the disease under study. In complex diseases, co-primary endpoints may be required by regulatory agencies as the cause of the disease may be multifactorial so that a drug will not be considered effective without the demonstration of a treatment effect on all of these disease features. For example, a typical clinical trial for Alzheimer's disease (AD) has cognitive, functional, and global endpoints so as to evaluate symptomatic improvements in dementia symptoms caused by the disease. The Committee for Medicinal Products for Human Use (CHMP) (2008) has recommended demonstrating statistical significance on two co-primary endpoints of these three (i.e., cognitive, functional, and global) for drug development for AD treatment; clinical trials with co-primary endpoints are designed to evaluate if the effect of a test treatment is superior (or non-inferior) to that of a control treatment on all primary endpoints. Failure to achieve a better treatment response in any endpoint implies that superiority over a control treatment cannot be confirmed (CHMP 2016; Food and Drug Administration 2017). These endpoints are as follows:

DOI: 10.1201/9781003109785-17

a. Objective cognitive tests [e.g., AD Assessment Scale Cognitive Subscale (ADAS-Cog) and Severe Impairment Battery (SIB)];

b. Self-care and activities of daily living [e.g., AD Cooperative Study Activities of Daily Living (ADCS-ADL) and its modified version for severe AD];

c. Global assessment of change [e.g., Clinician's Interview-Based Impression of Change-plus (CIBIC-Plus) and Clinical Global Impression of Improvement (CGI-I)].

The use of multiple endpoints increases difficulties for statisticians in terms of handling multiplicity in the design and analysis of clinical trials, particularly in controlling Type I and Type II error rates when the endpoints are potentially correlated. When a trial is designed to evaluate a joint effects on all primary endpoints, as in AD clinical trials, no adjustment is required to control the Type I error rate. However, the Type II error rate increases as the number of endpoints increases. This issue with having co-primary endpoints are related to the intersection–union problem (Offen et al. 2007; Hung and Wang 2009). In many such trials, the sample size is often unnecessarily large and impractical. Recently, to overcome the issue, many researchers have used a fixed-sample (size) design for co-primary endpoint trials and related analyses (see extensive references in Offen et al. 2007, Sozu et al. 2015, and Hamasaki et al. 2018). In addition to conducting conventional clinical trials within one region, MRCTs can provide a solution to this issue; this involves reducing the number of participants from one region. For example, in the recently completed clinical trial "Effect of LY450139 on the Progression of Alzheimer's Disease as Compared with Placebo (IDENTITY-2) (NCT00762411)," 1,111 participants were enrolled from 18 regions, including Taiwan and Japan (http://www.clinicaltrials.gov/ct2/show/NCT00762411). In fact, in ICH E17 guideline on "General Principles for Planning and Design of Multi-Regional Clinical Trials" (International Council for Harmonisation of Technical Requirements for Pharmaceuticals for Human Use ICH 2017 five approaches are recommended for overall sample size allocation to regions. In the first approach, regional sample sizes are determined such that similar trends in treatment effects across regions can be demonstrated. The second approach is to determine the sample size required in one or more regions such that region-specific treatment effects preserve a prespecified proportion of the overall treatment effect. In the third approach, participants are enrolled in proportion to region size. The fourth approach is to determine regional sample sizes so that significant results within one or more regions can be obtained. The last approach requires having a fixed minimum number of participants in one or more regions.

In this chapter, we focus on the design and evaluation of an MRCT with co-primary endpoints (Huang et al. 2017). The aim of an MRCT is to demonstrate the efficacy of a treatment in various regions worldwide and evaluate the possibility of applying the overall trial results to each region. In addition, we also consider the number of participants in a specific region to determine the consistency of treatment effects between participants in a specific region and the entire group.

17.2 Sample Size Calculation

For simplicity, we focused on a situation in which an MRCT is designed to evaluate treatment superiority over a placebo control on K (≥ 2) continuous co-primary efficacy endpoints, and the effect size for each co-primary endpoint is assumed to be uniform across M (≥ 2) regions. Let X_{ikj} and Y_{ikl} be efficacy responses related to the kth primary endpoint for the jth and lth participants in the ith region receiving the test product (T) and the control (C), respectively ($i = 1, ..., M$; $j = 1, ..., N_i^T$; $l = 1, ..., N_i^C$; $k = 1, ..., K$). Let $X_{ij} = (X_{i1j}, ..., X_{iKj})^T$ and $Y_{il} = (Y_{i1l}, ..., Y_{iKl})^T$ be the outcome vectors of K co-primary endpoints for the jth and lth participant in the ith region receiving the test product and the control, respectively ($j = 1, ..., N_i^T$; $l = 1, ..., N_i^C$). N_i^T and N_i^C are the sample sizes of the product (T) and the control (C) groups, respectively, for the ith region.

Because the effect size for each co-primary endpoint is uniform across regions, we can assume that X_{ij} and Y_{il} have multivariate normal (MVN) distributions with population mean vectors $\mu^T = (\mu_1^T, ..., \mu_K^T)$ and $\mu^C = (\mu_1^C, ..., \mu_K^C)$, respectively, and a known common covariance matrix $\Sigma = (\rho_{kk'}\sigma_k\sigma_{k'})$, where $(a_{kk'})$ denotes the matrix whose (k, k')th element is $a_{kk'}$, $\rho_{kk'} = \text{corr}\left[X_{ikj}, X_{ik'j}\right] = \text{corr}\left[Y_{ikj}, Y_{ik'j}\right]$ ($k \neq k'$) and $\sigma_k^2 = \text{Var}[X_{ikj}] = \text{Var}[Y_{ikj}]$. Let $\Delta_k = \mu_k^T - \mu_k^C$ for $k = 1, ..., K$. A positive population mean difference value for each co-primary endpoint represents a superior outcome for the product (T). The hypothesis for co-primary endpoints is given as follows:

$$H_0: \Delta_k \leq 0 \text{ for at least one } k \text{ vs. } H_A: \Delta_k > 0 \text{ for all } k. \quad (17.1)$$

The null hypothesis (H_0) can be expressed as the union of a hypothesis family $H_0 = \cup_{k=1}^K H_{0k}$, H_{0k}: $\Delta_k \leq 0$, and the alternative hypothesis (H_A) as the intersection of an alternative hypothesis family $H_A = \cap_{k=1}^K H_{Ak}$, H_{Ak}: $\Delta_k > 0$. The hypothesis for each co-primary endpoint is tested at the same significance (α) level with H_{0k}: $\Delta_k \leq 0$ versus H_{Ak}: $\Delta_k > 0$, and the null hypothesis (H_0) is rejected if (and only if) all of the null hypotheses (H_{0k}) are rejected; hypothesis test for co-primary endpoints is a test of statistical significance (α). Although the hypothesis is one sided, the proposed method can be easily extended to a two-sided one. Let

$$
\bar{X}_k = \frac{\sum_{i=1}^{M} \sum_{j=1}^{N_i^T} X_{ikj}}{\sum_{i=1}^{M} N_i^T} \quad \text{and} \quad \bar{Y}_k = \frac{\sum_{i=1}^{M} \sum_{j=1}^{N_i^C} Y_{ikj}}{\sum_{i=1}^{M} N_i^C}
$$

for $k = 1, \ldots, K$. Also, let

$$
Z_k = \frac{\bar{X}_k - \bar{Y}_k}{\sigma_k \sqrt{\frac{1}{\sum_{i=1}^{M} N_i^T} + \frac{1}{\sum_{i=1}^{M} N_i^C}}},
$$

for $k = 1, \ldots, K$. Subsequently, we reject H_0 at α if $Z_k > z_{1-\alpha}$ for all k, where $z_{1-\alpha}$ is the $100(1 - \alpha)$ percentile of the standardized normal distribution.

Let $N^T = \sum_{i=1}^{M} N_i^T$ and $N^C = \sum_{i=1}^{M} N_i^C$. In the design stage, we assume that groups are equally sized, that is, $N^T = N^C = N$. Let $\mathbf{Z} = (Z_1, \ldots, Z_K)'$. Then, under H_A, $\mathbf{Z}$ has an MVN distribution with mean vector $\sqrt{N/2}\boldsymbol{\delta}$ and covariance matrix $\boldsymbol{\rho} = (\rho_{kk'})$, where $\boldsymbol{\delta} = (\delta_1, \ldots, \delta_K)^T$, $\delta_k = \Delta_k / \sigma_k$.

On the basis of the results of Sozu et al. (2006, 2011), the power for rejecting the null hypothesis H_0 can be written as follows:

$$
1 - \beta = Pr\left[\bigcap_{i=1}^{K} \left\{ Z_k > z_{1-\alpha} \mid H_A \right\} \right].
$$

This power is referred to as conjunctive power (Senn and Bretz 2007) or complete power (Westfall et al. 2011). The sample size required for achieving the desired power of $1 - \beta$ at α for a one-sided test can be identified using the minimum N that satisfies

$$
\int_{z_{1-\alpha}}^{\infty} \cdots \int_{z_{1-\alpha}}^{\infty} f(z_1, \ldots, z_K;\ \sqrt{N/2}\boldsymbol{\delta},\ \boldsymbol{\rho}) dz_1 \cdots dz_K \geq 1 - \beta, \qquad (17.2)
$$

where $f(z_1, \ldots, z_K;\ \sqrt{N/2}\boldsymbol{\delta},\ \boldsymbol{\rho})$ represents the MVN distribution density with mean $\sqrt{N/2}\boldsymbol{\delta}$ and covariance matrix $\boldsymbol{\rho}$ corresponding to $z_1, \ldots, z_K$. An iterative procedure is required to determine the required sample size, with the most straightforward method being a grid search to increase N gradually until the power under n exceeds the desired power of $1 - \beta$, where the maximum value of sample sizes separately calculated for each endpoint can be used as the initial value for sample size calculation. However, this process often requires too much computing time. Sugimoto et al. (2012) and Hamasaki et al. (2013) have provided efficient and practical algorithms for sample size calculation.

17.3 Application of MRCT Results to a Specific Region

According to the ICH E17, MRCTs should enable the investigation of treatment effects on an overall population and allow researchers to study consistency in treatment effects across populations. In other words, the aim of an MRCT should be to demonstrate the efficacy of a treatment in various regions worldwide and evaluate the possibility of applying the overall trial results to each region. Suppose we aim to determine whether a treatment is effective in a specific region (e.g., the sth region, where $1 \le s \le M$). For the kth co-primary endpoint, let D_{ik} be the observed mean difference in the ith region, let D_k^{SC} be the observed mean difference from regions other than the sth region, and let D_k be the observed mean difference from all regions, i.e.,

$$D_{ik} = \frac{\sum_{j=1}^{N_i^T} X_{ikj}}{N_i^T} - \frac{\sum_{j=1}^{N_i^C} Y_{ikj}}{N_i^C},$$

$$D_k^{SC} = \frac{\sum_{\substack{i=1 \\ i \ne s}}^{M} \sum_{j=1}^{N_i^T} X_{ikj}}{\sum_{\substack{i=1 \\ i \ne s}}^{M} N_i^T} - \frac{\sum_{\substack{i=1 \\ i \ne s}}^{M} \sum_{j=1}^{N_i^C} Y_{ikj}}{\sum_{\substack{i=1 \\ i \ne s}}^{M} N_i^C}, \text{ and}$$

$$D_k = \bar{X}_k - \bar{Y}_k,$$

where

$$\bar{X}_k = \frac{\sum_{i=1}^{M} \sum_{j=1}^{N_i^T} X_{ikj}}{\sum_{i=1}^{M} N_i^T} \text{ and } \bar{Y}_k = \frac{\sum_{i=1}^{M} \sum_{j=1}^{N_i^C} Y_{ikj}}{\sum_{i=1}^{M} N_i^C}.$$

Given that the overall result is significant, we established the following criteria to determine whether the treatment is effective in the sth region:

i. $D_{s1} > \gamma_1 D_1, \dots, D_{sK} > \gamma_K D_K$ for $0 < \gamma_i < 1, i = 1, \dots, K$;

ii. $D_{s1} > \gamma_1 D_1^{SC}, \dots, D_{sK} > \gamma_K D_K^{SC}$ for $0 < \gamma_i < 1, i = 1, \dots, K$;

iii. $\gamma_1 < D_{s1}/D_1 < 1/\gamma_1, \dots, \gamma_K < D_{sK}/D_K < 1/\gamma_K$ for $0 < \gamma_i < 1$, $i = 1, \dots, K$;

iv. $\gamma_1 < D_{s1}/D_1^{SC} < 1/\gamma_1, \dots, \gamma_K < D_{sK}/D_K^{SC} < 1/\gamma_K$ for $0 < \gamma_i < 1$, $i = 1, \dots, K$.

The first two criteria are used to evaluate whether the treatment effect in the region of interest is as large as the overall treatment effect [i.e., in all regions) (criterion (I)) or that in the other regions (criterion (ii)]. The final two criteria are employed to investigate the consistency between treatment effects in a specific region, in all regions [criterion (iii)], or in other regions [criterion (iv)].

In the design stage, once N has been determined, consideration should be given to the number of participants from a specific region in the MRCT. According to ICH E17, for MRCTs, it is crucial that the regional sample size allocations be determined such that clinically meaningful differences in treatment effects among regions can be elucidated. Because data analyses of a specific region in the MRCT may not have sufficient statistical power, the number of participants required for that region should be adequate for establishing the consistency of treatment effects between that region and all regions.

Similar to the second approach suggested by ICH E17 in section 17.1, we suggest that the selected sample size should ensure the assurance probabilities of consistency criteria (i), (ii), (iii), and (iv) given δ are maintained at the desired level (i.e., 80%).

Let p_i denote the proportion of patients out of $2N$ in the ith region, $i = 1, \ldots, M$, where $0 < p_i < 1$ and $\sum_{i=1}^{M} p_i = 1$. Also, let N_i be the number of patients per group in the ith region. That is, $N_i = p_i N$. The assurance probabilities of criteria (i)–(iv) given δ and all co-primary endpoints are statistically significant can be represented as

$$AP_1 = P_\delta[D_{s1} > \gamma_1 D_1, \ldots, D_{sK} > \gamma_K D_K \,|\, Z_1 > z_{1-\alpha}, \ldots, Z_K > z_{1-\alpha}],$$

$$AP_2 = P_\delta[D_{s1} > \gamma_1 D_1^{SC}, \ldots, D_{sK} > \gamma_K D_K^{SC} \,|\, Z_1 > z_{1-\alpha}, \ldots, Z_K > z_{1-\alpha}],$$

$$AP_3 = P_\delta\left[\gamma_1 < \frac{D_{s1}}{D_1} < \frac{1}{\gamma_1}, \ldots, \gamma_K < \frac{D_{sK}}{D_K} < \frac{1}{\gamma_K} \,\middle|\, Z_1 > z_{1-\alpha}, \ldots, Z_K > z_{1-\alpha}\right] \quad (17.3)$$

and

$$AP_4 = P_\delta\left[\gamma_1 < \frac{D_{s1}}{D_1^{SC}} < \frac{1}{\gamma_1}, \ldots, \gamma_K < \frac{D_{sK}}{D_K^{SC}} < \frac{1}{\gamma_K} \,\middle|\, Z_1 > z_{1-\alpha}, \ldots, Z_K > z_{1-\alpha}\right],$$

where P_δ is the probability measure with respect to δ. Next, we must determine p_s to ensure that the assurance probabilities of criteria (i)–(iv) given δ are maintained at the desired level (e.g., 80%). These assurance probabilities can be calculated using normal distributions and some algebraic changes.

17.4 Numerical Results

Without loss of generality, assume that we wish to determine whether the overall results can be applied to the first region, that is, $s = 1$. To illustrate our

TABLE 17.1

Sample size and assurance probabilities for criteria (i), (ii), (iii), and (iv) given $\alpha = 0.025$, $1 - \beta = 0.9$, $(\Delta_1, \Delta_2) = (3, \ 0.45)$, and $(\sigma_1, \ \sigma_2) = (6, 1)$, $(\gamma_1, \ \gamma_2) = (0.5, 0.5)$, and $\rho_{12} = 0.1$

p_1	N	AP_1	AP_2	AP_3	AP_4
0.05	117	0.46	0.45	0.22	0.19
0.10	117	0.55	0.53	0.38	0.32
0.15	117	0.62	0.59	0.51	0.40
0.20	117	0.68	0.64	0.61	0.46
0.25	117	0.73	0.67	0.69	0.51
0.30	117	0.78	0.71	0.75	0.54
0.35	117	0.82	0.73	0.80	0.56
0.40	117	0.86	0.75	0.85	0.58
0.45	117	0.89	0.77	0.88	0.59
0.50	117	0.92	0.79	0.91	0.59
0.55	117	0.94	0.80	0.94	0.59
0.60	117	0.96	0.80	0.96	0.58
0.65	117	0.97	0.81	0.97	0.56
0.70	117	0.98	0.81	0.98	0.54
0.75	117	0.99	0.80	0.99	0.51
0.80	117	0.99	0.79	0.99	0.46
0.85	117	0.99	0.76	0.99	0.40
0.90	117	0.99	0.71	0.99	0.31

approach, let $K = 2$ and assume that $(\Delta_1, \Delta_2) = (3, 0.45)$ and $(\sigma_1, \sigma_2) = (6, 1)$, i.e., $\delta = (0.5, 0.45)^T$. With $\alpha = 0.025$, $1 - \beta = 0.9$ and $(\gamma_1, \gamma_2) = (0.5, 0.5)$. Tables 17.1–17.3 show the total sample size required per group and the assurance probabilities of criteria (i)–(iv) for $\rho_{12} = 0.1$, 0.3, and 0.7, respectively, with various p_1 values. In Table 17.1, the total sample size per group required for the MRCT would be 117, which is calculated from formulas (17.1) and (17.2) for $\rho_{12} = 0.1$. The first line in Table 17.1 indicates that if the proportion of patients in Region 1 out of the total number of patients in the study is 0.05, the assurance probabilities of criteria (i)–(iv) are respectively 0.46, 0.45, 0.22, and 0.19. As detailed in Table 17.1, to achieve assurance probability at the 80% level, the sample size for the first region must be approximately 35% of the overall sample size for criteria (i) and (iii) and approximately 55% for criterion (ii). However, the assurance probabilities of criterion (iv) never reach 80% regardless of the p_1 value. The sample size required per group is the minimum N satisfying formulas (17.1) and (17.2).

From Tables 17.1 to 17.3, the following phenomena can be identified. First, we revealed that as p_1 increases, the assurance probabilities of criteria (i) and (iii) increase. This is because as p_1 increases, the observed overall D_k results are increasingly dominated by the observed result from the first region, D_{1k}.

TABLE 17.2

Sample size and assurance probabilities for criteria (i), (ii), (iii), and (iv) given $\alpha = 0.025$, $1 - \beta = 0.9$, $(\Delta_1, \Delta_2) = (3, 0.45)$, and $(\sigma_1, \sigma_2) = (6, 1)$, $(\gamma_1, \gamma_2) = (0.5, 0.5)$, and $\rho_{12} = 0.3$

p_1	N	AP_1	AP_2	AP_3	AP_4
0.05	115	0.48	0.48	0.23	0.20
0.10	115	0.57	0.55	0.39	0.33
0.15	115	0.64	0.61	0.52	0.41
0.20	115	0.69	0.65	0.62	0.47
0.25	115	0.74	0.69	0.70	0.52
0.30	115	0.79	0.72	0.76	0.55
0.35	115	0.83	0.74	0.81	0.57
0.40	115	0.86	0.76	0.85	0.59
0.45	115	0.89	0.78	0.89	0.60
0.50	115	0.92	0.79	0.91	0.60
0.55	115	0.94	0.80	0.94	0.60
0.60	115	0.96	0.81	0.96	0.59
0.65	115	0.97	0.81	0.97	0.57
0.70	115	0.98	0.81	0.98	0.55
0.75	115	0.99	0.81	0.99	0.52
0.80	115	0.99	0.79	0.99	0.47
0.85	115	0.99	0.77	0.99	0.41
0.90	115	0.99	0.72	0.99	0.33

Second, as p_1 increases, the assurance probabilities of criteria (ii) and (iv) first increase and then decrease. This phenomenon occurred because the observed results from regions other than the first region, D_k^{SC} is always D_{2k} for $K = 2$ regardless value of p_1. Obviously N_2 decreases as p_1 increases. In Tables 17.1 to 17.3, for given p_1 and γ_1 values, $AP_1 > AP_2$. This can be explained by the following equation

$$AP_2 = P_\delta[D_{1k} > \gamma_k D_k^{SC}, k = 1, ..., K \,|\, Z_k > z_{1-\alpha}, k = 1, ..., K]$$

$$= P_\delta\left[D_{1k} > \frac{\gamma_k}{1 - p_1 + \gamma_k p_1} D_k, k = 1, ..., K \,|\, Z_k > z_{1-\alpha}, k = 1, ..., K \right]$$

$$< P_\delta[D_{1k} > \gamma_k D_k, k = 1, ..., K \,|\, Z_k > z_{1-\alpha}, k = 1, ..., K] = AP_1$$

As

$$0 < 1 - p_1 + \gamma_k p_1 = 1 - (1 - \gamma_k)p_1 < 1.$$

TABLE 17.3

Sample size and assurance probabilities for criteria (i), (ii), (iii), and (iv) given $\alpha = 0.025$, $1 - \beta = 0.9$, $(\Delta_1, \Delta_2) = (3, 0.45)$, and $(\sigma_1, \sigma_2) = (6, 1)$, $(\gamma_1, \gamma_2) = (0.5, 0.5)$, and $\rho_{12} = 0.7$

p_1	N	AP_1	AP_2	AP_3	AP_4
0.05	111	0.55	0.54	0.28	0.25
0.10	111	0.63	0.61	0.45	0.38
0.15	111	0.68	0.66	0.57	0.47
0.20	111	0.73	0.70	0.66	0.52
0.25	111	0.78	0.73	0.73	0.57
0.30	111	0.82	0.76	0.79	0.60
0.35	111	0.85	0.78	0.83	0.62
0.40	111	0.88	0.80	0.87	0.63
0.45	111	0.91	0.81	0.90	0.64
0.50	111	0.93	0.82	0.92	0.64
0.55	111	0.95	0.83	0.94	0.64
0.60	111	0.96	0.84	0.96	0.63
0.65	111	0.98	0.84	0.98	0.62
0.70	111	0.98	0.84	0.99	0.60
0.75	111	0.99	0.83	0.99	0.56
0.80	111	0.99	0.82	0.99	0.52
0.85	111	0.99	0.80	0.99	0.46
0.90	111	0.99	0.76	0.99	0.38

Similarly, $AP_3 > AP_4$ for fixed p_1 and γ_k values. By definition, $AP_1 > AP_3$ and $AP_2 > AP_4$. Given p_1 and γ_k, the AP_1 value is the largest and the AP_4 value is the smallest. The assurance probabilities of all criteria increase as ρ_{12} increases. This is reasonable because these two co-primary endpoints are similar.

In this section, we further discuss the practical application of our method by using an example. A randomized, double-blind, active-controlled MRCT is to be conducted involving patients with mild-to-moderate AD to compare a new treatment and placebo control. For this trial, researchers plan to recruit patients aged 50 years and older and diagnosed as having uncomplicated AD from three regions: Taiwan, the European Union, and the United States. The primary endpoints are changes in ADAS-Cog and CIBIC-Plus scores from baseline to week 24. On the basis of results from a previous exploratory study, differences between the test drug and placebo of the change in the ADAS-Cog score from baseline to week 24 and of the CIBIC-Plus score at week 24 are expected to be 2.88 and 0.44, respectively. Furthermore, standard deviations for both the groups in terms of the change in the ADAS-Cog score from baseline to week 24 and the CIBIC-Plus score at week 24 are equal and assumed to be 6.15 and 0.92, respectively. With $\rho_{12} = 0$, 0.3, and 0.8, $\alpha = 0.025$, and $1 - \beta = 0.9$, the sample sizes required per group determined using formulas (17.1) and (17.2) are as follows:

$$n = \begin{cases} 116 \text{ if } \rho_{12} = 0, \\ 114 \text{ if } \rho_{12} = 0.3, \\ 107 \text{ if } \rho_{12} = 0.8. \end{cases}$$

In addition to demonstrating an overall treatment effect in all regions, the trial sponsor wishes to assess whether the overall results from this multi-regional trial can be applied to Taiwan after statistical significance is determined in the overall treatment effect. In this respect, the proportion of patients recruited in Taiwan must be determined at the design phase to preserve the ability to establish consistency between Taiwan and both other regions. Suppose that the similarity criterion (i) is used and $\gamma_1 = 0.5$ and $\gamma_2 = 0.5$ are chosen. To ensure the assurance probability of AP_1 is at the 80% level, the sample size required per group, n_S, of Taiwan patients with respect to $\rho_{12} = 0$, 0.3, and 0.8 is detailed as follows:

$$n_S = \begin{cases} 116 \times 33\% \approx 40 \text{ if } \rho_{12} = 0, \\ 114 \times 32\% \approx 38 \text{ if } \rho_{12} = 0.3, \\ 107 \times 27\% \approx 30 \text{ if } \rho_{12} = 0.8. \end{cases}$$

17.5 Different Endpoints

In some scenarios, the agreement cannot be reached among regulatory authorities on a single primary endpoint. ICH E17 suggests using a single protocol with endpoint-related subsections tailored toward respective regulatory requirements.

Without loss of generality, we examined a case in which an MRCT focuses on only two regions and two primary endpoints. For example, the European Medicines Agency guidance outlines the prevention of atrial fibrillation recurrence as the primary endpoint, whereas the US FDA prefers prevention of symptomatic recurrence as an endpoint (Girman et al. 2011). If no common primary endpoint is adopted in the two regions, questions would be raised regarding how to simultaneously assess the different primary endpoints of the regions. A possible solution is to prespecify two hypotheses for the different regulatory authorities within one study protocol. According to ICH E17, no multiplicity adjustment is necessary for individual regulatory decisions based on their respective primary endpoints. In addition, this is not a co-primary endpoint problem anymore, and thus the Type II error (power) adjustment is not required. The sample size can be just determined based on an endpoint with the smallest standardized effect size.

17.6 Discussion

The aim of an MRCT is to demonstrate the efficacy of a drug in various global regions and evaluate the possibility of applying the overall trial results to each region. However, sponsors face challenges in demonstrating consistency between results for a specific region and overall MRCT results. In this chapter, four criteria were established to assess the similarity between a specific region and overall regions in an MRCT with co-primary endpoints. Regulators and sponsors can easily adopt these criteria to statistically assess treatment effect consistency between a specific region and the entire trial region and facilitate new drug registration in that specific region.

At the 11th Q&A session for ICH E5, the following was stated: "It may be desirable in certain situations to achieve the goal of bridging by conducting a multiregional trial under a common protocol that includes sufficient numbers of patients from each of multiple regions to reach a conclusion about the effect of the drug in all regions..." Evidently, sample size determination for each region is a challenge for regulators and sponsors. With the four criteria established, the sample size required for the specific region can easily be determined, conferring a high probability of observing a consistent trend in treatment effects between a specific region and the entire MRCT. We do not recommend a particular criterion for evaluating the consistent trends of treatment effects between specific and entire regions. On the basis of our experience, given the same sample size for a specific region, of all criteria, criterion (i) has the highest assurance probability. When criterion (iv) is used, it may be difficult to achieve an assurance probability of 80%.

Although our approach is straightforward, one important issue arises from the selection of the magnitude γ_i of the consistency trend. Japanese guidance suggests that the magnitude be 0.5 or greater for the first criterion when the MRCT has only one primary endpoint. We suggest that the determination of γ_i be discussed between the regulatory agency in the specific region and the trial sponsor. Crucially, all differences in race, diet, environment, culture, and medical practices between regions should be considered.

When more than one primary endpoint is considered crucial in a clinical trial, a decision must be made on whether it is desirable to evaluate a joint effects on all endpoints or at least one endpoint. This decision defines the alternative hypothesis to be tested and provides a framework for trial design. Here, we only discuss a situation in which a trial is designed to evaluate the joint effect of a new treatment compared with any control treatment on all primary endpoints, as is the case in some AD-related clinical trials. However, for a trial designed to evaluate an effect on at least one primary endpoint (Offen et al. 2007), many methods for dealing with such endpoints have been proposed (see Dmitrienko et al. 2010). Similarly, for trials with co-primary endpoints, the power for detecting an effect on at least one endpoint, termed disjunctive power (Senn and Bretz 2007) or minimal power (Westfall et al. 2011), can be defined and extended to the APs.

The correlation is usually unknown and thus must be estimated using data from pilot studies or proceeding clinical trials (e.g., Phase II trials) or using external data when correlations are being incorporated into sample size calculation. In some disease areas, correlations among endpoints are known. For example, Offen et al. (2007) provided a list of known disease areas; the relevant regulatory agency required this list for a co-primary endpoint trial. The list includes possible correlations among endpoints for each disease area.

We assumed that the effect size for each co-primary endpoint and correlations among endpoints were uniform across regions. Because MRCTs involves recruiting participants from many countries worldwide, a difference in the treatment effect or in correlations among endpoints may be expected due to regional differences (e.g., ethnic differences). Thus, for sample size calculation for MRCTs, it might be impractical to assume that the effect size for each co-primary endpoint and correlations among endpoints are uniform across regions. Further exploration of alternative approaches" is ongoing. In addition, we only focus on the continuous endpoint in this chapter. However, the same concept can be easily extended to other endpoints, e.g., the binary endpoint or time-to-event endpoint.

References

Committee for Medicinal Products for Human Use (CHMP). 2008. *Guideline on medicinal products for the treatment of Alzheimer's disease and other dementias (CPMP/EWP/553/95 Rev.1)*. European Medical Agency, London, UK. http://www.ema.europa.eu/docs/en_GB/document_library/Scientific_guideline/2009/09/WC500003562.pdf. Accessed on April 12, 2020.

Committee for Human Medicinal Products (CHMP). 2016. *Guideline on multiplicity issues in clinical trials (Draft) (EMA/CHMP/44762/2017)*. London, UK: European Medicines Agency. https://www.ema.europa.eu/en/documents/scientific-guideline/draft-guideline-multiplicity-issues-clinical-trials_en.pdf. Accessed on April 12, 2020.

Dmitrienko, A., A.C. Tamhane, and F. Bretz. 2010. *Multiple testing problems in pharmaceutical statistics*. Boca Raton: Chapman & Hall/CRC.

Food and Drug Administration. 2017. *Guidance for industry: Multiple endpoints in clinical trials*. Rockville, MD, USA: U.S. Department of Health and Human Services Food and Drug Administration. https://www.fda.gov/media/102657/download. Accessed on April 12, 2021.

Girman, C.J., E. Ibia, S. Menjoge et al. 2011. Impact of different regulatory requirements for trial endpoints in multiregional clinical trials. *Drug Information Journal* 45(5):587–594.

Hamasaki, T., S.R. Evans, and K. Asakura. 2018. Design, data monitoring and analysis of clinical trials with co-primary endpoints: A review. *Journal of Biopharmaceutical Statistics* 28:28–51.

Hamasaki, T., T. Sugimoto, S.R. Evans, and T. Sozu. 2013. Sample size determination for clinical trials with co-primary outcomes: Exponential event-times. *Pharmaceutical Statistics* 12:28–34.

Huang, W.S., H.N. Hung, T. Hamasaki, and C.F. Hsiao. 2017. Sample size determination for a specific region in multiregional clinical trials with multiple co-primary endpoints. *PLoS One* 12(6):e0180405.

Hung, H.M., and S.J. Wang. 2009. Some controversial multiple testing problems in regulatory applications. *Journal of Biopharmaceutical Statistics* 19:1–11.

International Council for Harmonisation of Technical Requirements for Pharmaceuticals for Human Use (ICH). 2017. E17 General principles for planning and design of Multi-Regional Clinical Trials. ICH Harmonised Guideline, ICH. https://database.ich.org/sites/default/files/E17EWG_Step4_2017_1116.pdf.

Offen, W., C. Chuang-Stein, and A. Dmitrienko et al. 2007. Multiple co-primary endpoints: Medical and statistical solutions. *Drug Information Journal* 41:31–46.

Senn, S, and F. Bretz. 2007. Power and sample size when multiple endpoints are considered. *Pharmaceutical Statistics* 6:161–170.

Sozu, T., T. Kanou, C. Hamada, and I. Yoshimura. 2006. Power and sample size calculations in clinical trials with multiple primary variables. *Japanese Journal of Biometrics* 27:83–96.

Sozu, T, T. Sugimoto, and T. Hamasaki. 2011. Sample size determination in superiority clinical trials with multiple co-primary correlated endpoints. *Journal of Biopharmaceutical Statistics* 21:650–668.

Sozu, T., T. Sugimoto, T. Hamasaki, and S.R. Evans. 2015. *Sample size determination in clinical trials with multiple endpoints*. Cham: Springer International Publishing.

Sugimoto, T., T. Sozu, and T. Hamasaki. 2012. A convenient formula for sample size calculations in clinical trials with multiple co-primary continuous endpoints. *Pharmaceutical Statistics* 11:118–128.

Westfall, P.H., R.D. Tobias, and R.D. Wolfinger. 2011. *Multiple comparisons and multiple tests using SAS*, 2nd edition. Cary, NC: SAS Institute Inc.

18

Multi-regional Clinical Trials with Heterogeneous Regional Treatment Effects

Hsiao-Hui Tsou, Yu-Chieh Cheng, K.K. Gordon Lan, Hsiao-Yu Wu, Ya-Ting Hsu, Fang-Jing Lee, Chi-Tian Chen, Meng-Hsuan Wu, and Chin-Fu Hsiao

18.1 Treatment Effect Evaluation and Combination

18.1.1 Brief Review of Statistical Models for Evaluation and Combination of Treatment Effects

With the globalization of drug development, multi-regional clinical trials (MRCTs) have become a popular strategy in the development of new medicines. According to the draft ICH E17 (ICH E17, 2016), an MRCT incorporates subjects from several regions (which may refer to geographical regions, countries, or regulatory regions) under the same protocol and seeks regulatory approval for all participating regions. An estimand in a clinical trial usually reflects what is to be estimated to demonstrate the clinical benefit of a test treatment (Leuchs et al., 2015; ICH E9 (R1), 2017). In MRCTs, the overall treatment effect is the primary estimand. However, the treatment effects may be heterogeneous among regions due to ethnic factors (such as race, diet, environment, culture, medical practice, etc.) or other reasons. The definition of the overall treatment effect may be unclear and ambiguous when there is heterogeneity among regions. Therefore, how to model regional differences and assess the impact of regional differences are important challenges in the design and evaluation of MRCTs.

In a traditional clinical trial, the primary goal is to demonstrate the efficacy of a new treatment (T) compared with a control (C). Thus, the trial is designed to detect the treatment effect $\theta = \mu_T - \mu_C$ and determine the sample size based on power analysis, where μ_T and μ_C are the treatment effects of groups T and C. To be more rigorous, for testing the hypothesis of treatment effect (H_0: $\theta = 0$

DOI: 10.1201/9781003109785-18

versus H_A: $\theta \neq 0$), we evaluate the amount of statistical information required to reach a certain power for a θ given under a simple alternative. For the comparison of the two means, the amount of information is proportional to the sample size and the patient-allocation ratio. When the total sample size N is determined, the maximum power of the test statistic Z-test is reached at 1:1 patient-allocation ratio, where Z-test is a statistical test for difference in means between two intervention groups under known variance. This will be illustrated in detail later when we introduce the concept of "effective sample size" in Section 18.1.2.6. When the trial is completed, the key result is obtained to draw the conclusion about the targeted clinical benefit of a test product.

For a K-center clinical trial ($K \geq 2$) with comparisons between two treatments T and C, treatment effects in K centers are usually assumed to be equal ($\theta_1 = \theta_2 = \ldots = \theta_K = \theta$) The overall treatment effect θ is usually estimated by $\hat{\theta} = \sum_{k=1}^{K} w_k \hat{\theta}_k$, where $\hat{\theta}_k$ and w_k are the estimates of treatment effect and weight proportional to sample size for center k, respectively. Implicitly, we assume that the patient-allocation ratios are the same overall K centers. When the patient-allocation ratios are different, "sample size" and "statistical information" have quite different implications. Roughly speaking, the amount of information available depends on sample size and allocation ratio. This concept will be discussed later under the subject of "effective sample size." There are some differences between a traditional K-centers trial and an MRCT. In a traditional multi-center trial, the objective is to evaluate the overall treatment effect with all centers regulated by the same authority. On the other hand, MRCT has a different objective. It seeks approval by different regional authorities simultaneously using the MRCT trial design. Another major difference between a traditional K-centers trial and an MRCT is regional heterogeneity. In MRCTs, ethnic factors (intrinsic and extrinsic factors) and other reasons may have an impact on the drug's effect in each participating region. The concept of traditional K-center trials, such as the assumption of a common treatment effect across the center, could not be applied to MRCTs when regional heterogeneity is anticipated.

To account for heterogeneous treatment effects across regions, Lan et al. (2012) proposed a discrete random effects model (DREM) to estimate the overall treatment effect in an MRCT. Later, Lan et al. (2014) applied DREM from continuous endpoints to binary and time-to-event endpoints. Liu et al. (2016) derived an optimal sample size allocation over regions under DREM to maximize the power of consistency and provided some guidelines on the design of MRCTs with consistency.

18.1.2 Investigate the Insights of Random Effect Model

18.1.2.1 Estimation of Treatment Effect

How to combine information from participating regions to estimate an overall treatment effect is an increasingly important topic in MRCTs.

Traditionally, a common treatment effect across regions is assumed for the design and evaluation of an MRCT. Suppose that K regions participate in an MRCT for comparing a new treatment T with a control C. The numbers of subjects with T and C are $N_T = \sum_{k=1}^{K} N_{Tk}$ and $N_C = \sum_{k=1}^{K} N_{Ck}$, respectively. N_{Tk} and N_{Ck} represent the numbers of subjects for T and C in region k, respectively. In practice, N_T and N_C could be different which will be discussed later. For a simple illustration, equal allocation is considered, i.e., $N_T = N_C$ and $N = N_T + N_C$, and $N_{Tk} = N_{Ck}$ and $N_k = N_{Tk} + N_{Ck}$ for every k. Let X_{Tkj} and X_{Ckj} be the efficacy responses for the jth subject in the kth region receiving the test product and control, respectively, $j = 1,\ldots, N_k/2$, $k = 1, 2, \ldots, K$. The efficacy responses can be expressed as $X_{Tjk} = \mu_{Tjk} + \varepsilon_{Tjk}$ and $X_{Cjk} = \mu_{Cjk} + \varepsilon_{Cjk}$, where ε_{Tkj} and ε_{Ckj} are both normally distributed with mean 0 and variance σ^2. Let treatment difference in region k be $\theta_k = \mu_{Tk} - \mu_{Ck}$, for $k = 1, 2,\ldots, K$, where μ_{Tk} and μ_{Ck} are the treatment effects of groups T and C, respectively, in region k. Naturally, θ_k is estimated by $\hat{\theta}_k = \bar{X}_{Tk} - \bar{X}_{Ck}$, where $\bar{X}_{Tk}$ and $\bar{X}_{Ck}$ are the sample means of T and C in region k, respectively.

18.1.2.2 Equal Treatment Effect: FEM

Traditionally, the treatment effects from different regions are regarded as a constant, i.e., $\theta_1 = \theta_2 = \ldots = \theta_K = \theta$ where θ is the common treatment effect. As noted in Hung et al. (2010), the global estimate would be a good estimate of the drug effect for each participating region when regional effect estimates are similar. The fixed-effects model (FEM) is widely applied to global trials, including an approach to rationalize for partitioning sample size into regions (Kawai et al., 2008), a sample size determination for a specific region (Ko et al., 2010), statistical consideration with Asian perspective for a specific region (Tsou et al., 2010), and the establishment of consistency among all regions (Tsou et al., 2012).

Under FEM, the testing hypothesis of the overall treatment effect is

$$H_0\colon \theta = 0 \text{ vs. } H_A\colon \theta \neq 0. \tag{18.1}$$

We are interested only in $\theta > 0$. For normal or continuous responses, a standard two-sample test statistic is

$$Z_{FEM} = \frac{\hat{\theta}_{FEM}}{\sigma\sqrt{4/N}}, \tag{18.2}$$

where $\hat{\theta}_{FEM} = \sum_{k=1}^{K} N_k \hat{\theta}_k / N$ is the estimate of θ under FEM. When responses are not normally distributed, the test statistic still follows an approximately normal distribution in large sample cases. Note that when $\sigma = 1$, Fisher's information for θ_{FEM} is $[Var(\theta_{FEM})]^{-1} = [4/N]^{-1} = N/4$.

18.1.2.3 Regional Heterogeneity in MRCTs and Model Violation of FEM

In practice, regional differences in treatment effects are often seen and discovered because of ethnic factors and other reasons. A well-known example is the Platelet Inhibition and Patient Outcomes (PLATO) trial (Wallentin et al., 2009; Mahaffey et al., 2011). The objective of the PLATO trial was to compare ticagrelor and clopidogrel in the treatment of 18,624 patients with acute coronary syndromes (ACS) for the prevention of cardiovascular events. The PLATO trial was conducted across 43 countries and 4 pre-defined geographic regions (North America, Asia/Australia, Central/South America, and Europe/Middle East/Africa). The primary endpoint was the time to CV death, myocardial infarction, or stroke. Ticagrelor significantly reduced the risk of major adverse cardiovascular events, with an overall hazard ratio of 0.84 and 95% CI = (0.77, 0.92). However, the observed hazard ratio for patients in North America was 1.25 and in the opposite direction of the overall hazard ratio. The hazard ratio favored ticagrelor in all regions but North America. The statistical interaction between treatment and regions was significant, with $p = 0.045$ for the four regions (Carroll et al., 2013). The result seems to suggest that North America was directionally inconsistent with the other geographic regions in terms of the treatment effect of ticagrelor relative to clopidogrel. Consequently, the applicability of FEM, in this case, is highly questionable. In addition, if such inconsistency is anticipated, FEM is hardly appropriate for planning and evaluating an MRCT. DREM may be an alternative approach to consider when there is inconsistency among regions.

18.1.2.4 Unequal Regional Treatment Effect: DREM

In practice, regional differences have been observed and may have an impact upon the assessment of a medicine's effect. Thus, the assumption of an unequal regional treatment effect may be appropriate for designing an MRCT when regional heterogeneity is anticipated. Lan et al. (2012) proposed a DREM, which assumes that treatment effects over regions are different to account for the regional differences. To evaluate the treatment effect in a population Ω, we consider a new treatment T being compared with a control C. The total sample size is N, and the patient-allocation ratio to T versus C is 1:1. The responses are expressed as X_{T1}, X_{T2}, ... and X_{C1}, X_{C2}, ... The total treatment effect difference can be re-written as $\Sigma X_{Ti} - \Sigma X_{Ci} = \Sigma(X_{Ti} - X_{Ci}) = \Sigma Y_i$. For simplicity, this pairing enables us to treat the comparison as a one-sample problem. Section 18.1.2.6 (effective sample size) gives detailed conversions for when the treatment assignment is not 1:1.

18.1.2.5 Insights of DREM

First of all, what is the patient population Ω and what are the subpopulations being considered in an MRCT under DREM? Let us write

$\Omega = \Omega_1 + \Omega_2 + ...+ \Omega_K$, where the subpopulation Ω_k stands for Regions k, $k = 1, 2, ..., K$. Denote the population size M as the sum of the subpopulation sizes $M_1, M_2, ..., M_K$. In the following, we assume that $\{M_1, M_2, ..., M_K\}$ are large, which implies that M is also large, and there will be little difference between sampling with replacement and without replacement. When we take a random sample $X = X(\omega)$ from Ω, the chance that this patient taken from Ω_k is $P(\omega \in \Omega_k) = M_k/M = W_k$, $k = 1, 2,..., K$. Denote θ_k as the treatment effect in region k, $k = 1,..., K$. These θ_k are non-random parameters. Under DREM, θ_k could be different. Then a random response Y can be expressed as $\mu + \varepsilon$, where $\mu = \theta_k$ if Y is taken from Ω_k, and ε is $N(0, 2\sigma^2)$. We assume that the within-region variation $2\sigma^2$ is the same over regions.

The first random component μ follows a multinomial distribution with mean $\theta = \Sigma W_k \theta_k$ and variance $\tau^2 = E(\mu^2) - \theta^2$, as shown in Lan et al. (2012). Under normality, each $Y \sim N(\theta, \tau^2 + 2\sigma^2)$ and the estimate of population treatment effect is

$$\hat{\theta} = \frac{\Sigma\Sigma Y_{ik}}{N/2} = \sum W_k \hat{\theta}_k \sim N\left(\theta, \frac{2(\tau^2 + 2\sigma^2)}{N}\right). \tag{18.3}$$

Without normality assumption on the random response Y, we apply the central limit theorem to obtain the normal approximation of $\hat{\theta}$.

In an ideal situation, we take a fixed proportion, say 0.1%, of patients from Ω. Then the sample sizes $\{N_1, N_2,..., N_K, N\}$ with $\Sigma N_k = N$ will be close to $\{0.001M_1, 0.001M_2, ..., 0.001M_K, 0.001M\}$. We expect $\{N_k/N\}$ to provide excellent approximates for $\{W_k\}$ in the large sample case. In practice, we may not take the same proportions from all regions. For example, PLATO was not designed to follow the plan with 18,624 patients selected randomly from 43 countries in 4 regions with the known sample to region proportion. The assumption of taking a fixed proportion from Ω or $\Omega(k)$ may be unpractical. Thus, there are two different ways to assign weights and consequently define and estimate average treatment effects. The first one is

$$\theta = \sum W_k \theta_k \text{ with } W_k = M_k/M; \text{ and } \hat{\theta} = \sum M_k \hat{\theta}_k / M. \tag{18.4}$$

The second one is given as

$$\theta = \sum W_k \theta_k \text{ with } W_k = N_k/N; \text{ and } \hat{\theta} = \sum N_k \hat{\theta}_k / N. \tag{18.5}$$

If the subpopulation sizes are known, we take subpopulation proportion weights (Eq. (18.3)). Unfortunately, the subpopulation sizes are usually unknown. To employ sample size weights (Eq. (18.4)), we provide two different arguments. The first one is a "naïve" argument. We use sample size weights since this is natural and well accepted by both clinicians and statisticians. The second is from the point of view of re-sampling.

After all, data are collected, we may perform inference by taking random samples from the combined data set, which leads to the use of sample size weights. Correspondingly, the overall within-region variation and the between-region variation are $\sum_{k=1}^{K} W_k 2\sigma^2 = 2\sigma^2$ and $\tau^2 = \sum_{k=1}^{K} W_k (\theta_k - \theta)^2$, respectively. The test statistic for the null hypotheses of Eq. (18.1) is

$$Z_{DREM} = \frac{\hat{\theta}}{\sqrt{\text{Var}(\hat{\theta})}} = \frac{\hat{\theta}}{\sqrt{(4\sigma^2 + 2\tau^2)/N}} \qquad (18.6)$$

which is approximated to a normal distribution with a sufficiently large sample size N. The new treatment T would be claimed beneficial to patients if $Z_{DREM} > z_{1-\alpha}$, where $z_{1-\alpha}$ denotes the $(1-\alpha)$th percentile of the standard normal distribution. Under an alternative hypothesis where $\theta = \delta.$, the power function for benefit is

$$PB = \Pr(Z_{DREM} > z_{1-\alpha} \mid N, \delta) = \Phi \left[\frac{\delta}{\sqrt{(4\sigma^2 + 2\tau^2)/N}} - z_{1-\alpha} \right], \qquad (18.7)$$

where Φ is the cumulative distribution function of the standard normal distribution. At the design stage, given significance level α and power $1 - \beta$, the total required sample size to detect $\theta = \delta > 0$ is

$$N_{DREM} = (4\sigma^2 + 2\tau^2) \left(\frac{z_{1-\alpha} + z_{1-\beta}}{\delta} \right)^2. \qquad (18.8)$$

18.1.2.6 Effective Sample Size

Practically, the treatment assignment in each region of an MRCT may not be 1:1. Sometimes—for reasons of cost, learning curves, ethics, etc.—it is desirable to have more patients in one arm than the other (Dumville et al., 2006). For example, more participants in the new treatment may encourage people to participate in a trial because their chance of receiving the new treatment is higher than 50% (Wittes, 2002). On the other hand, more participants may be assigned to the control group for studies investigating a new therapy in very short supply (Wittes, 2002).

In Section 18.1.2.5, we introduced DREM under the setting of equal patient allocation to the treatment group and the control group. Now we derive the relationship between the patient-allocation ratio and effective sample size. Suppose the Z statistic takes the form following for comparing the treatment effect between group A and group B:

$$Z = \frac{\bar{X}_A - \bar{X}_B}{\sigma\sqrt{1/N_A + 1/N_B}}. \tag{18.9}$$

Two examples are considered. Example 1: A total of 800 patients, $N_A = N_B = 400$. Then the Fisher information for $\sigma = 1$ is $(1/N_A + 1/N_B)^{-1} = 200$. For a 1:1 allocation, the two-sample factor is $\frac{1}{2} \times \frac{1}{2} = \frac{1}{4} = \frac{200}{800}$. Example 2: A total of 900 patients, $N_A = 300$, $N_B = 600$. Then the Fisher information for $\sigma = 1$ is $(1/N_A + 1/N_B)^{-1} = 200$. For a 1:2 allocation, the two-sample factor is $\frac{1}{3} \times \frac{2}{3} = \frac{2}{9} = \frac{200}{900}$. The Z-tests in examples 1 and 2 have the same distribution under H_0 and H_A. For power evaluations, if we recruit 900 patients with a 1:2 allocation ratio, the power would be the same as recruiting 800 patients with a 1:1 ratio.

What do we learn from this? There is a heuristic way to interpret the relationship between information and sample size. For a 1:1 allocation and total sample size N ($=N_A + N_B$), the number of information is

$$I = \frac{N}{2} \times \frac{1}{2} = \frac{N}{4} \tag{18.10}$$

For a 1:r allocation to group A and group B, the number of information is

$$I = \frac{N}{1+r} \times \frac{r}{1+r} = \frac{rN}{(1+r)^2}. \tag{18.11}$$

In many published manuscripts, we assume a 1:1 patient-allocation ratio. In general, for a 1:r allocation, we may replace the total sample size N by

$$N^e = \frac{4r}{(1+r)^2}N, \tag{18.12}$$

which is smaller than N when $r > 1$. The N^e is called the effective sample size for the 1:r allocation ratio. For additional details about information and information fractions for the design of clinical trials, see Lan et al. (1994).

In an MRCT, we may use the effective sample size N^e, replacing N, for the design and data analysis. More specifically, in an MRCT, suppose some regions use a 1:1 allocation for the control group (C) and treatment group (T), some regions use a 1:2 allocation, and some regions use a 1:r allocation. For the region k using a 1:r ratio with sample size N_k, we can replace N_k by the effective sample size $N_k^e = N_k \times 4r/(1+r)^2$ and treat this region as if the sample size is N_k^e and the ratio is 1:1. Then we can apply DREM with regional sample size N_k^e and equal treatment allocation as described in the above section to design the MRCT. Thus, the overall treatment effect under DREM is $\theta^e = \sum_{k=1}^{K} W_k^e \theta_k$, and W_k^e can be estimated by the effective sample size ratio N_k^e/N^e. The estimate of the population treatment effect is

$\hat{\theta}^e = \sum_{k=1}^{K} W_k^e \hat{\theta}_k$. Correspondingly, the overall within-region variation and the between-region variation are $\sum_{k=1}^{K} W_k^e 2\sigma^2 = 2\sigma^2$ and $\tau^2 = \sum_{k=1}^{K} W_k^e (\theta_k - \theta^e)^2$, respectively. The test statistic for hypotheses Eq. (18.1) is

$$Z_{DREM} = \frac{\hat{\theta}^e}{\sqrt{Var(\hat{\theta}^e)}} = \frac{\hat{\theta}^e}{\sqrt{(4\sigma^2 + 2\tau^2)/N^e}}. \qquad (18.13)$$

which is approximated to normal distribution with sufficiently large sample size N^e. According to ICH E17, MRCT is defined as a clinical trial conducted in more than one region under a single protocol. Thus, each region should have the same treatment allocation ratio in an MRCT. At the end of the trial, however, we often encounter the situation of patients lost to follow-up. That is, the ratio of the numbers of patients in the treatment group compared to the control group $n_{Tk}: n_{Ck}$ in region k often differs from the ratio $n_{Tl}: n_{Cl}$ in region l at the final data analysis stage. In this case, the application of effective sample size and the test statistic Z_{DREM} in Eq. (18.5) can be used for the data analysis.

In the case of unbalanced design in an MRCT, the effective sample size can be still applied to design the MRCT. According to an example in Quan et al. (2010), an MRCT was designed to evaluate the effect of an investigational drug on change from baseline in HbA_{1c}. In order to have more safety data for the investigational drug, the trial used an unbalanced design with 2:1 ratio for the active treatment and placebo groups. Thus, for region k with sample size N_k, we can replace N_k by the effective sample size $N_k^e = N_k \times 4r/(1+r)^2 = \frac{8}{9} \times N_k$, where $r = 2; k = 1, \ldots, K$. Therefore, this trial can be treated as an equal treatment allocation for the active treatment and placebo groups with regional sample size N_k^e. Then we can apply DREM as described in Section 18.3 to design the MRCT.

In practice, a region may use an allocation ratio different from other regions due to medical insurance policies in that particular region. Other reasons such as cost or patients' acceptability might also cause different allocation ratio in different regions in an MRCT. Note that we rephrase the allocation ratio through an effective sample size in this section. Therefore, a change of allocation ratio can be viewed as a change of sample size.

18.2 Explore a Two-stage Design of MRCT under a Random Effect Model

18.2.1 Sample Size Re-estimation for MRCTs under DREM

For a long time, we have been struggling with the definition of overall treatment effect in an MRCT. Traditionally, we designed clinical trials under the fixed (equal) treatment effect model where the overall treatment effect θ $(= \theta_1 = \theta_2 = \ldots = \theta_K)$ is well-defined. Behind this assumption, we may consider that observations are independent, identically distributed (i.i.d.). When there is no inconsistency among regions, we may perform traditional inferences, and changing the regional sample sizes will not cause biased with no or little theoretical concern (Cui et al., 1999; Chen et al., 2017). However, regional differences might be anticipated in reality. The definition of the overall treatment effect is unclear and ambiguous when there is heterogeneity among regions. In this case, we usually do not have good solutions for defining the overall treatment effect. The overall treatment effect could be an average effect using some kind of weights. DREM may provide a solution to address the overall treatment effect in MRCTs.

When designing an MRCT, the power evaluation is usually estimated from limited information and under uncertain assumptions. It would be desirable to modify total sample size or adjust sample size allocation to some regions using accumulating data at an interim time during this trial for increasing the efficiency of the trial. We discuss the following two scenarios without changing size allocation to regions usually adopted at an interim data.

> *Scenario 1* Sample size re-estimation based on interim results by using the conditional power approach (Li et al., 2002). Specifically, if the interim results present less treatment effect than planned in the design stage, total sample size would be increased to achieve sufficient power. For this scenario, after the sample size re-estimation (without changing sample size allocation to regions) based on the interim results, we can estimate treatment effect parameters and calculate the Z-score.

> *Scenario 2* An additional region wants to joint this MRCT at the interim results stage. The parameter of interest has been changed from K to $K + 1$ regions.

We do not change the critical values for the final test in these two scenarios. The type I error rate does not be effected by increased sample size in the scenario 1. Hence, we focus the impact of the type I error rate by increased regional number in the scenario.

18.2.2 Increase Region Number from K to $K+1$

The second scenario is that we consider a two-stage design for an MRCT under DREM for showing the impact on the type I error rate when adding a new region into an MRCT. To simplify, suppose that there are $K = 3$ regions in stage 1 and then 4 regions will be studied in stage 2. An interim analysis was conducted after stage 1. We add a new region into the MRCT due to political or other reasons. We have a new overall treatment effect θ' for the $K + 1$ regions, we discuss the detail scenario below.

As an example, we start with three regions (Japan, Korea, and Taiwan) in stage 1 and a new region Vietnam is added in stage 2. The testing hypothesis of the overall treatment effect is H_0: $\theta = 0\ vs\ H_0$: $\theta \neq 0$ in stage 1, and we are interested only in $\theta > 0$. Let (W_1, W_2, W_3) be the region weights in three regions. The total sample size for the original design is $N = \sum_{k=1}^{3} N_k$ with equal allocation for a control group and a treatment group, $N_{Ck} = N_{Tk} = N_k/2$. We assume that $\hat{\theta}_1, \hat{\theta}_2, \hat{\theta}_3$ are the estimators of treatment effects $\theta_1, \theta_2, \theta_3$, respectively. Let $\hat{\theta}_k = \bar{Y}_k = \sum_{i=1}^{N_k} Y_{ik}/N_k/2$, $k = 1, ..., 3$, where $Y_{ik} \sim N(\theta_k, 2\sigma^2 + \tau^2)$ and σ^2 is the common variance and τ^2 is the between-region variance. A test statistic under DREM for stage 1 is

$$Z = \frac{\hat{\theta}}{\sqrt{(4\sigma^2 + 2\tau^2)/N}}, \qquad (18.14)$$

where

$$\hat{\theta} = \sum_{k=1}^{3} W_k \bar{Y}_k = \sum_{k=1}^{3} \sum_{i=1}^{N_k} W_k Y_{ik}/(N_k/2) = \sum_{k=1}^{3} \sum_{i=1}^{N_k} Y_{ik}/(N/2) \qquad (18.15)$$

is an estimator of the overall treatment effect $\theta = \sum_{k=1}^{3} W_k \theta_k$ and $\tau^2 = \sum_{k=1}^{3} W_k (\theta_k - \theta)^2$ under DREM. In addition, we determine the required sample size N by Eq. (18.14) with given type I error rate α and type II error rate β.

After a period of time, we conduct an interim and decide to add a new region, Vietnam, into this MRCT. Let $\hat{\theta}'_4$ be the natural estimator of treatment effect of θ'_4. The weight of this new region W'_4 is usually determined in a meeting of all regional participants or representatives, included Vietnam). The new weights of original regions becomes $W'_k = (1 - W'_4) \times W_k$, $k = 1, ..., 3$. The new overall treatment effect is $\theta' = W'_4 \theta'_4 + (1 - W'_4)\theta$. The new total sample size is $N' = N + N_4$. The new testing hypotheses are

$$H'_0: \theta' = 0 \ vs \ H_0: \theta' \neq 0 \qquad (18.16)$$

and we are interested only in $\theta' > 0$. The final test statistics is

$$Z' = \frac{\hat{\theta}'}{\sqrt{(4\sigma^2 + 2\tau'^2)/N'}} = \sqrt{\frac{N}{N'}} Z + \sqrt{\frac{N_4}{N'}} Z_4, \qquad (18.17)$$

where

$$Z_4 = \frac{\hat{\theta}'_4}{\sqrt{(4\sigma^2 + 2\tau'^2)/N_4}}, \tag{18.18}$$

$\hat{\theta}' = \sum_{k=1}^{4} W'_k \hat{\theta}'_k$ is an estimator of $\theta' = \sum_{k=1}^{4} W'_k \theta'_k, \hat{\theta}'_k = \hat{\theta}_k, k = 1, 2,3,$ and $\tau'^2 = \sum_{k=1}^{4} W'_k (\theta'_k - \theta')^2$. Here, we suppose that $\tau'^2 \approx \tau^2$ and that the treatment effects of Japan, Korea, and Taiwan are the same in the two-stage design, such that $\theta'_k = \theta_k, k = 1,..., 3$.

Comparing the probability density distributions of Z and Z' helps us understand the difference between them. Under the null hypothesis, H_0: $\theta = 0$ with $\theta = \sum_{k=1}^{3} W_k \theta_k$, we have

$$\hat{\theta}_k \sim N\left(\theta_k, \frac{2(2\sigma^2 + \tau^2)}{N_k}\right), k = 1, ...,3. \tag{18.19}$$

Then

$$\hat{\theta} = \sum_{k=1}^{3} W_k \hat{\theta}_k \sim N\left(0, \frac{2(2\sigma^2 + \tau^2)}{N}\right), \tag{18.20}$$

with, $N = \sum_{k=1}^{3} N_k$ and $Z \sim N(0, 1)$. Under the another null hypothesis, H'_0: $\theta' = 0$ with $\theta' = \sum_{k=1}^{4} W'_k \theta'_k$, we have $\hat{\theta}'_k \sim N\left(\theta'_k, \frac{2(2\sigma^2 + \tau^2)}{N_k}\right), k = 1, ..., 4$.

Then,

$$\hat{\theta}' = \sum_{k=1}^{4} W'_k \hat{\theta}'_k \sim N\left(0, \frac{2(2\sigma^2 + \tau^2)}{N'}\right), \tag{18.21}$$

with $N' = \sum_{k=1}^{4} N_k$ and $Z' \sim N(0, 1)$. Although we add a new region, there is no difference between the distributions of Z and Z'. These two test statistics have the same probability density function. Hence, if we add a new region into a processing MRCT, then we still control the type I error rate without any adjustment. However, the power based on N' is greater than the power based on N due to the larger sample size.

Here, we show the performance of empirical type I error rates based on the above-described Z. To simplify, we consider $\theta_1 = 0.9$, $\theta_2 = \theta_3 = 0.8$, with $\sigma = 3$ in the design stage. The sample size is determined by $N = 2\left(\frac{z_{1-\beta} + z_{1-\alpha}}{\delta}\right)^2 (\sigma^2 + \tau^2)$, where $\tau^2 = \sum_{k=1}^{3} W_k (\theta_k - \theta)^2$, and we consider

TABLE 18.1

The empirical α and the empirical α' based on the test statistic Z and Z', respectively, at $W'_4 = 0.1$

W_1	W_2	W_3	N	N'	α^{a}	α'^{b}
0.1	0.45	0.45	431	479	0.0244	0.0242
0.2	0.4	0.4	421	469	0.0250	0.0249
0.3	0.35	0.35	411	457	0.0263	0.0259
0.4	0.3	0.3	401	447	0.0257	0.0254
0.5	0.25	0.25	392	436	0.0262	0.0259
0.6	0.2	0.2	383	427	0.0242	0.0247

a the empirical type I error rate based on Z.
b the empirical type I error rate based on Z'.

TABLE 18.2

The empirical α and the empirical α' based on the test statistic Z and Z', respectively, at $W'_4 = 0.1$, when we change sample allocation of three regions after an interim

W_1	W_2	W_3	N	N'	α	α'
0.1	0.45	0.45	431	479	0.0904	0.0531
0.2	0.4	0.4	421	469	0.071	0.039
0.3	0.35	0.35	411	457	0.051	0.0298
0.4	0.3	0.3	401	447	0.0326	0.0259
0.5	0.25	0.25	392	436	0.0162	0.0247
0.6	0.2	0.2	383	427	0.0048	0.0304

$\alpha = 0.025$ and $\beta = 0.2$. Here, we consider $W'_4 = 0.3$. The simulation times is 100,000 for calculating the empirical type I error rate.

Table 18.1 shows the empirical type I error rates based on Z and Z' at $W'_4 = 0.1$. This table shows the similar result of the empirical type I error rates based on Z and Z' under the same θ'_4.

However, if changing sample size allocation to regions is unavoidable, then the empirical type I error rate may not be controlled into expected value, such that less than 0.025. For instance, we conduct an MRCT in three regions, and a new region joins after an interim with $W'_4 = 0.1$. If we observe that the treatment effect of the first region is better than that of the other two regions in the interim, then we change the sample size allocation to regions, such that $(W'_1, W'_2, W'_3) = (0.4, 0.25, 0.25)$. Table 18.2 shows the result of empirical type I error rates based on Z and Z'. We find that the values of α or α' do not be controlled, such that less than 0.025 except $(W_1, W_2, W_3) = (0.5, 0.2, 0.2)$.

Hence, if we change sample size allocation to regions, then the corresponding type I error rate may be adjusted and the method of drop-minimum data analysis may provide an adjustment (Chen et al., 2017). Generally, a regulatory body may not suggest changing sample size allocations across regions because it lost the fair for patient's safety and efficacy.

18.3 Discussion

In an MRCT, the definition of overall treatment effect depends on how the population parameter is estimated. In other words, the treatment effect depends on the regions chosen. For example, the treatment effect for all patients in "China, Thailand, Malaysia, and Singapore" may be different from the treatment effect in "China and Thailand" or the treatment effect in "Malaysia and Singapore." To be more specific, consider regions: $\Omega = \Omega_1 + \Omega_2 + \Omega_3 + \Omega_4$ with regional treatment effects $\theta_1, \theta_2, \theta_3, \theta_4$; population sizes M_1, M_2, M_3, M_4.

> (Ex 1) The treatment effect θ for Ω is $(M_1\theta_1 + M_2\theta_2 + M_3\theta_3 + M_4\theta_4)/(M_1+M_2+M_3+M_4)$.
> (Ex 2) The treatment effect θ for $\Omega_1 + \Omega_2$ is $(M_1\theta_1 + M_2\theta_2)/(M_1+M_2)$.
> (Ex 3) The treatment effect θ for $\Omega_3 + \Omega_4$ is $(M_3\theta_3 + M_4\theta_4)/(M_3+M_4)$.

More generally, we cannot estimate the treatment effect in "Asia" by conducting an MRCT in only "China, Thailand, Malaysia, and Singapore," since Asia contains more than those four countries. The treatment effect is associated with the combined regions in the trial. Different region combinations represent different populations.

In practice, we often do not have an equal number of patients in each treatment group at the end of the trial due to medical insurance policy, cost, or patients' acceptability in that particular region even though the trial is designed under the setting of equal treatment allocation ratio. In this paper, we illustrate the relationship between treatment allocation ration and effective sample size. We provide a heuristic way to rephrase the allocation ratio through an effective sample size so that a change of allocation ratio can be viewed as a change of sample size. We further proposed an approach, applying DREM with regional sample size N_k^e and equal treatment allocation, to analyze the overall MRCT data in the case of unequal number of patients in treatment groups.

An application of the approach illustrated in the previous paragraph is drop-minimum data analysis (Chen et al., 2017). Drop-minimum data analysis was treated as an ad hoc data-analysis procedure. As considered in the drop-minimum approach (Chen et al., 2017), when $\hat{\theta}_1$ is smaller than $\hat{\theta}_2, \hat{\theta}_3$.

and a decision has been made to drop Ω_1 from the MRCT for $\Omega_1 + \Omega_2 + \Omega_3$, the population has been changed to $\Omega_2 + \Omega_3$ and the treatment effect should be modified accordingly. Note that we should not just delete the data from Region 1; the treatment effect estimate for the new population — Regions 2 and 3, after dropping Region 1 — should be modified (Chen et al., 2017).

Regional heterogeneity in MRCTs is often anticipated, and researchers are usually urged to re-estimate the sample size or re-allocate sample size to regions based on interim results. In such a situation, the definition of the overall treatment effect is unclear. Moreover, the originally pre-defined overall treatment effect may change after the adaptation. We usually do not have good solutions for defining the overall treatment effect in these cases. This article shares more insights into DREM and provides a solution to address these issues with MRCTs. The proposed approach may offer the first step to deal with the problems of bias resulting from adaptation.

References

Carroll, K. J. and T. R. Fleming. 2013. Statistical evaluation and analysis of regional interactions: the PLATO trial case study. *Statistics in Biopharmaceutical Research* 5:91–101.

Chen, F., L. Gang, and K. K. G. Lan. 2017. Inconsistency and drop-minimum data analysis. *Statistics in Medicine* 36(3):416–425.

Cui, L., H. M. Hung, and S. J. Wang. 1999. Modification of sample size in group sequential clinical trials. *Biometrics* 55(3):853–857.

Dumville, J.C., S. Hahn, J. N. V. Miles, and D. J. Torgerson. 2006. The use of unequal randomisation ratios in clinical trials: a review. *Contemporary Clinical Trials* 27(1):1–12.

Hung, H. M., S. J. Wang, and R. T. O'Neill. 2010. Consideration of regional difference in design and analysis of multi-regional trials. *Pharmaceutical Statistics* 9(3):173–178.

International Council for Harmonization of Technical Requirements for Pharmaceuticals for Human Use. 2017. ICH E9 (R1) addendum on estimands and sensitivity analysis in clinical trials to the guideline on statistical principles for clinical trials. *European Medicines Agency*. http://www.ema.europa.eu/docs/en_GB/document_library/Scientific_guideline/2017/08/WC500233916.pdf (accessed October 5, 2020).

International Council for Harmonization of Technical Requirements for Pharmaceuticals for Human Use. 2016. ICH E17: General Principles for Planning and Design of Multi-regional Clinical Trials (draft). http://www.ich.org/fileadmin/Public_Web_Site/ICH_Products/Guidelines/Efficacy/E17/ICH_E17_draft_Step_1.pdf (accessed October 5, 2020).

Kawai, N., C. Chuang-Stein, O. Komiyama, and Y. Li. 2008. An approach to rationalize partitioning sample size into individual regions in a multiregional trial. *Drug Information Journal* 42:139–147.

Ko, F. S., H. H. Tsou, J. P. Liu, and C. F. Hsiao. 2010. Sample size determination for a specific region in a multi-regional trial. *Journal of Biopharmaceutical Statistics* 20(4):870–885.

Lan, K. K. G., D. M. Reboussin, and D. L. DeMets. 1994. Information and information fractions for design and sequential monitoring of clinical trials. *Communications in Statistics-Theory and Methods* 23(2):403–420.

Lan, K. K. G., and J. Pinheiro. 2012. Combined estimation of treatment effects under a discrete random effects model. *Statistics in Biosciences* 4:235–244.

Lan, K. K. G., J. Pinheiro, and F. Chen. 2014. Designing multiregional trials under the discrete random effects model. *Journal of Biopharmaceutical Statistics* 24(2):415–428.

Leuchs, A. K., J. Zinserling, A. Brandt, D. Wirtz, and N. Benda. 2015. Choosing appropriate estimands in clinical trials. *Therapeutic Innovation & Regulatory Science* 49(4):584–592.

Li, G., W. J. Shih, T. Xie, and J. Lu. 2002. A sample size adjustment procedure for clinical trials based on conditional power. *Biostatistics* 3(2):277–287.

Liu, J. T., H. H. Tsou, K. K. G. Lan, C. T. Chen, Y. H. Lai, W. J. Chang, C. S. Tzeng, and C. F. Hsiao. 2016. Assessing the consistency of treatment effect under the discrete random effects model in multiregional clinical trials. *Statistics in Medicine* 35(14):2301–2314.

Mahaffey, K. W., D. M. Wojdyla, K. Carroll, R. C. Becker, R. F. Storey, D. J. Angiolillo, C. Held, C. P. Cannon, S. James, K. S. Pieper, J. Horrow, R. A. Harrington, and L. Wallentin. 2011. Ticagrelor compared with clopidogrel by geographic region in the platelet inhibition and patient outcomes (PLATO) trial. *Circulation* 124:544–554.

Quan, H., P. L. Zhao, J. Zhang, M. Roessner, and K. Aizawa. 2010. Sample size considerations for Japanese patients in a multi-regional trial based on MHLW Guidance. *Pharmaceutical Statistics* 9(2):100–112.

Tsou, H. H., S. C. Chow, K. K. G. Lan, J. P. Liu, M. Wang, H. D. Chern, L. T. Ho, C. A. Hsiung, and C. F. Hsiao. 2010 Proposals of statistical consideration to evaluation of results for a specific region in multi-regional trials—Asian perspective. *Pharmaceutical Statistics* 9(3):201–206.

Tsou, H. H., H. M. J. Hung, Y. M. Chen, W. S. Huang, W. J. Chang, C. F. Hsiao. 2012. Establishing consistency across all regions in a multi-regional clinical trial. *Pharmaceutical Statistics* 11(4):295–299.

Wallentin, L., R. C. Becker, A. Budaj, C. P. Cannon, H. Emanuelsson, C. Held, J. Horrow, S. Husted, S. James, H. Katus, K. W. Mahaffey, B. M. Scirica, A. Skene, P. G. Steg, R. F. Storey, and R. A. Harrington. 2009. Ticagrelor versus clopidogrel in patients with acute coronary syndromes. *The New England Journal of Medicine* 361:1045–1057.

Wittes, J. 2002. Sample size calculations for randomized controlled trials. *Epidemiologic Reviews* 24(1):39–53.

19

Regional Sample Size Calculation in Multi-regional Equivalence and Non-inferiority Trials

Jason J.Z. Liao, Yaru Shi, and Ziji Yu

19.1 Introduction

With the increasing globalization of drug development, the multi-regional clinical trial (MRCT) has gained extensive use. There are tremendous advantages to conducting an MRCT. To name a few, the MRCT provides the sponsors access to otherwise untapped pools of patients as well as early patient access to new medications, and can expedite global clinical development and facilitate registration in all regions across the globe, which helps in the expansion of clinical research into developing countries bringing medical care options to subjects who otherwise may not have access to them; it can bring new medicines to patients globally as fast as scientifically possible and reduce the drug lag and make the effective therapies available to patients all over the world simultaneously. In return, the investment in drug development increases potential benefits to local scientific and medical and paramedical professionals, which provides access to more advanced technologies and helps in the development of technical expertise.

To harmonize and expedite the drug development and registration in different regions, the ICH-E5 guideline [1] and recently developed ICH-E17 [2] recommended a systemic framework of evaluating the ethnic factors, such as the cultural and environmental differences, on drugs among different regions. To achieve this goal, participating in a global MRCT from the early design stage of the drug development to avoid delays in drug approval can be a feasible and simple solution. However, there are many challenges both

DOI: 10.1201/9781003109785-19

operationally and scientifically in conducting a drug development globally as outlined in the literature. One fundamental question for the design of an MRCT is how to partition sample size into each individual region. The sample size allocation method can be complicated. As documented in the literature [2,3], many approaches could be considered for allocating the overall sample size to regions each with its own limitations. One approach is to allocate equal numbers of patients to each region and show similar trends in treatment effects across regions, which may not be feasible or efficient in terms of enrollment and trial conduct. A second approach is to allocate the sample size needed in one or more regions based on the ability to show that the region-specific treatment effect preserves some pre-specified proportion of the overall treatment effect, which would be difficult if all regions have this requirement. A third approach can allocate subjects in proportion to region size and disease prevalence without adhering to a fixed allocation strategy for regions, which, however, could likely result in very small sample sizes within some countries and/or regions and therefore be insufficient alone to support any evaluation of consistency among region-specific effects.

Depending on the hypothesis of a clinical trial, the trial can be designed based on superiority, equivalence, or non-inferiority. The most common trial design is superiority and the related discussion on the sample size allocation of multi-regional studies can be found in the literature [3–7]. The most common approach for superiority trials is based on either a defined quantitative consistency or a defined qualitative consistency condition to derive the sample size allocation. However, there are many other studies involving equivalence or non-inferiority designs such as biosimilar studies [8–12]. In this chapter, the consistency conditions and sample size allocation rules are discussed for multi-regional equivalence or non-inferiority studies.

19.2 Sample Size Allocation for Multi-regional Equivalence Trials

Let Y_{ij} be the outcome of patient j receiving treatment i, ($i = 1$ for the test arm and $i = 0$ for the reference arm). Assume that Y_{ij} follows a normal distribution with mean μ_i and common standard deviation σ, and the treatment difference $\delta = \mu_1 - \mu_0$. The hypothesis setting for an equivalence trial can be formalized as

$$H_0: |\delta| \geq \Delta \quad vs. \quad H_a: |\delta| < \Delta \qquad (19.1)$$

where Δ is a pre-specified testing margin, δ is the treatment effect, i.e., the treatment difference between the test arm and reference arm. The equivalence is concluded if the

$$100 \times (1 - 2\alpha)\% \text{ confidence interval of } \hat{\delta} \subset (-\Delta, \Delta) \qquad (19.2)$$

with α as the two-sided significance level of the trial.

Similar to the consistency conditions for superiority trials [6], two consistency conditions were defined in Liao et al. [13] for equivalence trials. The quantitative consistency condition for an equivalence trial is defined as follow:

$$\Pr(|\hat{\delta}_J - \hat{\delta}_{all}| \leq \pi\Delta \,|\, \delta_J, \delta_{all}) \geq 1 - \beta', \qquad (19.3)$$

where δ_J, δ_{NJ}, and δ_{all} denote the true treatment effects of the Japanese patients, non-Japanese patients, and the overall population, respectively, $\hat{\delta}_J$ and $\hat{\delta}_{all}$ are the corresponding estimates for Japanese and overall patients, respectively; $\pi \leq 0.5$, $1 - \beta' \geq 80\%$. Note for convenience, Japanese patients are chosen as the regional patients throughout this chapter. This consistency condition can be illustrated as "the sample size for Japanese patients has to ensure at least $1 - \beta'$ probability to demonstrate that the difference between the treatment effect of the Japanese patient and the overall population is less than or equal to a pre-specified threshold value $\pi\Delta$."

The qualitative consistency condition for equivalence is defined as

$$\Pr(|\hat{\delta}_J| < \Delta, \,|\hat{\delta}_{NJ}| < \Delta \,|\, \delta_J, \delta_{NJ}) \geq 1 - \beta', \qquad (19.4)$$

with $1 - \beta' \geq 80\%$, where $\hat{\delta}_J$ and $\hat{\delta}_{NJ}$ are the corresponding estimates for Japanese and non-Japanese patients, respectively. The qualitative consistency condition can be explained as "the sample size of Japanese patients has to ensure at least $1 - \beta'$ probability to demonstrate that the treatment effects of both Japanese and non-Japanese patients are smaller than the pre-specified threshold Δ." The example and numerical results in Liao et al. [13] indicate that the quantitative consistency condition in (19.3) is more conservative than the qualitative consistency condition in (19.4), and the latter condition requires a smaller proportion of Japanese patients in the overall population.

Assume that $\delta_J - \delta_{NJ} = \mu\Delta$, with μ very close to 0, and f_μ as the corresponding minimum fraction of Japanese patients, then $\delta_{all} = f_\mu \delta_J + (1 - f_\mu)\delta_{NJ}$. As shown in Liao et al. [13], there is no closed mathematical expression for the minimum required number of Japanese patients. The minimum proportion of

Japanese patients f_μ based on the quantitative consistency condition in (19.3) can be obtained from the following equation numerically:

$$\Phi\left(\frac{(\pi - (1 - f_\mu)\mu)(Z_{1-\alpha/2} + Z_{1-\beta/2})}{\sqrt{(1 - f_\mu)/f_\mu}}\right)$$

$$- \Phi\left(\frac{-(\pi + (1 - f_\mu)\mu)(Z_{1-\alpha/2} + Z_{1-\beta/2})}{\sqrt{(1 - f_\mu)/f_\mu}}\right) \geq 1 - \beta' \qquad (19.5)$$

where $\Phi(\bullet)$ is the cumulative distribution function of the standard normal distribution, $1-\beta$ is the designed equivalence study power.

Similarly, the minimum proportion of Japanese patients f'_μ based on the qualitative consistency condition in (19.4) can be obtained numerically from (19.6)

$$[1 - 2\phi(-\sqrt{f'_\mu}(1 + \mu(1 - f'_\mu)(Z_{1-\alpha/2} + Z_{1-\beta/2})))]$$

$$\times [1 - 2\phi(-\sqrt{1 - f'_\mu}((1 + \mu f'_\mu)(Z_{1-\alpha/2} + Z_{1-\beta/2})))] \geq 1 - \beta' \quad (19.6)$$

Due to no closed form for the fraction of the regional sample size shown in (19.5) and (19.6), Table 19.1 presents the values of f_μ and f'_μ calculated from (19.5) and (19.6), respectively, for $\alpha = 0.05$, $1 - \beta = 0.8$, 0.9, $1 - \beta' \in (0.5, 0.9)$, $\pi \in (0.1, 0.5)$ and $\mu = 0$, 0.1, 0.2 for convenience. For both consistency conditions, the minimum proportion of Japanese patients for both consistency conditions does not depend on the outcome variability σ^2 and the equivalence threshold parameter Δ. The values of f_μ and f'_μ increase with respect to the consistency power $1 - \beta'$ and μ, while the values decrease with respect to the trial overall power $(1 - \beta)$. Note that this does not necessarily imply that the sample size for Japanese patients required by the trial decreases with respect to $(1 - \beta)$ since the sample size for the whole trial population increases with the trial overall power.

The relationships among f_μ, $1 - \beta'$ and π, for the quantitative consistency condition and that of f_μ' and $1 - \beta'$ from the qualitative consistency condition are further illustrated in Figure 19.2, for the special case $1 - \beta = 0.8$ and $\mu = 0$. The 3-D plot in Figure 19.1 indicates that the value of f_μ decreases significantly with respect to the quantitative consistency threshold parameter π.

Even though the sample size allocation for multi-regional equivalence studies in (19.5) and (19.6) was discussed for balanced normally distributed

TABLE 19.1

Numerical evaluations of the proportion of Japanese patients needed for multi-regional equivalence studies

μ^c	$1-\beta$	$1-\beta'$	f_μ Values of Quantitative Consistency Condition[a]					f'_μ Values of Qualitative Consistency Condition[b]
			$\pi=0.1$[d]	$\pi=0.2$	$\pi=0.3$	$\pi=0.4$	$\pi=0.5$	
0	0.90	0.50	0.78	0.47	0.28	0.18	0.12	0.04
0	0.90	0.60	0.84	0.58	0.38	0.25	0.18	0.06
0	0.90	0.70	0.89	0.67	0.48	0.34	0.25	0.08
0	0.90	0.80	0.93	0.76	0.58	0.44	0.34	0.13
0	0.90	0.90	0.95	0.84	0.70	0.57	0.45	0.21
0	0.80	0.50	0.81	0.52	0.32	0.21	0.15	0.04
0	0.80	0.60	0.87	0.63	0.43	0.30	0.21	0.07
0	0.80	0.70	0.91	0.72	0.53	0.39	0.29	0.10
0	0.80	0.80	0.94	0.80	0.64	0.49	0.38	0.16
0	0.80	0.90	0.96	0.87	0.74	0.62	0.51	0.26
0.10	0.90	0.50	0.78	0.48	0.28	0.18	0.13	0.03
0.10	0.90	0.60	0.85	0.58	0.38	0.26	0.19	0.04
0.10	0.90	0.70	0.89	0.68	0.49	0.35	0.27	0.07
0.10	0.90	0.80	0.93	0.76	0.59	0.45	0.36	0.11
0.10	0.90	0.90	0.95	0.84	0.70	0.57	0.46	0.18
0.10	0.80	0.50	0.82	0.53	0.33	0.22	0.15	0.04
0.10	0.80	0.60	0.87	0.63	0.43	0.30	0.22	0.06
0.10	0.80	0.70	0.91	0.72	0.54	0.40	0.30	0.09
0.10	0.80	0.80	0.94	0.80	0.64	0.50	0.39	0.13
0.10	0.80	0.90	0.96	0.87	0.74	0.62	0.51	0.23
0.20	0.90	0.50	0.79	0.50	0.30	0.19	0.13	0.02
0.20	0.90	0.60	0.85	0.61	0.41	0.27	0.19	0.04
0.20	0.90	0.70	0.90	0.70	0.51	0.37	0.27	0.06
0.20	0.90	0.80	0.93	0.78	0.61	0.47	0.36	0.09
0.20	0.90	0.90	0.96	0.85	0.72	0.59	0.48	0.15
0.20	0.80	0.50	0.82	0.55	0.35	0.22	0.15	0.03
0.20	0.80	0.60	0.88	0.65	0.45	0.32	0.22	0.05
0.20	0.80	0.70	0.91	0.73	0.56	0.41	0.31	0.07
0.20	0.80	0.80	0.94	0.81	0.66	0.52	0.41	0.11
0.20	0.80	0.90	0.96	0.87	0.76	0.64	0.53	0.19

[a] f_μ is calculated iteratively from (19.5)

[b] f'_μ is calculated iteratively from (19.6)

[c] $\mu\Delta = \delta_J - \delta_{NJ}$;

[d] π is the qualitative threshold parameter defined in (19.6)

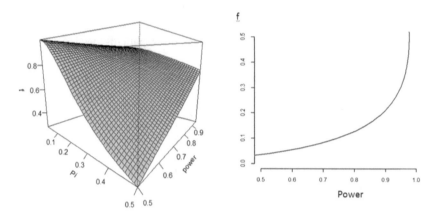

FIGURE 19.1
A three-dimensional plot for f_μ calculated from (19.5) against different values of π and the quantitative consistency power $1 - \beta'$ (left panel) and the scatter plot for f'_μ calculated from (19.6) against the qualitative consistency power $1 - \beta'$ (right panel) given the overall trial power $1 - \beta = 0.8$ and $\mu = 0$.

data. Because of the fact that both f_μ in (19.5) and f'_μ in (19.6) are independent of σ^2, which implies that the proportions of Japanese patients required by both consistency conditions remain the same for the normally distributed data in the unbalanced design, the unequal variance situation, and Binomial endpoints. Detail can be found in Liao et al. [13].

19.3 Sample Size Allocation for Multi-regional Non-inferiority Trials

The hypothesis test for a non-inferiority trial can be formalized as

$$H_0: \delta \le -\Delta \text{ vs } H_a: \delta > -\Delta$$

where $-\Delta$ is a prespecified negative margin and δ is the treatment effect. The non-inferiority is concluded if the

lower bound of the 2 − sided $100 \times (1 - \alpha)\%$ confidence interval of $\hat{\delta}$

being $> -\Delta$

where $\alpha/2$ is the 1-sided significance level of the trial.

Following the same thinking along with the equivalence studies, the quantitative consistency condition for a non-inferiority trial can be defined as

$$\Pr(\widehat{\delta}_J - \widehat{\delta}_{all} \geq -\pi\Delta \mid \delta_J, \delta_{all}) \geq 1 - \beta' \tag{19.7}$$

Similarly, the qualitative consistency for a non-inferiority trial can be defined as

$$\Pr(\widehat{\delta}_J > -\Delta, \widehat{\delta}_{NJ} > -\Delta \mid \delta_J, \delta_{all}) \geq 1 - \beta' \tag{19.8}$$

Following Liao et al. [13], let $\widehat{\theta} = \widehat{\delta}_J - \widehat{\delta}_{all}$, $\delta_J - \delta_{NJ} = -\mu\Delta$, $\delta_{all} = f_\mu \delta_J + (1 - f_\mu)\delta_{NJ}$, then

$$var(\widehat{\theta}) = var(\widehat{\delta}_J - \widehat{\delta}_{all}) = var(\widehat{\delta}_J - f_\mu \widehat{\delta}_J - (1 - f_\mu)\widehat{\delta}_{NJ})$$
$$= var((1 - f_\mu)(\widehat{\delta}_J - \widehat{\delta}_{NJ}))$$
$$= \frac{1 - f_\mu}{f_\mu} \cdot \frac{\Delta^2}{(z_{1-\alpha/2} + z_{1-\beta})^2}$$

Formula (19.7) can be rewritten as

$$1 - \Phi\left(\frac{-\pi\Delta - \theta}{\sqrt{var(\widehat{\theta})}}\right) \geq 1 - \beta'$$

where $var(\widehat{\theta}) = \frac{1 - f_\mu}{f_\mu} \cdot \frac{\Delta^2}{(z_{1-\alpha/2} + z_{1-\beta})^2}$ and $\theta = -(1 - f_\mu)\mu\Delta$. Thus, f_μ can be solved by the following equation

$$1 - \Phi\left(\frac{-(z_{1-\frac{\alpha}{2}} + z_{1-\beta})(\pi - (1 - f_\mu)\mu)}{\sqrt{(1 - f_\mu)/f_\mu}}\right) \geq 1 - \beta' \tag{19.9}$$

Similarly, formula (19.8) for the qualitative consistency condition can be rewritten as

$$\left(1 - \Phi\left(\frac{-\Delta - \delta_J}{\sqrt{var(\widehat{\delta}_J)}}\right)\right)\left(1 - \Phi\left(\frac{-\Delta - \delta_{NJ}}{\sqrt{var(\widehat{\delta}_{NJ})}}\right)\right) \geq 1 - \beta'$$

TABLE 19.2

Numerical evaluations of the proportion of Japanese patients needed for multi-regional non-inferiority trials

			f_μ Values of Quantitative Consistency Condition[a]					f'_μ Values of Qualitative Consistency Condition[b]
μ^c	$1-\beta$	$1-\beta'$	$\pi=0.1^d$	$\pi=0.2$	$\pi=0.3$	$\pi=0.4$	$\pi=0.5$	
0	0.9	0.6	0.38	0.13	0.06	0.04	0.02	0.01
0	0.9	0.7	0.72	0.4	0.23	0.14	0.09	0.03
0	0.9	0.8	0.87	0.63	0.43	0.3	0.21	0.07
0	0.9	0.9	0.94	0.8	0.63	0.49	0.38	0.16
0	0.8	0.6	0.45	0.17	0.08	0.05	0.03	0.01
0	0.8	0.7	0.78	0.47	0.28	0.18	0.12	0.04
0	0.8	0.8	0.9	0.69	0.5	0.36	0.27	0.09
0	0.8	0.9	0.95	0.84	0.7	0.57	0.46	0.22
0.1	0.9	0.6	0.62	0.27	0.12	0.06	0.04	0.01
0.1	0.9	0.7	0.8	0.53	0.33	0.2	0.13	0.03
0.1	0.9	0.8	0.89	0.7	0.52	0.37	0.27	0.08
0.1	0.9	0.9	0.95	0.82	0.68	0.55	0.44	0.19
0.1	0.8	0.6	0.66	0.32	0.15	0.08	0.05	0.01
0.1	0.8	0.7	0.83	0.58	0.38	0.25	0.17	0.04
0.1	0.8	0.8	0.92	0.75	0.58	0.43	0.33	0.11
0.1	0.8	0.9	0.96	0.86	0.74	0.62	0.51	0.26
0.2	0.9	0.6	0.73	0.44	0.23	0.11	0.06	0.01
0.2	0.9	0.7	0.85	0.63	0.43	0.28	0.19	0.04
0.2	0.9	0.8	0.91	0.75	0.59	0.45	0.33	0.1
0.2	0.9	0.9	0.95	0.85	0.72	0.6	0.5	0.22
0.2	0.8	0.6	0.76	0.48	0.26	0.14	0.08	0.01
0.2	0.8	0.7	0.87	0.66	0.48	0.33	0.23	0.05
0.2	0.8	0.8	0.93	0.79	0.64	0.5	0.39	0.14
0.2	0.8	0.9	0.96	0.87	0.77	0.66	0.55	0.3

[a] f_μ is calculated iteratively from (19.9)

[b] f'_μ is calculated iteratively from (19.10)

[c] $\mu\Delta = \delta_J - \delta_{NJ}$;

[d] π is the qualitative threshold parameter defined in (19.10)

where $var(\hat{\delta}_J) = \dfrac{2\sigma^2}{f_\mu N_{all}}$ and $var(\hat{\delta}_{NJ}) = \dfrac{2\sigma^2}{(1-f_\mu)N_{all}}$

Assume $\delta_J - \delta_{NJ} = -\mu\Delta$, and $f'_\mu \delta_J + (1 - f'_\mu)\delta_{NJ} = 0$ given that the expected difference between the new treatment and the placebo is 0, then

$\delta_J = -(1 - f'_\mu)\mu\Delta$ and $\delta_{NJ} = f'_\mu\mu\Delta$. Solving the following formula will yield the minimum f'_μ,

$$
(1 - (1 - \Phi(-\sqrt{f'_\mu}\,(1 - (1 - f'_\mu)\mu\,)(z_{1-\frac{\alpha}{2}} + z_{1-\beta})))\ (1
$$
$$
- \Phi(-\sqrt{1 - f'_\mu}\,(1 + f'_\mu\mu)(z_{1-\frac{\alpha}{2}} + z_{1-\beta})))
$$
$$
= \Phi(\sqrt{f'_\mu}\,(1 - (1 - f'_\mu)\mu\,)(z_{1-\frac{\alpha}{2}} + z_{1-\beta}))\ \Phi(\sqrt{1 - f'_\mu}\,(1 + f'_\mu\mu)(z_{1-\frac{\alpha}{2}} + z_{1-\beta}))
$$
$$
\geq 1 - \beta'
$$

(19.10)

Table 19.2 presents the numeric evaluations of the proportions of Japanese patients needed under a non-inferiority test. Note that both f_μ in (19.9) and f'_μ in (19.10) are independent of σ^2. Thus, the proportions of Japanese patients required by both consistency conditions for the normally distributed data in a balanced design remain the same for the normally distributed data in the unbalanced design, the unequal variance situation, and binomial endpoints.

The relationships among f_μ, $1 - \beta'$ and π, for the quantitative consistency condition and that of f_μ' and $1 - \beta'$ from the qualitative consistency condition are further illustrated in Figure 19.2, for the special case

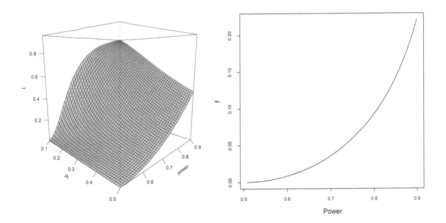

FIGURE 19.2
A three-dimensional plot for f_μ calculated from (19.9) against different values of π and the quantitative consistency power $1 - \beta'$ (left panel) and the scatter plot for f'_μ calculated from (19.10) against the qualitative consistency power $1 - \beta'$ (right panel) given the overall trial power $1 - \beta = 0.8$ and $\mu = 0$.

$1 - \beta = 0.8$ and $\mu = 0$. The 3-D plot in Figure 19.2 indicates that the value of f_μ decreases significantly with respect to the quantitative consistency threshold parameter π.

Similarly, both f_μ in (19.9) and f'_μ in (19.10) for balanced normally distributed data are independent of σ^2, which implies that the proportions of Japanese patients required by both consistency conditions remain the same for the normally distributed data in the unbalanced design, the unequal variance situation, and Binomial endpoints in a non-inferiority trial.

19.4 An Illustration: A Vaccine Trial

Pneumococcal disease, an umbrella term for all diseases caused by the bacteria streptococcus pneumoniae, leads to conditions as varied as ear infections, pneumonia, and meningitis. As with many dangerous illnesses, those most susceptible people are the elderly, young children, and those with weakened immune systems. Each year, more than 150,000 people will be hospitalized with one of these pneumococcal diseases [14]. Widespread use of Pneumococcal Conjugate Vaccines (PCV) has reduced the burden of pneumococcal disease caused by the serotypes contained in the vaccines.

Consider a phase 3, randomized, double-blind trial to compare the immunogenicity and safety of an experimental vaccine against an active comparator in healthy adults at elevated risk for pneumococcal diseases. The primary objective is to demonstrate the non-inferiority of new generation PCV compared with a currently licensed PCV, Prevnar 13™. Because Prevnar 13™ contains 13 serotypes, the immunogenicity endpoint of this trial is serotype-specific OPA responses for 13 shared serotypes at Day 30 post-vaccination. The non-inferiority margin $-\Delta$ for was fixed at $\log(0.5)$, meaning the logarithm of OPA GMT ratios for each serotype is $\log(0.5)$. Also, the standard deviation of the GMT ratios in log titer was assumed to be 3.7 for all 13 serotypes. It is noted that all 13 serotypes need to reject the null hypotheses to declare the success of this trial. Therefore, no multiplicity adjustment was needed. With the overall trial power fixed at 90% and the 1-sided significance level of the trial fixed at 0.025, the overall sample size was planned at 1200 under 90% of the evaluability rate. As this trial was also planned to be used for the potential Japan filling, the proportion of Japanese participants was calculated using both quantitative and qualitative conditions define in previous sections.

According to the result presented in Table 19.2, given $1 - \beta = 0.9$, $1 - \beta' = 0.8$, and $\pi = 0.5$, it yields $f_\mu = 21\%$ and $f'_\mu = 7\%$, which indicates that 252 and 84 Japanese participants are needed by the quantitative consistency and by the qualitative consistency conditions, respectively. It is also observed that the number of participants needed for quantitative consistency is more than that of qualitative consistency. Note that the calculated number using the qualitative consistency was well aligned with the Agency's independently proposed number.

19.5 Summary

To speed up the patient enrollments and drug approval for delivering efficacious medicines to needed patients, MRCTs have gained extensive use and the data from MRCT could be accepted by regulatory authorities across regions and countries as the primary sources of evidence to support global marketing drug approval simultaneously. The recently issued ICH-E17 "General Principals for Planning and Design of Multi-regional Clinical Trials" listed some challenges both operationally and scientifically in conducting drug development globally. The distinct and sometimes conflicting regulatory requirements may post very strong operational challenges for sponsors. Scientifically, a scientifically sound trial needs to be thoughtfully designed for the overall trial populations with multiple ethnic factors as well as investigating consistency in treatment effects across populations. The overall sample size should be appropriately determined with a reasonable regional sample size allocation scheme to address regional regulatory requirements and assess regional treatment effects.

Regional sample size allocation was considered in this chapter for an equivalence trial and a non-inferiority trial. The minimum proportion of Japanese patients in multi-regional studies was discussed so that the chance of observing significant treatment differences across regions is controlled. Two consistency conditions, namely the quantitative and qualitative consistency conditions, were proposed for both an equivalence trial and a non-inferiority trial, with the former focusing on ensuring that the treatment effect on Japanese patients is not much different from the overall effect, and the latter focusing on establishing the specified treatment effect per the design for both Japanese and non-Japanese patients. As demonstrated in both the equivalence trial and the non-inferiority trial, in general, the quantitative consistency condition is more conservative and requires more regional patients than that from the qualitative consistency condition. For both consistency conditions, no closed mathematical expression for the minimum proportion of Japanese patients is available, but the values can be obtained numerically. However, it is strongly recommended to have an early direct communication between the sponsor and regional health authority to reach a consensus about the proportion of regional subjects in a global trial.

References

[1]. ICH International Conference on Harmonization Tripartite Guidance E5, Ethnic factor in the acceptability of foreign data. The US Federal Register, 1998, Vol. 83: 31790–31796.

[2]. ICH Harmonized Guidance E17, General principles for planning and design of multi-regional clinical trials, US Department of Health and Human Resources Services, 2016. https://www.fda.gov/downloads/Drugs/GuidanceComplianceRegulatoryInformation/Guidances/UCM519603.pdf

[3]. Chen, J. and Quan, H. *Multiregional Clinical Trials for Simultaneous Global New Drug Development*. April 2016. Chapman and Hall/CRC.

[4]. Ministry of Health Labour and Welfare of Japan, Basic principles on global clinical trials. September 28, 2007.

[5]. Usesaka, H., Sample size allocation to regions in a multiregional trial. *Journal of Biopharmaceutical Statistics*, 2009, Vol. 19: 580–594.

[6]. Quan, H., Zhao, P.L., Zhang, J. Roessner, M. and Aizawa, K., Sample size considerations for Japanese patients in a multi-regional trial based on MHLW guidance. *Pharmaceutical Statistics*, 2010, Vol. 9: 100–112.

[7]. Kawai, H., Chuang-Stein C., Komiyama, O. and Li, Y., An approach to rationalize partitioning sample size into individual regions in a multiregional trial. *Drug Information Journal*, 2007, Vol. 42: 139–147.

[8]. Food and Drug Administration of U.S.A., Guidance for industry: Scientific considerations in demonstrating biosimilarity to a reference product. *US Department of Health and Human Resources Services*, 2012.

[9]. Liao, J.J.Z., A constrained non-inferiority approach for assessing clinical efficacy to establish biosimilarity. *International Journal of Clinical Biostatistics*, 2015, Vol. 1: 008, 1–7.

[10]. Julious, S.A., Sample sizes for clinical trials with normal data. *Statistics in Medicine*, 2004, Vol. 23: 1921–1986

[11]. Food and Drug Administration of U.S.A., Guidance for industry: Quality considerations in demonstrating biosimilarity to a reference product. *US Department of Health and Human Resources Services*, 2012.

[12]. Food and Drug Administration of U.S.A., Guidance for industry: Biosimilars: Questions and answers regarding implementation of the biologics price competition and innovation act of 2009. *US Department of Health and Human Resources Services*, 2012.

[13]. Liao, J.J.Z., Yu, Z. and Li, Y., Sample size allocation in multi-regional equivalence studies. *Pharmaceutical Statistics*, 2018, Vol. 17: 570–577.

[14]. Center for Disease Control and Prevention, Fast facts you need to know about pneumococcal disease. Available from: https://www.cdc.gov/pneumococcal/about/facts.html

Index

Note: **Bold** page numbers refer to tables and *italic* page numbers refer to figures.